Lecture Notes on
Clinical Biochemistry

Lecture Notes on Clinical Biochemistry

L.G. WHITBY
MD, PhD, FRCP(Lond & Edin), FRCPath, FRSEd
Emeritus Professor of Clinical Chemistry
University of Edinburgh

A.F. SMITH
MD, FRCPEdin, FRCPath
Senior Lecturer in Clinical Biochemistry
University of Edinburgh

G.J. BECKETT
BSc, PhD, MRCPath
Senior Lecturer in Clinical Biochemistry
University of Edinburgh

S.W. WALKER
DM, MB, BS
Senior Lecturer in Clinical Biochemistry
University of Edinburgh

FIFTH EDITION

OXFORD

BLACKWELL SCIENTIFIC PUBLICATIONS

LONDON EDINBURGH BOSTON

MELBOURNE PARIS BERLIN VIENNA

First published 1975
Revised reprint 1977
Reprinted 1978
Second edition 1980
Third edition 1984
Reprinted 1987
Fourth edition 1988
Reprinted 1989, 1991
Fifth edition 1993

Set by Semantic Graphics, Singapore
Printed and bound in Great Britain
at the University Press, Cambridge

DISTRIBUTORS

Marston Book Services Ltd
PO Box 87
Oxford OX2 0DT
(*Orders*: Tel: 0865 791155
         Fax: 0865 791927
         Telex: 837515)

USA
Blackwell Scientific Publications, Inc.
238 Main Street
Cambridge, MA 02142
(*Orders*: Tel: 800 759–6102
         617 876–7000)

Canada
Times Mirror Professional Publishing, Ltd
130 Flaska Drive
Markham, Ontario L6G 1B8
(*Orders*: Tel: 800 268–4178
         416 470–6739)

Australia
Blackwell Scientific Publications Pty Ltd
54 University Street
Carlton, Victoria 3053
(*Orders*: Tel: 03 347–5552)

A catalogue record for this title
is available from the British Library

ISBN 0–632–03687–7

Library of Congress
Cataloging in Publication Data

Lecture notes on clinical biochemistry/
  L.G. Whitby . . . [*et al*.].—5th ed.
        p.   cm.
  Rev ed. of: Lecture notes on clinical
  chemistry/L.G. Whitby,
  A.F. Smith, G.J. Beckett. 4th ed. 1988.
  Includes bibliographical references and
  index.
  ISBN 0–632–03687–7
  1. Clinical chemistry.
  2. Clinical biochemistry.
  I. Whitby, L.G. (Lionel Gordon)
  II. Whitby, L.G. (Lionel Gordon)
  Lecture notes on clinical chemistry.
    [DNLM: 1. Biochemistry.   QU 4 L471]
  RB40.L4 1993
  616.07′56—dc20

Contents

Preface, vii

Units, ix

Abbreviations, xi

1   Using Laboratories Responsibly, 1

2   Chemical Tests Performed Close to the Patient, in the Ward or Clinic Environment, 12

3   Interpreting and Using Laboratory Data, 21

4   Disturbances of Water, Sodium and Potassium Balance, 35

5   Acid–base Balance and Oxygen Transport, 57

6   Plasma Enzyme Tests in Diagnosis, 72

7   Abnormalities of Proteins in Plasma, 86

8   Liver Disease, 105

9   Renal Disease, 124

10   Gastrointestinal Tract Disease, 144

11   Disorders of Carbohydrate Metabolism, 162

12   Disorders of Plasma Lipids and Lipoproteins, 182

13   Disorders of Calcium, Phosphate and Magnesium Metabolism, 195

14   Disorders of Iron and Porphyrin Metabolism, 216

15   Nutrition, 229

16   Disorders of Purine Metabolism, 243

17   Abnormalities of Thyroid Function, 249

18   Disorders of the Adrenal Cortex and Medulla, 267

19   Hypothalamic and Pituitary Hormones, 293

20   Gonadal Function and Pregnancy, 303

21   Clinical Biochemistry in Paediatrics and Geriatrics, 321

22   Molecular Biology in Clinical Biochemistry, 346

23   The CNS and CSF, 364

24   Therapeutic Drug Monitoring and Chemical Toxicology, 367

25   Revision: Examination Questions, 376

     Appendix A: Multiple Choice Questions: Key to the Answers, 409

     Appendix B: SI Units and 'Conventional' Units, 411

     Appendix C: References, 414

     Index, 423

Preface

This edition differs considerably from the previous edition for several reasons. It reflects, firstly, the many contributions and growing influence of our two younger co-authors, Dr Geoff Beckett who joined Dr Alistair Smith and me in preparing the fourth edition, and Dr Simon Walker who has now joined the team. We recognize that considerable changes are likely to stem from the General Medical Council's most recent recommendations about the undergraduate medical curriculum. This has meant that the text of the fourth edition (1988) has been completely reviewed and extensively revised, processes that were in any case needed to enable us to include much new material.

Whether curricular change in some medical schools results in Clinical Biochemistry becoming one of the options in a 'core and options' pattern of undergraduate curriculum (with only limited representation in the core), or whether it retains its rightful place as an important core constituent, most doctors, shortly after qualifying in Medicine, will very soon come to realize that they will be very dependent on the local clinical biochemistry department (or departments with equivalent title). Recently qualified doctors comprise the principal users of the diagnostic services provided by these departments and it seems reasonable to expect that they should possess sufficient knowledge and understanding of Clinical Biochemistry to be able to make informed use of the diagnostic services available to them, whether their long-term aim be to make a career in hospital practice or in primary medical care (general practice). In preparing this edition, we have therefore had the needs of senior medical students and doctors in their early postgraduate years particularly in mind. To meet these needs we have set as our objectives the aims of helping our readers:

1 to acquire knowledge and understanding of the potential value and the limitations of commonly available chemical investigations, including those that readers of this book might be required to perform themselves, or be responsible for ensuring their reliable performance and proper interpretation;

2 to develop the ability to select chemical investigations that are appropriate to the diagnosis of disease and for the management of treatment in individual patients, and to be able to interpret the results of these investigations correctly;

3 to maintain a responsible and critical attitude in the use they make of the diagnostic services provided by Clinical Biochemistry and the other laboratory-based specialties.

Among the new material in this edition, we have included several case histories. We have not attempted to provide examples relating to every subject covered in the book, nor even to include case histories for every one of its chapters. In many instances, furnished with the information in the main text, the interpretation of the results of biochemical investigations should prove to be relatively straightforward. We have, therefore, mostly selected cases for their ability to serve as examples of conditions where, in our experience, many students and junior doctors, even some senior doctors, encounter difficulties in interpreting laboratory data, or are unaware of the pitfalls to be avoided. Another reason for our limited use of case descriptions as illustrative examples is that every patient should be thought of as an individual, whether presenting a diagnostic or therapeutic problem.

Other completely new material includes an introductory chapter on Molecular Biology and its applications in Clinical Biochemistry, and a revision chapter consisting of examination questions based on the information available in the main body of the text. In the past, Dr Alistair Smith and I prepared a separate book of multiple choice questions. However, in a developing subject like Clinical Biochemistry, the MCQ book soon suffered from the disadvantage of becoming out of phase with the corresponding textbook, as the latter moved on to its next edition. In effect, therefore, this edition combines two books in one.

This is the last edition with which I expect to be closely involved. In looking to the future, my colleagues and I decided that it would be appropriate now for the title of the book to be changed, to reflect the fact that the titles of the department and of the appointments held by its academic staff changed in 1991, following my retirement. Also, the emphasis within the book has changed in several places more towards the medically oriented specialty of Clinical Biochemistry, and away from the analytically oriented subject of Clinical Chemistry.

In conclusion, I wish to express my particular thanks to my most senior colleague and co-author, Dr Alistair Smith, and to my former secretary, Miss Doreen Fisher, who has once again undertaken the lion's share of the work involved in the preparation of the various drafts, ably assisted by Mrs Evelyn Ward. I also wish to thank my two younger co-authors, Dr Geoff Beckett and Dr Simon Walker, Dr Alan Westwood for his help with the chapter on Paediatric Biochemisty, Dr Peter Rae and Dr Elaine Turner for the provision of illustrative case histories and various other contributions, as well as the staff of Blackwell Scientific Publications, who have all proved so helpful since this book was added to the list of their *Lecture Notes* titles nearly 25 years ago.

L.G. Whitby

Units

The results of chemical investigations are mostly numerical. In their interpretation, it is very important to realize that the units of measurement may differ between laboratories. It is easy to fall into the trap of focussing on numbers and to assume that the units in which the results are expressed are those with which the doctor is familiar. If, however, the units of measurement should happen to be different from the accustomed units, for whatever reason, this can have serious consequences for the patient, as will be apparent from the following examples:

1 A plasma [glucose] of '30' in a known diabetic admitted to hospital in coma would indicate that the patient was in *hyper*glycaemic coma if the units of measurement were assumed to be expressed in Système International (SI) units, i.e. in mmol/L, or that the diagnosis was *hypo*glycaemic coma if the result was assumed to be expressed in 'conventional' or mass units, e.g. mg/dL (dL = 100 mL). Inappropriate therapy, based on incorrect assumptions about units, could all too easily have rapidly fatal consequences for this patient.

2 A lumbar CSF [total protein] of '300' would be interpreted very differently by a doctor accustomed to seeing CSF results expressed in SI units, i.e. in mg/L, for whom the result would be within the reference range, from a doctor accustomed to seeing such results reported in 'conventional' units, e.g. mg/dL, for whom the result would be interpreted as being of pathological significance.

3 Comparable opportunities for seriously incorrect interpretations of numerical data often arise when considering reports of plasma drug concentrations.

These examples should suffice to illustrate the dangers of doctors wrongly assuming that results of chemical analyses are always expressed in familiar units. Specifically, *there are important differences between the units with which most doctors are familiar when engaged in medical practice in the UK as compared with the corresponding units that are in everyday use in medical practice in the USA.*

One way of overcoming the difficulties described above is for results of analyses always to be reported in two different sets of units. This 'solution' has been tried and found to be unsatisfactory. We have, therefore, decided not to give two sets of figures and units every time reference ranges or other quantitative data are mentioned in this book (e.g. we do not state that 'the reference range for blood [urea] in males is 2.5–6.6 mmol/L, or 7.0–18.5 mg/dL expressed as blood urea nitrogen or BUN'). Instead, in Appendix B (p. 411), we provide Tables that interrelate the values for reference ranges, mostly given in this book in SI units, with their numerical equivalents in 'conventional' units; we also give general equations that enable interconversions between these two types of unit to be made.

We suggest that readers accustomed to receiving results of chemical analyses expressed in 'conventional' units should delete SI values and units wherever these appear in the text, and annotate the adjacent margin with those values and units to which they are accustomed in their medical practice.

Abbreviations

The following list mostly consists of abbreviations that are used frequently in this book. Other abbreviations are defined in the text at the appropriate places.

Concentrations are indicated by means of square brackets. For example, plasma [urea] means 'the concentration of urea in plasma'.

The following *atomic symbols* are used without further explanation in this book:

C	Carbon	H	Hydrogen	Na	Sodium
Ca	Calcium	I	Iodine	O	Oxygen
Cl	Chloride	K	Potassium	P	Phosphorus
Fe	Iron	N	Nitrogen	S	Sulphur

Units of measurement (examples)

Abbreviation	mmol/L	μmol/L	nmol/L	pmol/L
Molar concentration	10^{-3}	10^{-6}	10^{-9}	10^{-12}
Prefix to mole	milli	micro	nano	pico

Similarly with units of mass concentration (e.g. g/L, mg/L, etc.) and international units (IU/L, mIU/L, etc.) and with certain other units (e.g. U/L, mU/L, etc.).

ACTH	adrenocorticotrophic hormone
ADH	antidiuretic hormone (AVP preferred)
AFP	α_1-fetoprotein
AIDS	acquired immune deficiency syndrome
ALA	5-aminolaevulinic acid
ALT	alanine aminotransferase
AMP	adenosine monophosphate
AST	aspartate aminotransferase
AVP	arginine vasopressin (or vasopressin)
Bq	becquerel (the SI unit of radioactivity)
CAH	congenital adrenal hyperplasia
cal	calorie (and kcal, one thousand calories)
CBG	cortisol-binding globulin
CEA	carcinoembryonic antigen
CF	cystic fibrosis
CK	creatine kinase
CRH	corticotrophin-releasing hormone

Da	dalton (a measure of molecular mass); also *see* k for kDa
DDAVP	desaminocys-1-8-D-arginine vasopressin
DHA	dehydroepiandrosterone (S is added when referring to its sulphate)
DHCC	dihydrocholecalciferol (e.g. 1 : 25-DHCC)
DNA	deoxyribonucleic acid (and cDNA for copy DNA)
ECF	extracellular fluid
*Eco*R1	*Escherichia coli* restriction endonuclease 1
EDTA	ethylenediaminetetra-acetate
FSH	follicle-stimulating hormone
g	gram
GI	gastrointestinal
GFR	glomerular filtration rate
GGT	gamma-glutamyl transferase
GH	growth hormone
Gn-RH	gonadotrophin-releasing hormone
GTT	glucose tolerance test (oral)
h	hour
Hb	haemoglobin
HCC	hydroxycholecalciferol (e.g. 25-HCC)
hCG	(human) chorionic gonadotrophin
HDL	high density lipoprotein
HGPRT	hypoxanthine-guanine phosphoribosyltransferase
5-HIAA	5-hydroxyindoleacetic acid
HIV	human immunodeficiency virus
HLA	human leucocyte antigens
HMG-CoA	β-hydroxy-β-methylglutaryl-coenzyme A
HMMA	4-hydroxy, 3-methoxy mandelic acid
HPA	hypothalamic–pituitary–adrenal (axis)
hPL	(human) placental lactogen
5-HT	5-hydroxytryptamine or serotonin (P is added when referring to its phosphate)
ICF	intracellular fluid
Ig	immunoglobulin (the class is often specified, e.g. IgG, IgM)
IMP	inosine $5'$-phosphate
IU	international unit
k	kilo, as in kg, kDa (one thousand daltons), kPa
kb	1000 nucleotide bases (in a nucleic acid or polynucleotide fragment)
L	litre (the SI unit of volume in medicine)
LCAT	lecithin cholesterol acyltransferase
LD	lactate dehydrogenase (and isoenzymes LD_1, LD_2, etc.)
LDL	low density lipoprotein
LH	luteinizing hormone, and LH-RH for luteinizing hormone-releasing hormone
MEN	multiple endocrine neoplasia

min	minute
mol mass	molecular mass (also see M_r)
M_r	relative molecular mass
MSAFP	maternal serum α-fetoprotein
NAD (etc.)	nicotinamide-adenine dinucleotide, its phosphate (NADP) and their reduced forms (NADH and NADPH)
OHP	hydroxyprogesterone, and 17α-OHP for 17α-hydroxy progesterone
Pa	pascal (the SI unit of pressure)
PBG	porphobilinogen
P_{CO_2}	the partial pressure of CO_2 in the gas phase in equilibrium with CO_2 dissolved in blood (units kPa)
PCR	polymerase chain reaction
pK_a	the logarithm to the base 10 of the reciprocal of the ionization constant of an acid in a buffer solution. The pK_a of an acid is equal to the pH at which the [acid] and [base] are equal, and is the pH at which the buffering power is greatest
PKU	phenylketonuria
P_{O_2}	the partial pressure of O_2 in the gas phase in equilibrium with O_2 (units kPa)
PRPP	5-phosphoribosyl-1-pyrophosphate
PTH	parathyroid hormone
RFLP	restriction fragment length polymorphisms
RIA	radioimmunoassay
SHBG	sex hormone-binding globulin
SI	Système International
sp. gr.	specific gravity
T3	tri-iodothyronine (rT3 = reverse T3)
T4	thyroxine
Taq	*Thermus aquaticus*
TBG	thyroxine-binding globulin
TBP	thyroxine-binding proteins
TDM	therapeutic drug monitoring
TIBC	total iron-binding capacity
TRH	thyrotrophin-releasing hormone
TSH	thyroid-stimulating hormone
UDP	uridine 5'-pyrophosphate (formerly called uridine diphosphate, hence UDP)
VLDL	very low density lipoprotein

Chapter 1
Using Laboratories Responsibly

We strongly advise doctors to request investigations selectively, i.e. always to have a reason for asking to have each and every test, or group of interrelated tests, performed. However, predetermined patterns of selective requesting, or formal protocols, are sometimes appropriate, as in the orderly approach to the diagnosis of endocrine abnormalities or inherited metabolic disorders. Two very different ways of requesting chemical investigations will be considered:

1 *Selective requesting*. This involves choosing which tests to perform on the basis of the history of each patient's illness and the findings on clinical examination (including the results of extra-laboratory tests) as well as the results of previous laboratory investigations, X-ray studies, etc. This is often called *discretionary requesting*.

2 *Standardized requesting*. This involves performing a predetermined range of tests on everyone in a predefined group, even when there is no clinical indication for their performance, as when admission profiles are carried out on all patients attending some hospitals or clinics, or as part of programmes of well-population screening. These test-groupings are often called *screening tests*.

Selective or discretionary requests

In about 80% of patients presenting at out-patient departments or admitted to hospital wards, doctors will have made a provisional diagnosis after taking the history of each patient's illness; this percentage is greater in patients who have been seen before. The clinical examination, and possibly other tests such as 'side-room' tests on urine (Chapter 2), may further clarify the diagnosis.

Therefore, it is nearly always possible for doctors to adopt a logical approach to requesting tests, and to ask for investigations on a selective basis, as suggested by the information already available, as follows:

1 *To confirm a diagnosis*, e.g. plasma [free T4] and [TSH] to confirm a clinical diagnosis of hyperthyroidism.

2 *To aid differential diagnosis*, e.g. tests to distinguish between different forms of jaundice or between different possible causes of acute abdominal pain.

3 *To refine a diagnosis*. Chemical tests may help localize a lesion, e.g. plasma [ACTH] may differentiate pituitary from adrenal causes of Cushing's syndrome.

4 *To assess the severity of disease*, e.g. plasma [urea] or [creatinine] to indicate the severity of renal disease.

5 *To monitor progress*, e.g. plasma [glucose] and $[K^+]$ may be measured serially to follow the treatment of patients with diabetic ketoacidosis.

6 *To detect complications or side-effects*. This is especially important in patients

1

being treated with drugs that may damage the liver. These adverse effects may be detected by measuring plasma aminotransferase (ALT or AST) activity.

7 *To monitor therapy*, e.g. plasma drug concentrations may be determined to check a patient's compliance or to detect overdose.

The case for selective requesting

Most chemical investigations lack specificity (defined on p. 28), because abnormal results are only rarely diagnostic in themselves. Results of chemical investigations can most readily be interpreted if there was a clinical reason for selecting each investigation initially. Asher's catechism should be the doctor's guide:

1 Why do I request this test?
2 What will I look for in the result?
3 If I find what I am looking for, will it affect my diagnosis?
4 How will this investigation affect my management of the patient?
5 Will this investigation ultimately benefit the patient?

Unless doctors can answer one or more of the questions in this catechism at the time of initiating laboratory requests, it is unlikely that subsequently, when the results of the tests become available, the significance of the results will be fully understood, or that best use will necessarily be made of the information contained in the reports. Under these circumstances, abnormal results of laboratory investigations are all too liable to be ignored.

Standardized requests or screening tests

These are investigations carried out without a clinical indication for performing some, or possibly any, of the tests on a particular patient or apparently healthy person. The diagnostic yield from these tests on patients is nearly always considerably less than from investigations selected in the light of a doctor's provisional diagnosis, based on the patient's symptoms and on signs of disease. It is relatively unusual for a new or unexpected diagnosis to be made on the basis of the results of chemical tests carried out without there having been a clinical reason for requesting their performance.

Well-population screening

These are tests carried out to identify people who may possibly be sick, from among an apparently healthy population. They are intended to give people for whom results are normal grounds for believing that they are indeed healthy. All well-population screening programmes should:

1 Include measurements that will contribute to the early detection of diseases that are important in terms of their incidence or life-threatening nature, or that will offer other medical benefits to those who attend for screening.

2 Use tests or methods that are sensitive and specific (defined on p. 28), acceptable to the people to be screened, and able to be carried out in large numbers.

3 Be planned in the knowledge that the clinical, laboratory and other facilities required for following up abnormalities revealed by the programme exist, and that acceptable treatment is available for any disease discovered as a result of the screening programme.

4 Have had the financial aspects of the programme defined in advance.

The initial enthusiasm for large-scale complex multiphasic screening programmes on the apparently healthy ambulant population has waned. Case-finding programmes are, by their very nature, relatively selective and have more to offer.

Case-finding programmes

These depend on tests chosen to identify people with particular diseases, applied to high-risk groups or to definable components of the general population with known relatively high incidences of the diseases being sought. Case-finding programmes search for people who should benefit from being identified as having a specific abnormality and thereafter treated as patients (Table 1.1).

Screening of patients

Many laboratories analyse and report some tests as *functional or organ-related groups*. For example, a 'liver function test' group might comprise plasma bilirubin, ALT, alkaline phosphatase, GGT and albumin measurements. Such functional groupings, based on tests which are closely related clinically, ease requesting, reporting and interpretation procedures. The use of small groupings of inter-related tests in this way is *not* an example of screening.

Some laboratories use fixed-configuration multichannel analysers to perform physiologically-unrelated large groups of tests on every specimen analysed, with little or no additional trouble and little more expense than that involved in performing any single one of the tests in the *analytical group*. For example, in a

Table 1.1 Examples of tests used in case-finding programmes

Programmes to detect diseases in	Chemical investigations
Neonates	
Phenylketonuria	Serum [phenylalanine]
Hypothyroidism	Serum [TSH] and/or [thyroxine]
Adolescents and young adults	
Substance abuse	Drug screen
Pregnancy	
Diabetes mellitus in the mother	Plasma and urine [glucose]
Open neural tube defect in the fetus	Maternal serum [α-fetoprotein]
Industry	
Industrial exposure to lead	Blood [lead]
Industrial exposure to pesticides	Plasma cholinesterase activity
Elderly	
Malnutrition	Plasma [albumin] and/or [pre-albumin]
Thyroid dysfunction	Plasma [TSH] and/or [thyroxine]

specimen for which plasma [bilirubin] has been requested, not only may the results of other 'liver function tests' be available but also the results of 'electrolyte', 'bone' and perhaps other functional groups of tests. Thus, for reasons of analytical convenience, such laboratories may generate results for many tests few of which have been requested on clinical grounds. In these circumstances, the laboratory may report all results obtained, whether or not all the tests have been requested. Otherwise, once doctors know that the laboratory has a multichannel analyser which performs a fixed combination of tests, consciously or subconsciously they tend to request all the tests available on that analyser whether or not its total analytical repertoire relates closely to the real clinical needs of their patients.

Medical advantages and disadvantages of screening

The *advantages of screening* hospital patients at the time of their admission or first attendance at hospital are that hitherto unsuspected and potentially treatable disease may be detected at an early stage and perhaps thereby significantly influence the subsequent management of some patients. Theoretically, also, admission screening should save time and enable some patients to be discharged from hospital earlier than might otherwise have been the case. In practice, various studies have shown that this forecast is not correct.

Disorders detected by screening of hospital patients by means of chemical investigations that would not necessarily have been among the tests requested on clinical grounds include the occasional recognition of hitherto unsuspected cases of:

1 *Hyperparathyroidism*, suggested by the unexpected finding of a raised plasma [calcium]. This is the most frequent way in which this diagnosis is made nowadays (p. 202).

2 *Hypothyroidism*, suggested by the unexpected finding of a raised plasma [TSH] and/or a low [total T4] or [free T4]. However, other reasons for these findings must be carefully considered (p. 255–260).

3 *Diabetes mellitus*, suggested by the unexpected finding of an abnormal random plasma [glucose].

4 *Renal tract disease*, indicated as a possibility when a raised plasma [creatinine] or [urea] is unexpectedly reported.

5 *Liver disease*, suggested by the unexpected finding of increased plasma ALT, AST, GGT or alkaline phosphatase activity (depending on which screening test is used).

The *disadvantages of screening*, experienced in both hospital and general (community-based) medical practice, include:

1 Doctors receive large quantities of information on every patient, much or all of it without obvious clinical relevance to individual patients. Often they do not have time to review the data systematically, because of the amount.

2 Because of the difficulty of assimilating these 'floods' of results, information of clinical significance is liable to be missed among the other, in many cases less relevant, data.

3 Additional investigations may be needed in order to decide whether any unexpected abnormal results generated by screening tests are of diagnostic importance.

In short, the most useful applications of chemical tests in screening occur in case-finding studies (see above). We share the widely held view that performing a large range of chemical tests in the unselective screening of hospital patients is of relatively limited diagnostic value. Examples of screening and case-finding programmes of proven worth will be considered in later chapters.

Collection of specimens

Most quantitative chemical investigations are carried out on blood: the next most frequently examined specimens are urine. Other specimens sent for chemical analysis include CSF, intestinal secretions, faeces, calculi, sweat, amniotic fluid and fluids obtained by paracentesis, and occasionally saliva.

This section describes points that need to be observed to ensure that specimens for chemical analysis are always of good quality. Specimens collected or preserved under unsuitable conditions may appear to be suitable for analysis, but the results obtained with such specimens are often inaccurate, and fail to indicate the true condition of patients at the time they were collected.

Identification of patients and specimens

It is essential that every specimen be collected from the correct patient and that each specimen be identified unequivocally in relation to the corresponding patient on the request for investigations, whether the request be written on a form or entered via a computer terminal. The following points must be observed:

1   *Patient identification data (PID).* These must be unique, and must be used correctly with every request for investigations.

2   *Test request information.* Each request should include relevant clinical details and must specify the tests to be performed and state precisely where the report is to be sent.

3   *Collection of specimens.* These must be appropriate for the analyses to be performed, and preserved correctly, in accordance with the laboratory's requirements.

4   *Matching of specimens to requests.* Each specimen must be able to be easily and unequivocally matched to the corresponding request for investigations.

There is no fool-proof method of identifying patients and specimens, but most health-care PID systems can do so uniquely if properly used. With manually completed request forms, however, identification data often fail to be entered completely and correctly on the forms, even when the data are readily available. Under these circumstances, although it will often be possible to carry out the analyses, there may be insufficient PID information for the report to be matched up unambiguously with the patient from whom the specimen was collected or with that patient's medical records. It is just as important to label specimens unequivocally, as it can otherwise be difficult or even impossible for laboratory staff to match each specimen to the corresponding request for analyses.

Collection and preservation of blood specimens

It is important to think before collecting specimens of blood for chemical analysis. Many factors associated with specimen collection can adversely affect the results and thus impair their validity. The grossest examples of carelessness involve the collection of specimens from the wrong patients or labelling specimens incorrectly after collection. Other factors to bear in mind, since they might affect the timing of specimen collection or the need for the patient to be prepared prior to being investigated, include:

1 *Diet*. Dietary constituents may temporarily alter the concentrations of analytes in blood significantly. For instance, a carbohydrate-containing meal is likely to increase blood [glucose], and plasma [creatinine] and [urea] may sometimes rise considerably after a protein-containing meal. Other dietary constituents may interfere with the performance of some analyses (e.g. urinary catecholamine measurements). Any guidance that the laboratory provides about the timing of specimen collection in relation to food intake should be complied with.

2 *Drugs*. Many drugs influence the chemical composition of blood. Sometimes it may be possible to delay starting treatment, or to stop it temporarily, to enable essential investigations to be performed. More often, however, the effects of drug treatment have to be taken into account when interpreting test results, e.g. in patients on anti-epileptic drugs (p. 369) or in women taking oral contraceptives (p. 312). It is important to give details of relevant drug treatment when requesting chemical analyses, especially when toxicological investigations are to be performed (p. 370).

3 *Diurnal variation*. The concentrations of many substances in blood vary considerably at different times of day (e.g. cortisol, triglycerides). Specimens for these analyses must be collected at the times specified by the laboratory as there may be no reference ranges relating to their concentrations in blood at other times.

Care when collecting blood specimens

The posture of the patient, the choice of skin-cleansing agent, and the selection of a suitable vein (or other source) are the principal factors to consider before proceeding to collect each specimen. Technique is then important, including the amount of venous stasis, the steps to be taken to avoid causing haemolysis, and the need to bear in mind that blood is a potentially infective agent.

The *skin must be clean* over the site for collecting the blood specimen. However, it must be remembered that alcohol and methylated spirits can cause haemolysis, and that their use is clearly to be avoided if blood [ethanol] is to be determined.

Limbs into which intravenous infusions are being given must not be selected as the site of venepuncture unless particular care is taken. The needle or cannula must first be thoroughly flushed out with blood. Otherwise, the specimen will be diluted to an unpredictable extent by the infusion fluid, wherever the specimen is obtained (whether proximal or distal to the infusion site, or from the infusion site itself).

Arterial blood specimens, and arterialized capillary specimens, to be obtained for full acid–base studies, should be collected from patients who are suitably relaxed and no longer apprehensive (p. 59).

Venepuncture technique should be standardized as far as possible, to enable closer comparison of successive results obtained on patients who are being repeatedly investigated. Venous blood specimens should be obtained with minimal stasis. Prolonged stasis can markedly raise the concentrations of plasma proteins and other non-diffusible substances (e.g. protein-bound substances). It is advisable to release the tourniquet before withdrawing the sample of blood.

For routine specimens, these should ideally be collected from patients who have fasted overnight and who have been lying down for at least 20 minutes prior to specimen collection. These conditions should be attainable with hospital in-patients, but are only partially practicable with ambulant patients, and are inappropriate in the case of emergencies or urgently required investigations. When a patient's posture changes from lying to standing, there may be an increase of as much as 13% in the concentration of many components of the blood within 15 minutes (e.g. plasma proteins and constituents such as calcium or cortisol that are bound or partly bound to protein), due to redistribution of fluid in the extracellular space.

Haemolysis can occur for many reasons. It renders specimens unsuitable for plasma K^+, magnesium and many protein and enzyme activity measurements. Specimens should be collected with only moderate suction and the needle always removed from the syringe before emptying it slowly into the specimen container, leaving behind any froth in the syringe. No more than the appropriate amount of blood should be added to the specimen tube, and any anticoagulant or preservative then mixed with the blood by repeated gentle inversion; the tube must not be shaken. When collecting capillary specimens, the selected site must be warm and there should be a free flow of blood; squeezing dilutes the blood sample with tissue fluid and increases the risk of haemolysis.

Case 1.1

The resident doctor on a surgical ward was called at 2334 h by the nursing staff to see a 55-year-old patient whose condition was thought to have deteriorated 2 days after a hemicolectomy. After examining the patient, the doctor performed a venepuncture and requested plasma urea and electrolyte measurements as an emergency. The results (column B), together with those for the same analyses on a specimen collected earlier that day (column A) were as follows:

Analysis	Column A	Column B	Reference range
[Urea]	8.5	1.8	2.5–6.6 mmol/L
[Na$^+$]	131	142	132–144 mmol/L
[K$^+$]	3.2	1.4	3.3–4.7 mmol/L
[Total CO$_2$]	24	10	24–30 mmol/L

What is the most likely explanation for these changes in results? There was no obvious clinical reason for such changes. What should the doctor do next? This patient is discussed on p. 11.

Care of blood specimens after collection

Blood specimens should be transported to the laboratory as soon as possible after collection. Special arrangements are needed for some specimens (e.g. for acid–base measurements, p. 59) because of their lack of stability. Most other analytes are stable for at least 3 hours, and some blood constituents are stable for much longer if plasma or serum is first separated from the cells. Directions for storage of plasma or serum (e.g. in a refrigerator overnight) can be obtained from the laboratory. As a rule, whole blood specimens for chemical analysis must not be stored in a refrigerator. Several changes occur in blood specimens following collection unless proper precautions are observed. *The commoner and more important changes that occur prior to the separation of plasma or serum from the cells are*:

1   Glucose is converted to lactate; this process is inhibited by fluoride.
2   Several substances pass through the erythrocyte membrane, or may be added in significant amounts to plasma as a result of red cell destruction insufficient to cause detectable haemolysis. Examples include K^+ and lactate dehydrogenase.
3   Loss of CO_2 occurs since the P_{CO_2} of blood is much higher than in air.
4   Plasma [phosphate] increases due to hydrolysis of organic ester phosphates in the erythrocytes.
5   Labile plasma enzymes lose their activity, e.g. prostatic acid phosphatase.

Whenever a specimen is liable to present a particular *infection hazard* to laboratory staff (e.g. hepatitis B, HIV-related specimen), this must be clearly indicated as part of the request. Any special directions about transport to the laboratory and the labelling of the specimen must also be closely observed.

Collection and preservation of urine specimens

Many measurements can be performed on random (untimed) specimens of urine. However, their value is usually greatly increased if they can be performed on an aliquot of a *complete timed collection* of urine. To obtain such a collection, clear instructions must be given both to the patient and to the nursing staff (if the patient is in hospital); these must be obeyed, or the test abandoned and started again, as follows:

1   Just before the collection period is due to start, the patient empties his/her bladder. *This urine must be discarded.*
2   Thereafter, from the start (e.g. at 0800 h) to the end of the collection period, *all urine passed by the patient must be added to the container*. If this contains preservative, the specimen must be mixed gently each time more urine is passed and added to the collection.
3   At the end of the period (e.g. 0800 h the next day, in the case of a 24-hour collection), the patient empties his/her bladder. *This urine must be included* in the collection.
4   The period over which the collection was made must be recorded.

Urine specimens should be sent to the laboratory soon after the collection period is over. Where there is difficulty in transporting a large receptacle containing the complete collection of urine, the total volume should be measured and recorded. Then, after proper mixing, an aliquot (e.g. 25 mL) can be transferred to a small container and this sample sent to the laboratory, the volume of the complete 24-hour specimen being stated both in the request for analysis and on the label of the sample.

Urine specimens tend to deteriorate unless preservative is added from the start, or the specimen refrigerated throughout the collection period. The changes include:

1 Destruction of glucose by bacteria.
2 Conversion of urea to ammonia, by bacteria, with fall in $[H^+]$ and precipitation of phosphates.
3 Oxidation of urobilinogen to urobilin and porphobilinogen to porphyrins.

Collection and preservation of faecal specimens

Quantitative work with faecal specimens can only be performed with patients who are fully cooperative, and who are preferably being looked after by trained staff in a metabolic unit. Even then, it can be difficult to ensure complete faecal collections. Preservation of faecal specimens prior to their transport to the laboratory for chemical analysis is by refrigeration.

Urgent investigations when the laboratory is closed

Some analyses can be carried out by clinical staff, using the kind of equipment discussed in Chapter 2. Others depend on those laboratory staff who man an out-of-hours duty roster. Usually only one technician is rostered for this purpose, even in large hospitals, so it is essential that requests for urgent investigations be restricted to those tests that are needed for immediate diagnostic purposes or for the management of seriously ill patients. If non-urgent investigations will be required on specimens collected at these times, plasma or serum can be separated off and stored in a refrigerator until the laboratory is next open normally (e.g. the following weekday).

It is important to note that many laboratories use analytical techniques outside normal working hours that are different (quicker and often less specific) from those used when the laboratories are fully staffed. This can lead to difficulties if the results for analyses performed by out-of-hours emergency procedures are compared with results obtained later by the laboratory's routine procedures. Likewise, results for analyses performed, for example, on ward-based analysers may differ quite markedly from results obtained later on the same specimen for analyses carried out in the laboratory, because of differences between the techniques employed in the different locations.

Audit

All countries now have increasing concerns about the cost of health-care delivery. In particular, since the seemingly inexorable spiral in costs has to be contained, it is clear that expenditure has to be related to health outcomes such as mortality, morbidity, quality of life, etc. Audit is the process whereby the procedures involved in patient care are monitored in order to give high priority to the delivery of an efficient and cost-effective service. The *measure of health outcome is benefit to the patient.*

The value of audit can most readily be seen in those specialties concerned directly with patient care, but the principles are applicable to all clinical, investigational (e.g. Radiology) and laboratory-based specialties such as Clinical Biochemistry.

The audit process

There is an essential sequence to auditing activities consisting of the following steps:

1 Identify an area of concern or interest, particularly if it is felt that there is room for improvement in the service or if the same quality of service can be provided more economically.
2 Review and analyse the present procedures.
3 Identify specific aspects that might be capable of improvement.
4 Identify alternative procedures or standards which might lead to improvement.
5 Take the practical steps necessary to implement any changes proposed.
6 Compare the performance after the changes with those before them.

It must be emphasized that the final stage of analysis of the effects of any change is an integral part of the audit process; it is essential to know whether the measures taken have improved the service or made it more cost-effective. Sometimes, changes have no effect, or even adverse effects.

Audit in Clinical Biochemistry

Internal and external audit of quality have been practised widely in Clinical Biochemistry for many years. These procedures have involved extensive internal quality assessment procedures which monitor accuracy and precision of the assays performed every day in the laboratory, as well as National External Quality Assurance Schemes (NEQAS) which are available for most analyses, and which monitor their performance at fortnightly (or less frequent) intervals. These quality initiatives are now being widened to embrace the specific objectives of medical audit, i.e. those concerned with outcome and with cost. There are a number of broad areas which suggest themselves for review:

1 *Specimen collection and transport.* Is advice about the selection of suitable tests available? Are request forms easy to use? Are appropriate containers for specimens readily available? Is the specimen transport system convenient, rapid and efficient? Is there a phlebotomy service and, if so, how effective is it?
2 *Analytical aspects of the service.* Are good quality results being produced? Is there an acceptably small number of grossly inaccurate results (blunders) due, for example, to transcription errors? Is the test repertoire appropriate? Are there any tests which are now outmoded? Are there newer, more effective, tests which would enable more efficient diagnosis? Is equipment sited at the most appropriate place (e.g. in the ward) and capable of delivering results within the time-scale required for the optimal management of the patient?
3 *Reporting and interpretation.* Are reports being delivered to the right place within the necessary time-scale? Are clinical staff being provided with the appropriate information which will allow them to interpret results correctly, e.g. reference ranges and laboratory handbook? Is the system of monitoring and

commenting on reports adequate and helpful? Is expert advice on the interpretation of results always readily available?

4 *Emergency service.* Is this being provided in the most cost-effective manner?

5 *Clinical protocols.* Is there a case for introducing standardized clinical protocols for the investigation and treatment of well-defined clinical conditions? Such protocols would define the appropriate investigations, and their timing, in relation to patients with, for example, myocardial infarction, liver disease, thyroid disease, etc. Protocols that state the investigations appropriate for the pre-operative patient can also be defined for particular circumstances (e.g. the acute abdomen).

6 *Education and research.* Are users of the diagnostic service being educated in the proper use of laboratory facilities? Is the laboratory playing its part in fulfilling a more general educative role in the hospital and the community? Is there appropriate investment in research and development? Some of these aspects may be seen as fulfilling more long-term objectives.

Some of the areas defined above can be looked at from within the laboratory. Others require collaboration with clinicians and, sometimes, with other disciplines related to Medicine. Computer technology is often not required to complete many projects related to the sort of problems outlined above. However, more complex resource-management systems able to identify and monitor the investigation and management of individual patients will be required for proper analysis of some of the problems, e.g. the use of clinical protocols.

There may be many areas where laboratory diagnostic services can be altered in order to render the health service as a whole more cost-effective. It is important that programmes be not too ambitious initially and that all new measures be subject to rigorous scrutiny, to determine whether the service has, indeed, been improved by the changes introduced.

In many countries, laboratories are required to be accredited if they are to perform investigations related to patient care. Accreditation is dependent, in many cases, on a laboratory having in place appropriate audit procedures.

Comments on Case 1.1 (p. 7)

The results in column B are typical of those reported when a blood specimen has been obtained from a site close to where an intravenous infusion of 0.9% NaCl (150 mmol/L) is being given. The resident should obtain a satisfactory blood specimen and ask for the analyses to be repeated. When the plasma analyses were repeated in this patient, the results were as follows (data in mmol/L):

[Urea], 9.0; [Na^+], 130; [K^+], 3.4; Total CO_2, 22

Chapter 2
Chemical Tests Performed
Close to the Patient, in the Ward
or Clinic Environment

The range and complexity of chemical investigations able to be performed in the ward and clinic environment, and in general practitioners' surgeries, continue to grow. Wet chemistry methods, the techniques classically associated with 'side-room' methods, have been replaced by 'dipstick' technology and reagents in tablet form for testing urine and faecal specimens. For blood analyses, developments in systems that can perform chemical analyses on whole blood specimens (i.e. without the need for centrifuging and manual transfer operations), coupled with developments in microprocessor-controlled analytical procedures and digital read-out, now offer practical alternatives to having to send all specimens to hospital laboratories for analysis.

The advantages to doctors and patients of being able to have certain chemical analyses performed locally relate mainly to the speed with which the results become available. This can be of critical importance in intensive care areas, especially if these are sited at a considerable distance from the main hospital laboratory. Also, in out-patient clinics, the rapid availability of results can mean that the doctor is able to adjust a patient's treatment, if necessary, and give appropriate advice during the one attendance rather than having to recall the patient or give the advice by letter.

We recognize and accept that more and more chemical analyses will be performed at a distance from the hospital laboratory, which is sometimes situated off-site, several miles away. After considering the range of analyses already able to be performed in the ward or clinic environment, often by staff who are not professional laboratory workers, this chapter will describe those criteria that doctors must bear in mind, and regularly practise, if extra-laboratory analytical work is to be performed both safely and reliably.

'Side-room' tests on urine and faeces

Patients sometimes complain about the colour of their urine. In that case, it is important to enquire about their diet and to consider their possible drug intake (prescribed and self-administered). It is also essential to inspect a fresh specimen of urine before deciding which chemical investigations might be appropriate. Table 2.1 lists some abnormal colours and gives examples of their possible causes. Other patients may complain of passing very dark faeces, and these should be tested for occult blood before initiating further investigations.

Urine tests

Tests such as those listed in Table 2.2 can all be performed satisfactorily by doctors

Table 2.1 Examples of abnormal colours of freshly passed urine specimens

Colour*	Examples of possible causes of the abnormal colour	
	Pathological	Diet and drugs
Greenish-brown	Bile pigments, i.e. bilirubin (and biliverdin)†	
Grey or brown or blackish	Melanogens, homogentisic acid‡	Some parenteral iron preparations, L-dopa‡
Pinkish or red or reddish-brown	Haemoglobin, myoglobin, porphobilinogen,‡ porphyrins	Beetroot (anthocyanines), cascara, danthron and senna (examples of anthroquinone-containing laxatives), phenolphthalein (if urine alkaline)
Reddish-brown	Haemoglobin, methaemoglobin	
Yellow		Tetracyclines

* Urine is normally straw-coloured, but the depth of its colour can vary greatly; the natural colour of concentrated urine specimens can affect the hue developed in the presence of any abnormal colorant.
† Yellow froth, due to the presence additionally of bile salts, appears on shaking; the yellow colour is due to conjugated bilirubin.
‡ Colour appears or darkens on standing.

Table 2.2 'Side-room' tests on urine and faecal specimens (the chemical tests able to be performed with materials obtainable from one manufacturer*)

Components of multi-test reagent strips for testing urine

Bilirubin	Ketones	Protein
Blood	Nitrite†	Specific gravity
Glucose	pH	Urobilinogen

Single-test materials (strips or tablets) for testing urine

Bilirubin	Glucose	Ketones‡
Reducing substances		

Test material for testing faeces
Occult blood

* Bayer Diagnostics, Ames Technicon, Bayer plc, Evans House, Hamilton Close, Houndmills, Basingstoke, Hants RG21 2YE, UK. A comparable range of multi-test reagent strips for urine testing is available from Boehringer (address in Table 2.3).
† A non-specific chemical test for urinary tract infection.
‡ Also sometimes used on blood specimens from patients in diabetic coma.

and nurses and, in some instances, by patients or their relatives at home, after a limited amount of tuition. For a proper understanding of these tests, including their chemical basis as well as details of their interpretation and potential sources of interference that need to be avoided, it is incumbent upon doctors (as the people responsible for the quality of test performance, whether undertaken personally or delegated) to read the manufacturers' literature carefully. If points about the tests are still not clear, doctors should either consult a professional laboratory worker in their local hospital laboratory or ask the manufacturer's representative to clarify points of difficulty. It is not appropriate to regard dipsticks as fool-proof, as things that merely need to be dipped into a urine specimen and then compared against a set of standard colours. Some of these tests are potentially so important as to deserve brief consideration.

Glucose and reducing substances

It is worth testing the urine of any patient who complains of weight loss, or excessive thirst or undue frequency of micturition, for the presence of glucose and protein. These tests should also be performed as part of any full clinical examination, and are regularly included as part of medical examinations for insurance purposes.

Tests for glucose in urine (glucosuria) all depend on the use of dipsticks impregnated with glucose oxidase, an enzyme that is specific for glucose. Tests for reducing substances in urine (glycosuria) use chemicals that react with any compound that possesses a reducing group. For instance, copper sulphate in alkaline solution reacts with glucose (the reducing substance most often detectable in urine), as well as with fructose, galactose and lactose (but not sucrose) and with creatinine (if the urine specimen is concentrated).

The tests for glucosuria and glycosuria give semi-quantitative results. These can be used satisfactorily by some diabetic patients to monitor and regulate the control of their treatment between clinic visits.

The recognition of renal glucosuria requires the testing of urine specimens passed during a glucose tolerance test (p. 166) in which blood specimens have been collected at 30-minute intervals, in order to detect the occurrence of glucosuria at blood glucose concentrations below the normal renal threshold for glucose (10 mmol/L).

It is worth testing the urine of neonates routinely for reducing substances as many inborn errors of metabolism give rise to urinary metabolites that react positively in this test.

Protein

Tests for proteinuria are best carried out on an early morning specimen of urine, as this is normally the most concentrated specimen that can be readily obtained. The test materials do not detect all proteins with equal sensitivity; for instance, they often fail to detect Bence Jones protein, whereas they detect albumin if present in concentrations greater than 100 mg/L.

Special tests are required in order to detect Bence Jones protein (p. 98) and 'microalbuminuria', an early sign of diabetic nephropathy (p. 172). If proteinuria is found on 'side-room' testing of urine, it will then be necessary to distinguish between: (i) benign causes of proteinuria (e.g. postural proteinuria); (ii) patients who do not have renal disease but who may have a condition that can cause proteinuria (e.g. fever, congestive cardiac failure); and (iii) patients with organic renal disease (Chapter 9).

Ketones

The tests for ketones in urine are most sensitive for acetoacetic acid but they also detect acetone. However, they do not react with 3-hydroxybutyric acid, the 'ketone body' that is present in urine in greatest amount in poorly controlled diabetes mellitus, starvation, hyperemesis gravidarum, etc.

It is worth instructing diabetic patients to record results for urine ketones (and protein), if they are using multi-reagent dipsticks to test their own urine regularly for the presence of glucose. Testing urine for ketones is also important in the recognition of diabetic ketoacidosis (p. 172).

Some inborn errors of metabolism give rise to the excretion of ketones in urine, and it is worth testing for these at the same time as testing for reducing substances in neonatal urine. However, these urinary dipstick tests are not a substitute for the much more sensitive and specific tests on blood spots for phenylketonuria (p. 329).

Urobilinogen and bilirubin

The results of these tests, when considered in relation to a patient's history and the findings on clinical examination, are potentially very helpful in distinguishing pre-hepatic jaundice from hepatocellular and post-hepatic jaundice (Table 8.2, p. 109). They may also help with the recognition of acute hepatitis before the onset of jaundice, and in following the subsequent course of the disease.

It is essential to have a fresh specimen of urine when testing for urobilinogen.

Specific gravity (sp. gr.)

In patients complaining of thirst or frequency of micturition, it is worth measuring urinary sp. gr., having first tested the urine for the presence of glucose and protein. Specific gravity measurements provide an indication of renal concentrating power, if performed on early morning specimens, but determining the sp. gr. of a random sample of urine gives limited information. Urinary sp. gr. is usually directly proportional to osmolality, but the test gives misleadingly high results if there is significant glycosuria or proteinuria whereas osmolality measurements are not significantly affected (p. 36).

pH

Urine is normally acidic (as compared with plasma) in healthy subjects on a meat-containing diet. An alkaline urine may be found in vegans, in patients ingesting alkali, or in patients with urinary tract infections. 'Side-room' tests can be used to give a rough estimate of urine pH over the range 5–9 pH units. It is important to measure urine pH on freshly voided urine specimens.

Faeces

The detection of gastrointestinal blood loss may be very important for clinical diagnosis. The various chemical tests all depend on the pseudoperoxidase activity of haem. Unfortunately, interpretation of results is not simple because:

1 Up to 2 mL blood may be lost normally in the faeces each day.
2 The various 'side-room' tests differ widely in their sensitivity.

3 Meat and some vegetables, and certain iron preparations, may cause false-positive results as they also have pseudoperoxidase activity.
4 Reducing agents (e.g. ascorbic acid) cause false-negative results if ingested in sufficient quantity.
5 Bleeding from tumours into the gut lumen is often intermittent.
6 Blood lost into the lumen of the gastrointestinal tract is unlikely to be evenly dispersed. Unless faecal specimens are homogenized, sampling errors are likely.

All chemical tests for faecal occult blood yield some false-positive and some false-negative results. At present, there is no entirely satisfactory chemical test for occult blood. Despite all these disadvantages, however, these tests are cheap and easy to perform, and they still have a place in diagnosis.

False-positive results often occur with the more sensitive methods of blood detection, and are serious as they cause unnecessary further investigation with all the attendant worry for the patient. Their incidence can be reduced by repeating the occult blood test after the patient has been placed for 3 days on a diet that excludes meat and green vegetables, but even so the predictive value of a positive result in terms of screening for serious organic disease (e.g. carcinoma of the colon) is under 10%.

False-negative results occur with the less sensitive tests. Such results are dangerous. They give the doctor and the patient a misleading sense of security and can considerably delay diagnosis of potentially serious but often initially curable conditions. These less sensitive tests should not be used.

Requirements for performing all types of chemical 'side-room' tests

The satisfactory performance of 'side-room' tests on urine and faeces are:
1 A clean working area, properly ventilated.
2 Proper performance of the tests themselves.
3 Provision for the safe disposal of specimens and test materials.

Good technique is essential with precise adherence to the manufacturers' clear and simple instructions. If the directions are not strictly followed, false-positive and false-negative results will be obtained and the tests are then liable to fall into disrepute because of their apparent lack of reliability. Cleanliness is particularly important.

Medical students and doctors tend to rely on nurses to carry out the tests on urine and faeces. It is, nevertheless, important that they should themselves gain and retain experience in their performance since the quality of the results is normally the responsibility of clinical staff. Doctors may need to instruct others (e.g. patients, patients' relatives) in aspects of the performance of 'side-room' tests. It is also essential that they be able to discuss the records of 'side-room' test results, and to do so knowledgeably. It is the doctor's responsibility to deal with any difficulties in interpretation; these are often due to faulty technique.

The best results with urine 'side-room' tests are obtained with the single-test or limited multi-test materials. Recording several sets of results, all obtained within a very short time, tends to be inaccurate. Nevertheless, the multi-test urine-testing materials have many advantages, and are not difficult to use correctly.

Measurements on blood specimens in ward and clinic areas

There are several examples of equipment that can be used satisfactorily for the performance of quantitative chemical analyses on blood specimens and which do not require to be operated by professional laboratory staff. Accident and emergency departments, assisted ventilation units, special care baby units and post-operative recovery rooms are all examples of hospital locations where there are recurring and predictable needs for the urgent and rapid performance of a definable range of chemical measurements on blood specimens, if the results are to be available sufficiently quickly to provide maximum help in the management of patients.

It frequently happens that the hospital laboratory is a considerable distance away from some intensive care units, and may even be off-site. As it can take time to arrange even for urgent specimens to be transported to the laboratory, the needs of these units for rapid and reliable results are being met more and more by the purchase of analytical equipment for local use.

Examples of equipment that can be operated satisfactorily by clinical staff in intensive care units, and by other non-laboratory personnel, include the following:

1 *Bilirubinometers*. Their main use is in obstetric units for measuring plasma [bilirubin] in jaundiced infants to help with decisions about treatment.

2 *Blood-gas analysers*. In obstetric units, measurements of fetal blood $[H^+]$ prove helpful in the early detection of fetal distress, and existing equipment enables blood P_{CO_2}, P_{O_2} and plasma $[HCO_3^-]$ to be determined at the same time. Many operating theatres and other intensive care areas have automatic blood-gas analysers.

3 *Blood glucose analysers*. Reflectance meters are now widely used in neonatal and special care baby units, accident and emergency departments and other intensive care units as well as in less urgent situations such as diabetic clinics and doctors' consulting rooms.

4 *Other ion-selective electrode systems*. These have been developed mainly for the measurement of plasma $[Na^+]$ and $[K^+]$ on whole blood specimens, i.e. there is no need to centrifuge these specimens prior to analysis. However, seriously misleading results for plasma $[K^+]$ will be obtained if the specimen is even only slightly haemolysed; with these analysers, haemolysis is liable to go undetected. They are mostly used in intensive care areas in support of major surgery (e.g. cardiac bypass, organ transplant operations).

Recent developments

Single-test 'stick' technology for the measurement of blood [glucose] has been followed by major developments in the packaging of reagents, thereby rendering possible the performance of a much wider range of quantitative analyses. One system that uses these reagents no longer requires the initial centrifuging of blood specimens and manual separation of plasma; its analytical processes are all microprocessor-controlled, with results presented as a digital read-out (Table 2.3).

The growing range of analyses available on such equipment offers doctors a practical alternative to their having to send all blood specimens to hospital

Table 2.3 Tests on blood specimens in the clinic environment (the chemical tests able to be performed with a system obtainable from one manufacturer*)

Measurements of concentration		Enzyme activity measurements
Bilirubin	Haemoglobin	Alanine aminotransferase (ALT)
Cholesterol	Potassium	Amylase (total)
HDL-cholesterol	Triglycerides	Pancreatic amylase
LDL-cholesterol†	Urea	Aspartate aminotransferase (AST)
Creatinine	Uric acid	Creatine kinase
Glucose		Gamma-glutamyl transferase (GGT)

* BCL, Boehringer Mannheim House, Bell Lane, Lewes, East Sussex BN7 1LG, UK.
† By calculation from results of other lipid analyses.

laboratories for these analyses. However, the capital and operating costs of these systems, and the requirements that must be regularly observed (see below) if they are to be used safely and reliably, have to be weighed against the advantages to be gained from obtaining these results quickly. It seems likely that most doctors will continue to depend on hospital chemical laboratories for performing most of the investigative work that they require for the diagnosis and management of their patients' illnesses.

The tests listed in Table 2.3 do not represent the limits of the extra-laboratory techniques that can now be used to provide results of chemical investigations locally in real time. For instance, glycated haemoglobin (HbA_{1c}) can now be measured in the clinic by non-laboratory personnel and the results used to help determine the appropriate advice to be given to diabetic patients before they leave the clinic. Other developments of techniques for clinic use are being made in the field of drug-testing, but there can be difficulties in interpreting their results correctly.

Cholesterol screening

Screening strategies whereby members of the general public are encouraged, sometimes by commercial interests, to arrange for their own blood cholesterol measurements to be performed (e.g. in supermarkets or other retail outlets) can be less than satisfactory unless there are stringent safeguards. The quality of the results needs to be monitored regularly and appropriate counselling about diet, the implications of the result, etc., should accompany every cholesterol result. Without this advice, the screening process is largely valueless and may lead to inappropriate action or unwarranted anxiety on the part of the person screened.

Requirements for performing extra-laboratory blood tests

The requirements for the satisfactory performance of chemical analyses on blood specimens in the ward or clinic environment (including general practitioners' surgeries and office practice) are more demanding than for 'side-room' tests on urine and faeces, especially if these measurements are to be performed by other than professionally trained laboratory staff. These requirements will be briefly reviewed.

Health and safety

Working with blood specimens carries a significant risk of acquiring infection with, for instance, hepatitis B or HIV.

It is essential that a *workable* code of safe practice be drawn up by professional laboratory staff, and that all clinic staff who will use the equipment be given appropriate instruction before undertaking specimen-handling and analytical operations. These staff must be made to appreciate the need to conform thereafter to the code of practice *every time* they perform analyses.

Training

Non-laboratory staff require to be properly trained in the operation of chemical analysers purchased for ward or clinic use. Such training should be undertaken, for each member of staff, by professional laboratory staff. Although this can make great demands on the trainers' time, it is essential to eliminate the otherwise potentially dangerous practice of, for instance, clinical staff 'training' other doctors when rotas or appointments change.

Only properly trained staff should be permitted to use the equipment, following their training. They need to be provided with simple sets of written instructions, and must understand the need to obey these instructions.

Non-laboratory staff performing chemical analyses need to be made to appreciate the importance of carrying out at least some of the quality control procedures that are regularly practised by professional staff in hospital laboratories. They must be able to recognize when an instrument is giving unreliable results, and know what to do under these circumstances. The importance of proper calibration and quality control procedures should be explained and stressed as part of the initial training programme.

Record-keeping

There should be a clearly set out check-list that ward or clinic staff can easily follow so as to ensure their compliance with directions before, during and after making each set of observations. There must be a record book for entering results and any other essential data relating to the use of the equipment such as calibration readings and results for quality control specimens.

Clinic staff should be made aware of the importance of keeping proper written records of all their work. It is unfortunately all too true that, when analytical results are needed quickly on a patient, clinic staff tend to neglect essentials such as quality control and record-keeping procedures and, possibly as a consequence, to obtain invalid results.

Involvement of laboratory staff

Hospital staff and general practitioners should not hesitate to consult laboratory staff about the choice of analytical equipment for use in an extra-laboratory environment. When selecting such equipment, there is much to be said for including in the specification a printer that generates a continuous hard copy of all the analyses performed on the equipment, with a record of the time each set of results was generated. This helps with retrospective investigation of poor quality work.

It should normally be the responsibility of professional laboratory staff to train others in the use of extra-laboratory chemical equipment to be used for analyses on blood. They should also be the people responsible for carrying out regular checks (e.g. daily in intensive care units) on the equipment, and for examining the records of analytical performance for the period since their previous set of checks.

It is unlikely, even with the best extra-laboratory equipment, that its users will cease to depend from time to time on the hospital laboratory for performing some or all of the analyses normally performed on the equipment. As the analytical techniques used by the laboratory may differ in important respects from those used on the extra-laboratory equipment, different sets of reference ranges may apply; this is especially likely in the case of enzyme activity measurements, including results reported in 'international units' (p. 73).

Test selection and interpretation, and related considerations

The performance of chemical tests by clinical staff in any location needs to be subject to the same processes of disciplined test selection as are discussed in Chapter 1, and in the later chapters of this book, for tests that are to be performed on their behalf by staff in a hospital laboratory. Economic considerations are likely to demand this, even if other reasons for selectivity are discounted, as the costs of extra-laboratory analyses fall on clinicians' budgets. Likewise, the collection of specimens for extra-laboratory analytical work has to be undertaken with the same care and attention to detail.

The interpretation of the relatively simple 'side-room' dipstick and other tests on urine and faeces require good lighting, normal perception of colours and strict adherence to the suppliers' instructions about the time when observations of test results are to be made.

The interpretation of quantitative chemical investigations performed on extra-laboratory equipment demands consideration of the general questions discussed in Chapter 3 and of the aspects relating to particular analyses considered in the relevant subsequent chapters. Where difficulties in the interpretation of these analyses arise, it is advisable to consult a professionally trained laboratory member of staff.

As with all laboratory-based procedures, extra-laboratory analyses should be subjected to regular audit, and this should include so far as possible participation in External Quality Assurance Schemes, despite the additional expense that this involves.

In conclusion, it is important to draw the attention of clinical staff to the possible medicolegal implications of wrong results for chemical analyses, especially when these can be shown to be due to careless work such as might be implied by poor recording of results, including failure to record data for quality control specimens.

Chapter 3
Interpreting and Using Laboratory Data

Most reports issued by clinical biochemistry laboratories contain numerical, quantitative measures of concentration or activity expressed in the appropriate units. When interpreting these data, doctors should consider some or all of the following questions:

1 Is each result normal or abnormal? Reference ranges are needed in order to answer questions about quantitative data.

2 Does each result fit in with my previous assessment of this patient? If not, can I explain the discrepancy?

3 In a patient who has been investigated previously, has a significant change occurred in any of the results from those previously reported? To answer this question, information is needed about the laboratory's analytical standard deviation (SD) or coefficient of variation (CV) values.

4 Do any of the results alter my diagnosis of this patient's illness or influence the way in which the illness should be managed?

5 If I cannot explain a result, what do I propose to do about it?

This chapter discusses the interpretation of laboratory results and the factors that may cause them to vary under the following main headings:

1 *Analytical factors.* These cause errors in measurement.

2 *Biological and pathological factors.* Both these sets of factors affect the concentrations of analytes in blood, urine and other fluids sent for analysis.

The training and interests of doctors mainly direct their attention to the pathological causes of biochemical abnormalities (e.g. the reasons why plasma [calcium] might be abnormal). However, it is worth stressing that results also can and do vary for both analytical and biological (or physiological) reasons. Analytical factors will be considered first.

Analytical sources of variation

Analytical results are subject to both systematic and random error, no matter how good the laboratory and no matter how skilled the analyst. Inaccuracy and imprecision are terms used to describe these two types of error, best introduced by first defining their opposites, namely accuracy and precision:

1 *Accuracy.* The accuracy of a method is a function of its ability to yield results close to the true value of what is being measured. An accurate method has no systematic bias. Thus, plasma [glucose] used to be measured by methods that included other substances in addition to glucose; these methods were therefore inaccurate and gave results with a positive bias. Now, most laboratories use enzymic methods which measure only glucose and are, therefore, inherently accurate.

2 *Precision.* The precision of a method is related to its ability to yield the same result every time the same specimen is analysed. If multiple measurements are made on one specimen, the spread of results will be small for a precise and large for an imprecise method. For example, if a specimen has a true value for plasma [K$^+$] of 3.6 mmol/L, an imprecise method might yield values ranging from, say, 3.1 to 4.0 mmol/L whereas a precise method might yield values within the range 3.5 to 3.7 mmol/L. *The quantitative aspects of lack of precision, or imprecision, need to be considered in more detail.*

If a very large number of measurements of plasma [K$^+$] were to be made on the sample referred to in the previous paragraph, by both the imprecise method and the more precise method, a histogram of the scatter of results would in both cases be bell-shaped (approximating to a Gaussian or Normal distribution), but with the results of the precise method being clustered more tightly about the mean of 3.6 mmol/L.

The standard deviation is the usual measure of scatter around a mean value. If the spread of results is wide, the SD is large, whereas if the spread is narrow the SD is small. *For data which have a Gaussian distribution*, as is nearly always so for analytical errors, the shape of the curve (Fig. 3.1) is *completely defined by the mean and the SD*, and these characteristics are such that:
1 About 67% of results lie in the range mean ± 1 SD.

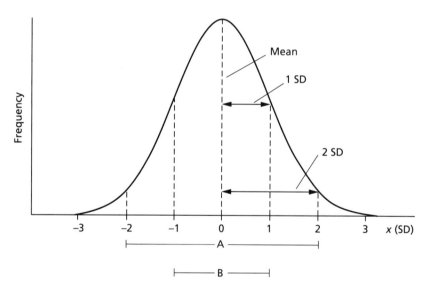

Fig. 3.1 Diagram of a Gaussian (Normal or symmetrical) distribution curve. The span (A) of the curve, the distance between the mean − 2 SD and the mean + 2 SD, includes about 95% of the 'population', whether this consists, for instance, of a set of analytical results (as discussed in the text and further exemplified in Fig. 3.2 for results of Na$^+$ analyses) or other types of quantitative measurement relating to large, homogeneous, groups of people. The narrower span (B), the distance between the mean − 1 SD and mean + 1 SD, includes about 67% of the 'population'.

2   About 95% of results lie in the range mean ± 2 SD.

3   Over 99% of results lie in the range mean ± 3 SD.

Most clinical biochemistry laboratories publish SD data for their analytical imprecision figures for various measurements. This allows clinicians to interpret results as far as potential analytical errors are concerned. For a method that is unbiased, the true result for a chemical measurement lies, in 95% of instances, within two (analytical) SD of the result reported; it will nearly always lie within three SD of the result reported.

In the example given above, the precise method for plasma [K$^+$] might have had an analytical SD of 0.1 mmol/L. If a result of 4.2 mmol/L, say, were obtained by this method for a sample from a patient, the true value for that plasma [K$^+$] would lie, in 95% of the repeated measurements, between $4.2 - 2 \times 0.1$ and $4.2 + 2 \times 0.1$, i.e. between 4.0 and 4.4 mmol/L. The imprecise method, however, might have had an analytical SD of 0.3 mmol/L and, in this case, for the same result of 4.2 mmol/L, we could only say that the true value lay between 3.6 and 4.8 mmol/L; this would clearly be totally unsatisfactory for diagnostic use.

Blunders

These are grossly inaccurate results that bear no constant or predictable relation to the true value. They arise, for instance, from mislabelling of specimens at the time of collection, or transcription errors when preparing or issuing reports.

If a very unexpected result is obtained from the laboratory, the doctor looking after the patient should *always discuss* the result with the laboratory *immediately* so that laboratory staff can check whether a blunder has been made in the laboratory. Blunders, when they occur, may be due to the hitherto undetected interchange of two specimens in which case results for *another* patient may *also* be grossly in error.

Serial results on the same patient

Doctors often have to interpret two or more sets of results for the same analysis or group of analyses performed on different occasions on the same patient. If the results differ, this raises the following question: *Is the difference between two measurements of the same analyte significant?*

We can illustrate this by the example of a patient who is found to have a plasma [urea] of 16.5 mmol/L one day and 18.0 mmol/L the next day. The question then is whether this change of 1.5 mmol/L represents a genuine rise in plasma [urea], possibly associated with deterioration in the patient's condition, or does the difference between the results merely reflect the inherent lack of precision of the analytical method? Assuming that the two specimens were collected under the same conditions, the answer to this question depends on knowing the analytical SD for the method, and applying the following rule:

> If results for analyses performed on specimens collected on different occasions, but *under otherwise identical conditions*, differ by more than 2.8 (i.e. $2\sqrt{2}$) analytical SD, it is very likely (i.e. there is over 95% chance) that a genuine change in concentration of the substance has occurred.

We can apply this rule to the example given above, assuming for this purpose an analytical SD of 0.35 mmol/L for urea measurements in this concentration range:

1   The difference between the two results is 1.5 mmol/L.

2   The change between the two results that is very likely to represent a genuine change is $0.35 \times 2.8 = 1.0$ mmol/L.

3   As the observed difference of 1.5 mmol/L exceeds 2.8 analytical SD, the increase from 16.5 to 18.0 mmol/L is an analytically genuine increase in plasma [urea]. Whether or not the change was important clinically would depend on the doctor's assessment of the patient's condition.

4   If instead of 18.0 the second value had been 17.4 mmol/L, this increase would be less than 2.8 analytical SD and it would not have been possible to say whether there had been a genuine increase in the plasma [urea].

Biological and pathological causes of variation

We can only begin to consider the possible biological significance of results after their analytical significance has been assessed. The key questions now are:

1   How do results vary in health?

2   How do results vary in different diseases?

How do results vary in health?

The concentrations of all analytes in blood vary with time due to diverse physiological factors *within* the individual. These will be considered first. In addition, there are differences *between* individuals.

Within-individual variation

Many of the factors listed below have been considered in a different context, in Chapter 1. The following may be important causes of within-individual variation:

1   *Diet.* Variations in diet can affect the results of many tests including plasma [cholesterol], the response to glucose tolerance tests, urinary calcium excretion.

2   *Time of day.* Several plasma constituents show diurnal variation (variation with the time of day), or a nychthemeral rhythm (variation with the sleeping–waking cycle). Examples include plasma iron, ACTH and cortisol concentrations.

3   *Posture.* Proteins and all protein-bound constituents of plasma show significant differences in concentration between blood collected from upright and from recumbent individuals. Examples include plasma calcium, cholesterol, cortisol and total thyroxine concentrations.

4   *Muscular exercise.* Recent exercise, especially if vigorous or unaccustomed, may increase plasma creatine kinase activity and blood [lactate], and lower blood [pyruvate].

5   *Menstrual cycle.* Several substances show variation with the phase of the cycle. Examples include plasma [iron], and the plasma concentrations of the pituitary gonadotrophins, ovarian steroids and their metabolites, as well as the amounts of these hormones and their metabolites excreted in the urine.

6   *Drugs.* These can have marked effects on chemical results. Attention should be drawn particularly to the many effects of oestrogen-containing oral contraceptives on plasma constituents (p. 312).

Table 3.1 Residual individual variation of some plasma constituents (expressed as the approximate day-to-day, within-individual coefficient of variation)

Plasma constituent	CV(%)	Plasma constituent	CV(%)
[Sodium]	1	ALT activity	25
[Calcium]	1–2	AST activity	25
[Potassium]	5	[Iron]	25
[Urea]	10		

Even after allowing for known physiological factors which may affect plasma constituents and for analytical imprecision, there is still considerable *residual individual variation* (Table 3.1). The magnitude of this variation depends on the analyte, but may be large and must be taken into account when interpreting successive values from a patient.

Between-individual variation

Differences between individuals can affect the concentrations of analytes in the blood. The following are the main examples:

1 *Age*. Marked physiological variation with age is a common finding. Examples include plasma [phosphate] and alkaline phosphatase activity, and plasma and urinary concentrations of the gonadotrophins and sex hormones.

2 *Sex*. Many substances show differences in concentration between the sexes. Examples include plasma creatinine, iron, urate and urea concentrations and GGT activity, and plasma concentrations and 24-hour urinary output of the sex hormones.

3 *Race*. Racial differences have been described for plasma [cholesterol] and [protein]. It can, however, be difficult to distinguish the supposed effects of race from effects of dietary and other factors.

Reference ranges

In any consideration of results, it is necessary to compare each result obtained with a set of results that might normally have been *expected* in a variety of circumstances. This set of results, which we can obtain from a particular *defined (or reference) population*, is known as a reference range. It is determined, in practice, by measuring a set of *reference values* from a group of individuals who are representative of that population. They will *usually* be healthy individuals and reference ranges carry the implicit assumption that they relate to the healthy state; however, they can relate to *any* definable population (e.g. patients with myocardial infarction). The important point is that the nature of the reference population should be given whenever reference ranges are quoted. In some circumstances, a single individual can serve as his or her own reference 'population' (see below).

To interpret results on a particular patient, the most suitable reference ranges would be results for analyses obtained for that individual before becoming ill. For example, in a patient undergoing elective surgery, a pre-operative set of values can be obtained, to compare with results obtained post-operatively. However, for most patients, baseline data obtained when they were healthy will not be available. In the absence of such personal data, results from patients have to be compared with results from healthy people, preferably of the same age group and sex since, as indicated above, both of these factors may affect biochemical results. Samples of blood from healthy individuals are not always easy to obtain, especially not in sufficient numbers to allow stratification for sex and age, and *blood donors* are very often selected as the most readily available reference population.

When results of analyses for a reference population are analysed, they are invariably found to cluster round a central value with a distribution that may be symmetrical (often Gaussian; Fig. 3.2, left) or asymmetrical (often log-Gaussian; Fig. 3.2, right). Parametric statistics, which assume a Gaussian or log-Gaussian distribution, are commonly used and ease the calculation of reference ranges from the data obtained for the reference population. However, reference ranges can also be calculated from these data without making any assumptions about the distribution of the data, using non-parametric methods.

Because of geographical, racial and other biological sources of variation between individuals, as well as differences in analytical methods, each laboratory should define and publish its own reference ranges. Conventionally, these include the central 95% of the results obtained for each analysis from the reference population. This 95% figure is arbitrary, selected in order to minimize the overlap between results from diseased populations and from healthy individuals. Reference ranges stratified for age and sex are preferable but this is often difficult, since a large reference population would be required to define each reference range; also, moderately sophisticated reporting procedures would be needed to enable linkage of details about the patient with each result to be reported and the relevant stratified reference range.

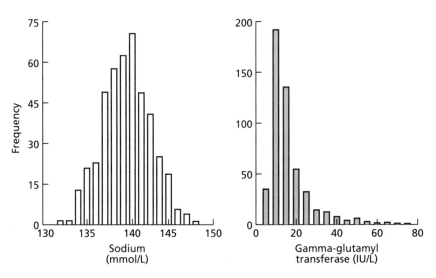

Fig. 3.2 Histograms that show the relative frequency with which results with the values indicated were obtained when plasma [Na^+] and GGT activities were measured in a reference population of healthy adult women. The sodium data are symmetrically distributed about the mean, whereas the GGT data show a log-Gaussian distribution.

Analytical factors can affect the reference ranges for individual laboratories. If, for instance, an *inaccurate* method with either a positive or a negative bias is used, the reference range will reflect the bias of the method. The effect of methodological *imprecision* is less obvious. Each observed reference range comprises two components, biological variability (BV) and analytical variability (AV). The effects of these on the observed variability (OV) are additive, such that:

$$OV = \pm \sqrt{(BV^2 + AV^2)}$$

If the precision of a method is poor, the observed variability will be significantly larger than the biological variability. In practice, most analytical methods are now sufficiently precise for analytical variability to have only a small effect on the reference ranges for laboratory methods.

'Normal ranges'

Many doctors and laboratory staff still use the expression 'normal range' for an analysis, and commonly equate it with the reference range. However, the term 'reference range' is to be preferred for two main reasons:

1 As defined above, about 5% of results from healthy people will be outside the reference range, so the term '*normal range*' is clearly inappropriate, if similarly defined, since it implies that 5% of healthy people are not normal.

2 The practice of relating the reference range to a defined reference population, without necessarily implying either health or disease, is a useful one.

We recommend that the term 'reference range' be used rather than 'normal range'. However, to avoid cumbersome phraseology, we shall from time to time use the terms 'abnormal' and 'normal' to denote results which are, respectively, outside or within the corresponding reference range.

How do results vary in disease?

Biochemical test results do not exist in isolation since, by the time that tests are requested, the doctor will often have made a provisional diagnosis and a list of differential diagnoses based on each patient's symptoms and signs. For example, in a patient with severe abdominal pain, tenderness and rigidity, there may be several possible explanations that must be differentiated one from another. These might include acute pancreatitis, perforated peptic ulcer and acute cholecystitis; in all three conditions, the plasma amylase activity may be raised, i.e. above the upper reference value for healthy adults. However, published reference ranges are largely irrelevant in this kind of example, since *we are not dealing here with a healthy adult*; healthy adults do not have abdominal pain, tenderness and rigidity. Instead, the doctor needs to know how the plasma amylase activity might vary in the disorders which are considered likely diagnostic possibilities from the clinical point of view. It would be useful to know, for instance, if very high plasma amylase activities were associated with one of these diagnostic possibilities, but not with the other two.

This example illustrates the point that, to interpret results properly, doctors need to know the pattern in which results of chemical measurements are likely to be distributed in patients at each stage of a wide variety of diseases, as well as in health. They also need to know the approximate incidence, in their practice, of the various diseases under consideration, but these basic data are often unknown.

To summarize the position, for diagnostic purposes, in order to interpret results on patients adequately, we need to know:

1 *The reference range for healthy individuals* of the appropriate age-range and of the same sex.

2 *The reference range for patients* with the disease, or diseases, under consideration.

3 *The prevalence of the disease*, or diseases, in the population to which the patient belongs.

The assessment of diagnostic tests

In evaluating and interpreting a test it is necessary to know how it behaves in health and disease. We shall use the following terms:

1 *Sensitivity (true-positive rate)*. This is the incidence (per cent) of positive results for a test in patients with the particular disease. A test which is always abnormal (or positive) in patients with the disease has 100% sensitivity.

2 *False-positive rate*. This is the incidence (per cent) of positive results in people known or subsequently proved to be free from the particular disease. If a test is always normal in individuals who do not have the disease, that test has a false-positive rate of 0%.[1]

3 *The predictive value of a positive test result*. This is the percentage of positive results that are true positives when a test is performed on a defined population containing both healthy and diseased individuals.

The ideal test is 100% sensitive and has a 0% false-positive rate, shown diagrammatically in Fig. 3.3 (A). This ideal is rarely achieved; there is usually overlap between the healthy and diseased populations (Fig. 3.3 (B)). In practice, we have to decide where to draw dividing lines which separate 'healthy' from 'diseased' groups, or which separate disease X from disease Y. We can illustrate this requirement for decisions by means of the following *hypothetical example*:

Suppose that we wish to distinguish patients with acute myocardial infarction from those with other causes of acute chest pain. In blood taken 24 hours after the onset of pain we know that plasma creatine kinase (CK) activity is usually raised in patients who have had a myocardial infarction, and that it is sometimes raised in patients without infarction. The overlap is illustrated in Fig. 3.4, which we here assume portrays results obtained from a study of very large numbers of patients in both categories.

---

[1] NB It should be noted that the term *specificity* (incidence of *negative* results in those without the disease) is very commonly used in the same context as the false-positive rate. The following relationship holds:

Specificity (%) = (100 − false-positive rate (%))

For example, if the false-positive rate is 5%, then the specificity is 95%. We think that it is conceptually easier always to think in terms of the incidence of *positive* results in the presence or absence of disease so we prefer to use the term 'false-positive rate'.

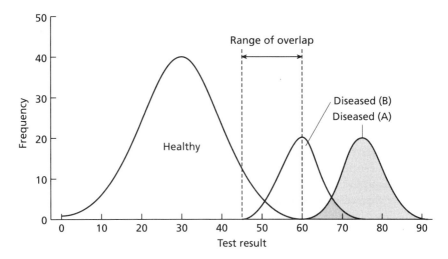

Fig. 3.3 Diagrammatic representations of the distributions of results obtained with a test (A) that completely separates healthy people from people with a disease without any overlap between the distribution curves (i.e. an ideal test with 100% sensitivity and 100% specificity), and a test (B) that is less sensitive and less specific with which there is an area of overlap between the distribution curves for healthy people and people with disease.

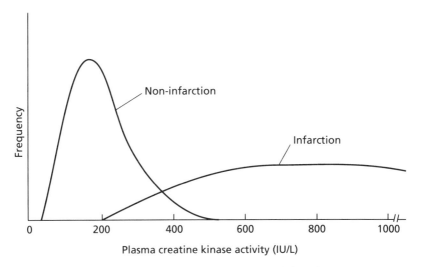

Fig. 3.4 The predictive value of a positive (abnormal) result for a diagnostic test, using the results of a hypothetical study in which plasma CK activity was measured in a very large number of patients admitted to hospital with acute chest pain. The enzyme activity measurements relate to 24 hours after the onset of the pain, i.e. a time when the results would usually be raised if the diagnosis of myocardial infarction is correct. The results have been subdivided into those relating to patients who had had a myocardial infarction and those who had another (non-cardiac) cause of their chest pain. The text describes the implications for the sensitivity, specificity and predictive value of an abnormal result of setting the cut-off value for abnormality at 200 IU/L and at 450 IU/L.

If we wish to identify *every* patient with myocardial infarction, we must take a *low* cut-off figure for plasma CK activity of about 200 IU/L. The test is then 100% sensitive but the false-positive rate is unacceptably high, since only about 70% of patients without infarction are correctly classified by the test. If, on the other hand, we wish to identify *only* patients who have had a myocardial infarct and to *exclude* all those without an infarct, then a *high* cut-off must be selected, at a plasma CK activity of about 450 IU/L. The false-positive rate is now 0% but the sensitivity has suffered, since only about 75% of patients with myocardial infarction have been identified with this higher cut-off figure.

In this example we have deliberately taken two extremes, to show that it is usually possible to increase the sensitivity of a test, but only at the expense of a high false-positive rate. Conversely, the false-positive rate can be decreased, but only at the expense of a loss of sensitivity. In practice, the bias towards sensitivity or a low rate of false positives will depend on clinical objectives. For example, if all patients with myocardial infarction are to be admitted to a coronary care unit, a low cut-off figure is needed to make the test 100% sensitive. The 'price' of this decision will be that more patients without myocardial infarction will also be admitted to the unit, thereby incurring additional expense and, very possibly, straining the specialist facilities unnecessarily and unacceptably.

Disease prevalence

Before discussing the effect of disease prevalence on diagnostic decision-making, *predictive values* need to be considered. These are defined as follows:

$$\text{Predictive value of a positive test result} = \frac{\text{True positives}}{\text{All positives}} \times 100$$

$$\text{Predictive value of a negative test result} = \frac{\text{True negatives}}{\text{All negatives}} \times 100$$

Predictive values are arrived at most easily if a table is constructed (Table 3.2).

Table 3.2 The predictive value of the results of analyses

Diagnostic category	Positive results	Negative results	Totals
Disease present	True positives (TP)	False negatives (FN)	Numbers with disease (TP + FN)
Disease absent	False positives (FP)	True negatives (TN)	Numbers without disease (TN + FP)
Totals	Total positives (TP + FP)	Total negatives (TN + FN)	Total numbers studied
Predictive value of a positive result =	$\dfrac{TP}{(TP+FP)} \times 100\%$	Predictive value of a negative result =	$\dfrac{TN}{(TN+FN)} \times 100\%$

Tables such as this are of great assistance in considering the diagnostic utility of any investigation. In practice, predictive values are very important diagnostically as they give the *probability* that an abnormal result, which is being interpreted by a doctor, comes from someone with disease.

Knowledge of the sensitivity and of the false-positive rate, combined with clinical considerations, can affect the cut-off values for any test. *Decisions about cut-off values are also crucially dependent on the prevalence of the disease* in question since this will affect the predictive value of the test. To illustrate this point, we shall again use the example of plasma CK activity measurements in the diagnosis of myocardial infarction:

1 *Coronary care unit.* We shall first assume that the test is to be used in the coronary care unit, where the incidence of myocardial infarction is high, i.e. about 50% of the patients admitted are assumed to have had an infarct. We shall also assume that 2000 patients have been admitted and that a cut-off plasma CK activity value of 350 IU/L has been selected, giving (for illustrative purposes) a sensitivity of 95% and a false-positive rate of approximately 10%. As expected (Table 3.3), most of the abnormal results come from patients with myocardial infarction, and most of the negative results from patients without myocardial infarction.

2 *General medical ward.* We shall next consider a general medical ward in which we assume that only 5% of admissions with chest pain are due to myocardial infarction. The same sensitivity and false-positive rate of CK measurements and the same cut-off value (350 IU/L) are assumed. Table 3.4 shows that an abnormal test result, after *changing only the prevalence* of the disease, is now twice as likely to be associated with the absence as with the presence of myocardial infarction, i.e. *the predictive value of the test is less in the general medical unit than in the coronary care unit.* In other words, in the general medical ward, plasma CK measurements by themselves are of relatively little diagnostic value for identifying patients who have had a myocardial infarction. If the test is to be used for this purpose, it may be appropriate to alter the cut-off value, for example by increasing it so that the test is less sensitive but gives rise to fewer false positives.

Table 3.3 A hypothetical set of results for plasma creatine kinase activity measurements in patients admitted to a coronary care unit with chest pain

Diagnostic category	Positive results (> 350 IU/L)	Negative results (< 350 IU/L)	Totals
Infarct confirmed	950	50	1000
No infarct	100	900	1000
Totals	1050	950	2000
Predictive value of a positive result =	$\frac{950}{1050} \times 100\% = 90.5\%$	Predictive value of a negative result = $\frac{900}{950} \times 100\% = 94.7\%$	

Assumptions: Sensitivity 95%, specificity 90%, prevalence of myocardial infarction 50%. The data relate to 2000 patients.

Table 3.4 A hypothetical set of results for plasma creatine kinase activity measurements in patients admitted to a general medical unit with chest pain

Diagnostic category	Positive results (> 350 IU/L)	Negative results (< 350 IU/L)	Totals
Infarct confirmed	95	5	100
No infarct	190	1710	1900
Totals	285	1715	2000
Predictive value of a positive result =	$\frac{95}{285} \times 100\% = 33.3\%$	Predictive value of a negative result = $\frac{1710}{1715} \times 100\% = 99.7\%$	

Assumptions: Sensitivity 95%, specificity 90%, prevalence of myocardial infarction 5%. The data relate to 2000 patients.

Screening for rare diseases

The above examples show that the interpretation to be placed on a positive result for a test depends heavily on the prevalence of the disease for which that test is being used. For diseases which are rare, tests of extremely high sensitivity and specificity are required. To illustrate this point, we shall consider an inherited metabolic disorder with an incidence of 1 : 5000; this is similar to that of some of the commoner, treatable, inherited metabolic diseases such as phenylketonuria or congenital hypothyroidism (Table 21.2, p. 323). We shall assume that we have a test with a good performance, i.e. a sensitivity of 99.5% and a false-positive rate of 0.5% (Table 3.5).

Table 3.5 shows that, for *every* neonate affected by the disorder and who has a positive test result, there will be about 25 (4999/199) neonates who also have a positive test but who do not have the disease. Two important points emerge:

1   Tests with very high sensitivity and with very low false-positive rates are required when screening for rare disorders.

2   A heavy investigative load will result from the screening programme, since all the false positives will have to be followed up to determine whether or not they indicate the presence of disease.

Table 3.5 A hypothetical set of results of a screening test for a relatively common inherited metabolic disorder in neonates

Diagnostic category	Positive results	Negative results	Totals
Disease present	199	1	200
Disease absent	4999	994 801	999 800
Totals	5198	994 802	1000 000
Predictive value	3.8%	100%	

Assumptions: Sensitivity of the test 99.5%, specificity 99.5%; prevalence of the disorder, 1 : 5000; 1000 000 neonates screened.
Note that the prevalence of phenylketonuria and of hypothyroidism in the UK are about 1 : 5000 live births (Table 21.2, p. 323), and that about 800 000 neonates in the UK are screened annually.

Very often, in designing large-scale population screening programmes, it is necessary to adjust the cut-off value for the screening test so that the numbers of false positives remain manageable, even if this means that a few people with the disorder that is being sought will be missed.

The clinical uses of laboratory data

To recapitulate, when provided with sets of results from the laboratory, doctors need to review each result and its relationship to the distribution of values in the healthy population. This is where reference ranges with all their present shortcomings have to be considered. Few laboratories, as already noted, report data on individual patients in relation to stratified reference ranges that take into account the effects of age, sex and possibly other factors.

The doctor also needs to consider the *distribution* of results for a particular measurement in defined disease groupings, and the approximate *prevalence* of the various diseases in the population with which he or she is concerned.

The screening of patients with large numbers of tests (e.g. all patients on first admission to hospital) has shown that doctors often have difficulty in assimilating large sets of data and discerning what is significant when faced with masses of figures. Some computer-assisted systems of reporting draw attention to results that can be classified as 'abnormal', defined arbitrarily as those which fall outside the reference range. No matter which method of reporting results is adopted, *doctors should always ask themselves the questions listed on p. 21.*

Unexpected or unexplained abnormal results are all too often dismissed as laboratory errors and ignored, or the test is repeated without further thought. The tendency to overlook or ignore unexplained abnormal results is greatest for screening investigations since, for many of these tests, there would have been no clinical reason for their performance in the first place. However, as it is possible that the laboratory has made an error or even a blunder, any unexplained abnormal result must be brought to its staff's attention, since:

1   The test may be able to be repeated on the original specimen or the result in question be corrected (e.g. if there has been a miscalculation).

2   The results of tests performed on specimens from one or more other patients (affected, for instance, by a transcription error) may also be found to need correction.

3   The information may provide the first evidence of a methodological problem in the laboratory, causing systematic bias of all results for that analysis from all patients.

The main uses of clinical biochemistry results

These were outlined on p. 1, and can be restated here as follows:

1   Assisting in the diagnostic process.

2   Helping to assess the severity of disease, and so helping to formulate the prognosis, e.g. peak enzyme activities after a myocardial infarction.

3   Monitoring the progress of patients and their response to treatment, e.g. weekly 'liver function tests' during the recovery phase from viral hepatitis.

4   Serving a precautionary function. Failure to perform certain investigations might result in a charge of professional negligence, e.g. plasma [digoxin] should be measured before increasing the dose in patients with congestive cardiac failure and renal functional impairment.

5 Providing data that may, in time, lead to better understanding of the disease.

These uses of clinical biochemistry data interrelate with the questions contained in Asher's catechism (p. 2) which should have been considered when initiating laboratory requests. Failure to take these questions properly into account when requesting investigations leads to misuse, overuse and even frank abuse of diagnostic services because of inability later on to make proper use of the results in the corresponding reports.

Chapter 4
Disturbances of Water, Sodium and Potassium Balance

Disorders of water and sodium homeostasis, their causes and their investigation by chemical methods, are described in this chapter. Disturbances of potassium metabolism are then discussed, but these must also be considered in association particularly with disturbances of acid–base balance, described in the next chapter.

Water and sodium balance

In considering the balance of any substance, two aspects must be borne in mind, external balance and internal balance:

1 *External balance.* This matches input with output. An example of external balance for water is given in Table 4.1. Dietary intakes of Na^+ (and Cl^-) are very variable worldwide, but are closely matched by their corresponding urinary losses under normal conditions. There is normally little loss of these ions through the skin or in the faeces. A typical 'Western' diet would provide 100–200 mmol of both Na^+ and Cl^- daily.

2 *Internal balance.* This relates to the distribution of water and solutes between different body compartments. In a 70 kg adult, the total body water is about 42 L, consisting of about 28 L of ICF water and 14 L of ECF water. The ECF water is distributed as 3 L plasma water and 11 L interstitial water. The total body Na^+ is about 4200 mmol of which about 50% is in the ECF, 40% in bone, and 10% in the ICF. Thus, Na^+ is mainly extracellular.

Disturbances of Na^+ and water balance causing large losses are very important. Movements of Na^+ and water between plasma and glomerular filtrate, or between plasma and gastrointestinal (GI) secretions, provide the potential for large losses with serious and rapid alterations in internal balance. Signs and symptoms attributable to the expansion or contraction of cells, particularly of the brain, or to alterations in neuromuscular excitability, may develop. For example, about 25 000 mmol Na^+ are filtered at the glomerulus over 24 hours with

Table 4.1 Average daily water intake and output of a normal adult in the UK

Intake of water	mL	Output of water	mL
Water drunk	1500	Urine volume	1500
Water in food	750	Water content of faeces	50
Water from metabolism of food	250	Losses in expired air and insensible perspiration	950
Total intake	2500	Total output	2500

subsequent reabsorption normally of more than 99%; also, 1000 mmol Na^+ enter the GI tract in various secretions each day, but less than 0.5% (5 mmol) is normally lost in the faeces.

Internal distribution of water and sodium

There are two important factors which influence the distribution of fluid between the ICF and the intravascular and extravascular compartments of the ECF:

1 *Osmolality*. This affects movement of water across cell membranes.

2 *Colloid osmotic pressure*. Together with hydrodynamic factors, this affects the movement of water and low mol mass solutes (predominantly NaCl) between the intravascular and extravascular compartments.

Osmolality, osmolarity and tonicity

Osmolality is the osmotic pressure exerted by a solution across a membrane. It is proportional to the number of solute particles per unit weight of water, irrespective of the size or nature of the particles. The units are mmol/kg.

Most laboratories measure *plasma osmolality* directly, in those relatively few patients where such measurements are required. It is also possible to calculate the osmolality of plasma approximately using formulae exemplified by the following (all concentrations must be in mmol/L):

1 Calculated osmolality $= 2[Na^+] + 2[K^+] + [glucose] + [urea]$

2 Calculated osmolality $= 1.89[Na^+] + 1.28[K^+] + 1.08[glucose]$
$+ 1.03[urea] + 7.45$

In the first of these formulae, the values for Na^+ and K^+ are doubled so as to allow for their associated anions, always present in equivalent amount. The second, more complex, empirical formula is said to be more accurate although neither formula is a complete substitute for direct measurement. In most instances, calculated osmolality is close to measured osmolality, but the two may differ considerably when there are gross increases in plasma protein or lipid concentrations, both of which decrease the plasma water per unit volume. They also differ considerably when unmeasured low mol mass solutes (e.g. ethanol) are present in plasma in substantial amount.

Urine osmolality can also be measured directly, or it can be calculated using the same formula as the first of the two given above for calculating plasma osmolality, but excluding the glucose term unless the patient is diabetic. Urine osmolality is also linearly related to its specific gravity (sp. gr.), unless there are significant amounts of glucose, protein or X-ray contrast media present, all of which are liable to increase the sp. gr. considerably but have relatively little effect on the osmolarity.

Osmolarity is the number of particles of solute per litre of solution. Its units are mmol/L. Its measurement or calculation has been largely replaced by osmolality.

Tonicity is a term often used interchangeably with osmolality. However, it should only be used in relation to the osmotic pressure due to those solutes (e.g. Na^+) which exert their effects across cell membranes, thereby causing movement of water into or out of the cells. Substances which can diffuse into the cells (e.g. urea, alcohol) contribute to plasma osmolality but *not* to plasma tonicity.

The osmolality of ICF and ECF equilibrate with one another by movement of

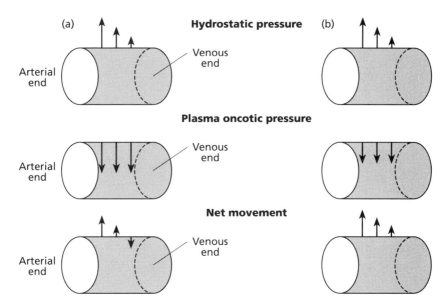

Fig. 4.1 Movements of water and low mol mass solutes across the capillary wall when the plasma [protein] concentration is (a) normal and (b) low. The effects shown are: hydrostatic pressure which drives water and low mol mass solutes *outwards* and decreases along the length of the capillary; and plasma oncotic pressure which attracts water and low mol mass solutes *inwards* and is constant along the length of the capillary. The net movement of water and low mol mass solutes across the capillary wall is governed by the net effect of hydrostatic and plasma oncotic pressures.

water across cell membranes. An increase in ECF tonicity causes a reduction in ICF volume as the tonicity of the two compartments equalizes when water moves from the ICF to the ECF. Conversely, decrease in ECF tonicity causes an increase in ICF volume; the tonicity of ICF and ECF equilibrate likewise.

Colloid osmotic pressure (oncotic pressure)
    The osmotic pressure exerted by plasma proteins across cell membranes is negligible compared with the osmotic pressure of a solution containing NaCl and other small molecules. However, whilst small molecules diffuse freely across the capillary membrane (i.e. are not osmotically active at this site), plasma proteins cross the capillary membrane poorly. Thus, plasma [protein] and hydrodynamic factors together influence the distribution of water and solutes between the intravascular and interstitial compartments (Fig. 4.1).

Regulation of external water balance
    The intake of water is normally controlled by the sensation of thirst, and its output by the secretion of arginine vasopressin (AVP), also known as antidiuretic hormone (ADH). In states of pure water deficiency, plasma osmolality increases, causing a sensation of thirst and stimulating AVP secretion, both mediated by hypothalamic osmoreceptors. In turn, AVP promotes water reabsorption in the

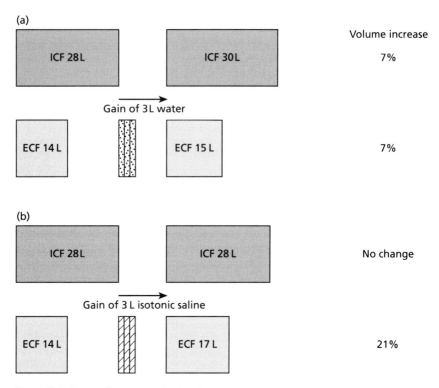

Fig. 4.2 Different effects on the body's fluid compartments of fluid gains of 3 L of (a) water and (b) isotonic saline. The volumes shown relate to a 70 kg adult. Gains of fluids, respectively, are represented thus: (▨) and (▨).

distal nephron and production of a concentrated urine of small volume. Conversely, a large intake of water suppresses thirst and reduces AVP secretion, leading to a brisk diuresis.

Secretion of AVP is normally controlled by small changes in ECF tonicity, but it is important to note that it is also under tonic inhibitory control from baroreceptors in the left atrium and great vessels on the left side of the heart. Where haemodynamic factors (e.g. excessive blood loss, heart failure) reduce the stretch on these receptors, a reduction in tonic inhibitory control stimulates AVP secretion. Water retention is relatively ineffective in expanding the intravascular compartment, since water diffuses freely throughout all compartments (Fig. 4.2). However, its contribution may become important under conditions of more severe intravascular volume depletion, when the normal osmolar regulation of AVP is overridden. This can lead to the fall in plasma osmolality and the hyponatraemia that are observed as a result of ECF volume depletion or altered distribution of fluid between the interstitial and the intravascular spaces.

Regulation of external sodium balance

The ECF volume is controlled by varying the amount of Na^+ excreted in the urine since, when osmoregulation is normal, the amount of extracellular water is maintained in a constant quantitative relationship to the amount of extracellular Na^+. At least four mechanisms are probably important regulators of Na^+ excretion, namely: (i) the renin–angiotensin–aldosterone system; (ii) the glomerular filtration rate (GFR); (iii) the atrial natriuretic peptides (ANP); and (iv) dopamine release in the kidney. These will be briefly considered:

1 *Renin*. This is secreted in response to a fall in renal afferent arteriolar pressure or to a reduction in supply of Na^+ to the distal tubule. It acts on angiotensinogen (renin substrate) in plasma, converting it to angiotensin I (AI), which is then converted to angiotensin II (AII) by angiotensin-converting enzyme (ACE). Both AII and its metabolic product angiotensin III (AIII) are pharmacologically active, and stimulate the release of aldosterone. Acting on the distal tubule, aldosterone promotes Na^+ reabsorption in exchange for urinary loss of H^+ or K^+. Since Na^+ cannot enter cells freely, its retention (with isosmotically associated water) contributes solely to ECF volume expansion, unlike pure water retention (Figs 4.2 and 4.3). Although the renin–angiotensin–aldosterone system causes relatively slow responses to Na^+ deprivation or Na^+ loading, evidence suggests that *this is the main regulatory mechanism* for Na^+ excretion.

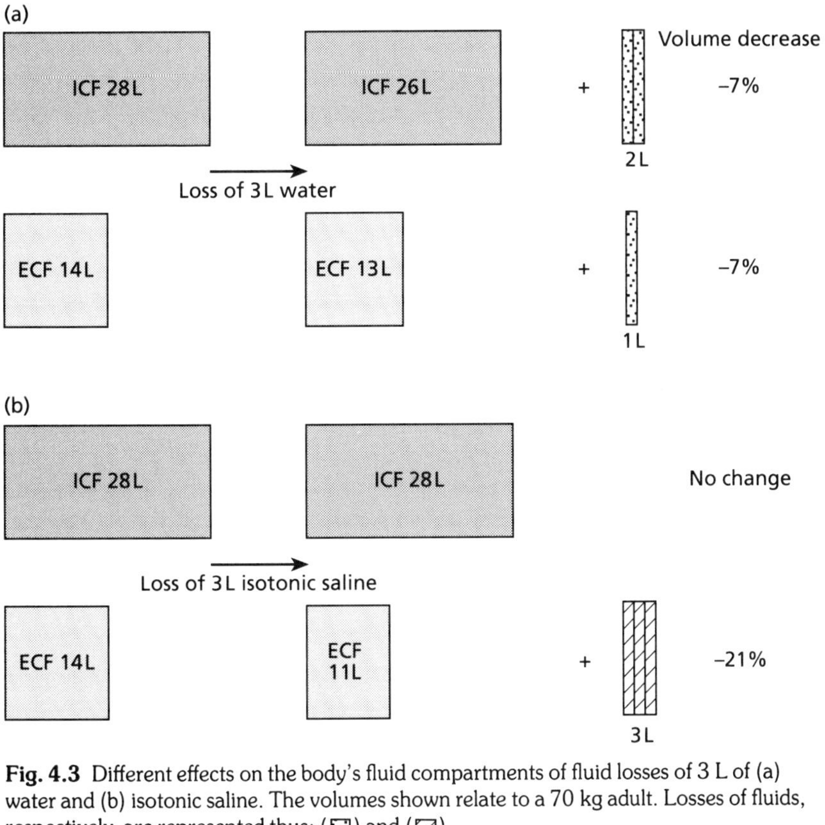

Fig. 4.3 Different effects on the body's fluid compartments of fluid losses of 3 L of (a) water and (b) isotonic saline. The volumes shown relate to a 70 kg adult. Losses of fluids, respectively, are represented thus: (⚃) and (▨).

2 *GFR.* The rate of Na^+ excretion is often related to the GFR. When the GFR falls acutely, less Na^+ is excreted, and vice versa.

3 *ANP,* several similar peptides in the atrium of the heart, promote Na^+ excretion by the kidney, apparently by causing a marked increase in GFR. These ANP also antagonize other actions of the renin–angiotensin–aldosterone system but the importance of the ANP regulatory mechanism is not yet clear.

4 *Dopamine.* Local renal synthesis of dopamine by proximal tubular cells is increased in response to an increase in the filtered load of Na^+. Dopamine released into the proximal tubular lumen acts in the distal tubule to stimulate Na^+ excretion.

Disorders of water and sodium homeostasis

In patients who lose or gain water, the losses or gains are distributed throughout all compartments, whereas in *patients who lose or gain Na^+ and water, as isotonic fluid,* the losses or gains of fluid are borne by the much smaller ECF compartment (Figs 4.2 and 4.3). The body is, therefore, less able to withstand acute losses or gains of isotonic fluid than losses or gains of water, and it is usually more urgent to replace losses of isotonic fluid than losses of water. For the same reason, circulatory overload is more likely with isotonic Na^+-containing solutions than with isotonic dextrose (the dextrose is metabolized, leaving water behind).

Determinations of plasma $[Na^+]$, whether the results be normal, high or low, cannot be used as simple measures of body Na^+ status. The plasma $[Na^+]$ *must* be interpreted in relation to the patient's history and findings on clinical examination and, where appropriate, other investigations.

The main causes of depletion and excess of water are summarized in Table 4.2, and of Na^+ in Table 4.3. Although some of these conditions may be associated with abnormal plasma $[Na^+]$, it must be emphasized that this is not necessarily the case. For example, patients with *acute losses* of isotonic fluid (e.g. plasma, blood) may be severely and dangerously hypovolaemic and Na^+-depleted, and

Table 4.2 Causes of depletion and of excess of water

Categories	Examples
Depletion of water	
Inadequate intake	Infants, patients in coma or who are very sick, or have symptoms such as nausea or dysphagia
Abnormal losses via	
Lungs	Inadequate humidification in mechanical ventilation
Skin	Fevers and in hot climates
Renal tract	Diabetes insipidus, lithium therapy
Excess of water	
Excessive intake	
Oral	Psychogenic polydipsia
Parenteral	Hypotonic infusions after operations
Renal retention	Excess of AVP (SIADH, Table 4.5), hypoadrenalism, hypothyroidism

Table 4.3 Causes of depletion and of excess of sodium

Categories	Examples
Depletion of sodium	
Inadequate oral intake	Rare, by itself
Abnormal losses via	
Skin	Excessive sweating, dermatitis, burns
GI tract	Vomiting, aspiration, diarrhoea, fistula, paralytic ileus, blood loss
Renal tract	Osmotic diuresis, diuretic therapy, renal tubular disease, mineralocorticoid deficiency
Excess of sodium	
Excessive intake	
Oral	Sea water (drowning), salt tablets, hypertonic NaCl administration (this is rare)
Parenteral	Post-operatively, infusion of hypertonic NaCl
Renal retention	Acute and chronic renal failure, primary and secondary hyperaldosteronism, Cushing's syndrome

very possibly in shock, but their plasma $[Na^+]$ may nevertheless be normal or even raised.

Hyponatraemia

The reference range for plasma $[Na^+]$ is 132–144 mmol/L. Most patients with hyponatraemia also have a low plasma osmolality (reference range, 280–290 mmol/kg). Unless an unusual cause of hyponatraemia is suspected (see 'Other causes of hyponatraemia', p. 45), measurement of plasma osmolality contributes little or no extra information.

Patients with hyponatraemia can be divided into three clinical categories, depending on whether the ECF volume is low, normal or increased. In turn, the ECF volume reflects a total body Na^+ which is low, normal or increased, respectively. The value of this classification is twofold. Firstly, from the clinical history and examination, it is often possible to assess the ECF volume and, therefore, the total body Na^+ status. Secondly, treatment depends on the category appropriate for the patient.

Hyponatraemia with low ECF volume (Table 4.4)

The patient has lost Na^+ and water in one or more body fluids (e.g. GI tract secretions, urine, inflammatory exudate). This leads to characteristic and predictable clinical manifestations including tachycardia, orthostatic hypotension, reduced skin turgor and oliguria. The hypovolaemia causes secondary aldosteronism with a low urinary $[Na^+]$ (usually less than 20 mmol/L) and a 'volume stimulus' to AVP secretion, resulting in oliguria and a concentrated urine. The consequent water retention contributes to the hyponatraemia.

Treatment requires administration of isotonic saline (150 mmol/L), and volume expanders (albumin, dextran) if there is hypotension.

Table 4.4 Causes of hyponatraemia

ECF volume	Categories	Examples
Decreased total body Na^+ (loss of $Na^+ > H_2O$)	Extra-renal losses of Na^+ (urine $[Na^+] < 20$ mmol/L)	
	GI tract	Vomiting, diarrhoea
	Skin	Burns, severe dermatitis
	'Internal'	Paralytic ileus, peritoneal fluid
	Renal losses of Na^+ (urine $[Na^+] > 20$ mmol/L)	
	Diuretics	p. 51, 135
	Kidneys	Renal tubular acidosis
	Adrenals	Mineralocorticoid deficiency
Normal or near-normal total body Na^+	Acute conditions	Parenteral administration of water, after surgery or trauma, or during or after delivery
	Chronic conditions	
	Antidiuretic drugs	Opiates, chlorpropamide
	Kidneys	Chronic renal failure
	Adrenals	Glucocorticoid deficiency
	AVP excess	SIADH (Table 4.5)
	Osmoregulator	Low setting in carcinomatosis
Increased total body Na^+	Acute conditions	Acute renal failure
	Chronic conditions	Oedematous states (p. 43)

Hyponatraemia with normal ECF volume (Table 4.4)

The hyponatraemia results from excessive water retention, due to inability to excrete a water load. This may develop acutely or it may be chronic:

1 *Acute water retention.* Plasma [AVP] is acutely increased after trauma or major surgery, and during delivery and post-partum, as part of the metabolic response to trauma. Administration of excessive amounts of water (e.g. as 5% dextrose) in these circumstances may exacerbate the hyponatraemia and cause acute water intoxication (p. 55).

2 *Chronic water retention.* Perhaps the most widely known chronic 'cause' of this form of hyponatraemia is the *syndrome of inappropriate secretion of ADH (SIADH)*. Whether this concept is of value in understanding its aetiology, or valid in terms of altered physiology, is uncertain. Its characteristics are listed in Table 4.5. As the name implies, ADH (or rather AVP) is being secreted in the absence of an 'appropriate' physiological stimulus, in the absence of either hypernatraemia or fluid depletion.

There are many causes of SIADH (Table 4.5). These are often transient, in which case plasma $[Na^+]$ returns to normal when the primary disorder (e.g. pneumonia) is treated. In patients with cancer, however, the hyponatraemia is presumably due to production of AVP or a related substance by the tumour, and is usually persistent. Treatment depends on the severity of the condition. For

Table 4.5 The syndrome of inappropriate secretion of ADH (SIADH)

Characteristics of the syndrome	Causes (and examples)
1 Low plasma [Na$^+$] and osmolality	Malignant disease of the bronchus, prostate, pancreas, etc.
2 Inappropriately high urine osmolality	Chest diseases, e.g. pneumonia, bronchitis, tuberculosis
3 Excessive renal excretion of Na$^+$	CNS diseases including brain trauma, tumours, meningitis
4 No evidence of volume depletion	Drug treatment, e.g. carbamazepine, chlorpropamide, opiates
5 No evidence of oedema	Miscellaneous conditions including porphyria,
6 Normal renal and adrenal function	psychosis, post-operative states

mildly symptomatic patients, severe fluid restriction (i.e. 500 mL/day or less) is often effective. However, if this is not effective, treatment with a drug that antagonizes the renal effects of AVP (e.g. lithium carbonate, demeclocycline) may be tried.

Other causes of chronic retention of water

Chronic renal disease. Damaged kidneys may be unable to achieve normal levels of urine concentration or dilution. Whereas the normal kidney can produce a urine with an osmolality as low as 60 mmol/kg, in chronic renal disease the lowest osmolality able to be achieved may be as high as 250 mmol/kg (this should be compared with the normal plasma osmolality of 280–290 mmol/kg). Consequently, the ability to excrete a water load is severely impaired and excess water intake (oral or intravenous) readily produces a dilutional hyponatraemia. These patients may also be overloaded with Na$^+$ (p. 134).

Glucocorticoid deficiency. Abrupt withdrawal of long-term glucocorticoid therapy, or anterior pituitary disease, can lead to selective glucocorticoid deficiency. Under these circumstances, patients may be unable to excrete a water load, leading to hyponatraemia.

Resetting of the osmostat. These patients have a plasma [Na$^+$] that is chronically low, generally 125–130 mmol/L, but they respond normally to a water load. The inference is that the osmostat is 'reset' at a lower level. This has been described in association with malnutrition, carcinomatosis and tuberculosis. Deficiency of intracellular K$^+$, with reduced intracellular solute, has been suggested as being responsible for the 'resetting' of the osmostat.

Hyponatraemia with increased ECF volume (Table 4.4)

Significant increases in total body Na$^+$ give rise to clinically manifest oedema. Generalized oedema is usually associated with secondary aldosteronism, caused by a reduction in renal blood flow which stimulates renin production. Patients fall into at least three categories:

1 *Renal failure.* Excess water intake in a poorly controlled patient with chronic renal disease, with pre-existing Na$^+$ retention, can lead to hyponatraemia with oedema. Patients with acute renal failure can also become overloaded with Na^+ and water. These patients do not normally pose diagnostic problems.

2 *Congestive cardiac failure.* The failing heart leads to reduced renal perfusion and 'apparent' volume deficit, registered by atrial baroreceptors and the great arteries of the chest and neck. Increased venous pressure also alters fluid distribution between the intravascular and interstitial compartments (Fig. 4.1). The consequent secondary aldosteronism and increased AVP secretion produce Na^+ overload and hyponatraemia.

3 *Hypoproteinaemic states.* Low plasma [protein], especially low [albumin], leads to excessive losses of water and low mol mass solutes from the intravascular to the interstitial compartments (Fig. 4.1). Hence interstitial oedema is accompanied by reduced intravascular volume, with consequent secondary aldosteronism and stimulation of AVP release.

'Sick cell syndrome'

Patients with oedema and hyponatraemia may be very ill and are often very resistant to treatment. Although the total ECF volume is increased, the effective arterial plasma volume is often contracted. Secondary hyperaldosteronism (which causes further Na^+ retention) and AVP secretion (which causes water retention) may not be the whole explanation since plasma [aldosterone] and [AVP] are not always raised. Some attribute the hyponatraemia, at least in part, to the 'sick cell syndrome'. In this, cell membrane permeability to intracellular solutes increases, leading to movements of solute and water from the intracellular to the extracellular compartments, with resultant hyponatraemia.

Case 4.1

A 63-year-old coal miner had had a persistent chest infection, with cough and sputum, for the previous 2 months. Clinical examination of his chest was consistent with this history, but otherwise clinical findings were unremarkable. Examination of a blood specimen and a random urine specimen yielded the following results:

Plasma analysis	Result	Reference range	Units
[Urea]	2.3	2.5–6.6	mmol/L
[Na^+]	118	132–144	mmol/L
[K^+]	4.3	3.3–4.7	mmol/L
[Total CO_2]	32	24–30	mmol/L
Osmolality	260	280–290	mmol/kg

Analyses on urine: [Na^+], 74 mmol/L; osmolality, 625 mmol/kg

What is the most likely cause of this man's low plasma [Na^+] and osmolality? This patient is discussed on p. 56.

Other causes of hyponatraemia

In all the examples of hyponatraemia discussed above, the low plasma [Na$^+$] occurs in association with reduced plasma osmolality. Other possibilities that may need to be considered include:

1 *Artefact.* Misleading or 'apparent' hyponatraemia is often caused by collection of a blood specimen from a vein close to a site at which fluid is being administered intravenously. This explanation needs to be excluded.

2 *Pseudohyponatraemia.* This is due to a reduction in plasma water caused by marked hyperlipidaemia or hyperproteinaemia (e.g. multiple myeloma). The diagnosis can be confirmed by measuring plasma [Na$^+$] in undiluted plasma, using a direct ion-selective electrode, or by measuring plasma osmolality. In the absence of another cause of true hyponatraemia, the results of these measurements will be normal.

3 *Hyperosmolar hyponatraemia.* This may be due to hyperglycaemia, administration of mannitol, or occasionally other causes. The hyponatraemia mainly reflects the shift of water out of the cells into the ECF in response to osmotic effects, other than those due to Na$^+$, across cell membranes. Treatment should be directed to the cause of the hyperosmolality rather than to the hyponatraemia.

Hypernatraemia

This is the commonest cause of increased tonicity of body fluids. It is nearly always due to water deficit rather than Na$^+$ excess. The ICF volume is decreased due to movement of water out of the cells.

Hypernatraemia with decreased body sodium (Table 4.6)

This is the commonest group. It is usually due to extra-renal loss of hypotonic fluid. The nature and severity of the disturbance of fluid balance is conveniently thought of as comprising two components, losses of water and losses of isotonic fluid:

1 *Loss of water* causes volume reduction of both ICF and ECF and consequent hypernatraemia.

2 *Loss of isotonic fluid* causes reduction in ECF volume, with hypotension, shock and oliguria. Urine osmolality is high and urine [Na$^+$] less than 20 mmol/L.

Table 4.6 Causes of hypernatraemia

Body sodium	Categories	Examples
Decreased body Na$^+$ (loss of H$_2$O > Na$^+$)	Extra-renal Renal	Sweating, diarrhoea Osmotic diuresis (e.g. diabetes)
Normal body Na$^+$ (loss of H$_2$O only)	Extra-renal Via kidneys	Fever, high-temperature climates Diabetes insipidus (p. 301)

Increased body Na$^+$ (retention of Na$^+$ > H$_2$O)	Steroid excess
	
	Intake of Na$^+$
		Steroid treatment, Cushing's
		   syndrome, Conn's syndrome
		Self-induced or iatrogenic, oral
		   or parenteral

Urinary loss of *hypotonic* fluid sometimes occurs, due to renal disease or to osmotic diuresis; in these patients, urine [Na$^+$] is likely to be greater than 20 mmol/L. The commonest cause of hypernatraemia associated with an osmotic diuresis is hyperglycaemia.

Hypernatraemia is not dangerous in this group of patients and treatment should, initially, aim to replace the deficit of isotonic fluid by infusing 150 mmol/L (isotonic) saline.

Hypernatraemia with normal body sodium (Table 4.6)

These patients have a pure water deficit, as may occur when insensible water losses are very high (e.g. in hot climates or in patients with a high fever) and insufficient water is drunk as replacement. The urine has a high osmolality; its Na$^+$ content depends on Na$^+$ intake.

Hypernatraemia with normal body Na$^+$ also occurs in diabetes insipidus (p. 301) due to excessive renal water loss; this loss is normally replaced by drinking. However, dehydration may develop if the patient is unable, for any reason, to drink, as may occur in very young children or in unconscious patients. The urine has a low osmolality; its Na$^+$ content depends on Na$^+$ intake.

Treatment should aim to rehydrate these patients fairly slowly, to avoid causing acute shifts of water into cells, especially the brain, which may have accommodated to the hyperosmolality by increasing its intracellular solute concentration. Water, administered orally, is the simplest treatment. Intravenous therapy may be necessary, with 5% glucose or glucose–saline.

Hypernatraemia with increased body sodium (Table 4.6)

This is relatively uncommon. Mild hypernatraemia may be caused by excess of mineralocorticoids or glucocorticoids. More often, it occurs if excess Na$^+$ is administered therapeutically (e.g. NaHCO$_3$ during resuscitation). Treatment may be with diuretics or, rarely, by renal dialysis.

Other chemical investigations in fluid balance disorders

Several other chemical investigations, in addition to plasma [Na$^+$], may prove of value in patients in whom the history or clinical examination suggests that there is a disorder of fluid balance.

Blood specimens

Plasma albumin

This measurement may help to assess acute changes in intravascular volume. It is also often useful in following changes in patients with fluid balance disorders over time. Plasma [albumin] should be measured in patients with oedema, to find out whether hypoalbuminaemia is present and to determine its severity.

Plasma urea and plasma creatinine

These measurements may be of value since hypovolaemia is usually associated with a reduced GFR, and so with raised plasma [urea] and [creatinine]. As

---

Case 4.2

A 45-year-old man was brought into the accident and emergency department late at night in a comatose state. It was impossible to obtain a history from him, and clinical examination was difficult, but it was noted that he smelt strongly of alcohol. The following analyses were requested urgently:

Plasma analysis	Result	Reference range	Units
[Glucose]	4.2		mmol/L
[Urea]	4.7	2.5–6.6	mmol/L
[Na^+]	137	132–144	mmol/L
[K^+]	3.3	3.3–4.7	mmol/L
[Total CO_2]	10	24–30	mmol/L
Osmolality	465	280–290	mmol/kg

What is the calculated osmolality on this patient (formulae on p. 36)? Why might the *measured* osmolality differ so markedly from the *calculated* osmolality? This patient is discussed on p. 56.

---

explained elsewhere (p. 127), plasma [urea] may increase before plasma [creatinine] in the early stages of water and Na^+ depletion.

Plasma osmolality

Plasma osmolality is measured much less often than plasma [Na^+] since it is usually adequate to estimate the osmolality from the calculated osmolarity (p. 36). However, plasma osmolality measurements are of value when it seems likely that the calculated osmolarity and measured osmolality might differ significantly. This occurs when:

1 There is marked hyperproteinaemia or hypertriglyceridaemia. In these patients, the plasma water concentration is abnormally low.

2 Significant amounts of foreign low mol mass materials (e.g. ethanol, ethylene glycol) are present in plasma.

In both these examples, the finding of a marked discrepancy between the measured osmolality and the calculated osmolarity may be of diagnostic value.

Plasma chloride

Alterations in plasma [Cl^-] parallel those in plasma [Na^+], except in the presence of some acid–base disturbances (p. 65). Chloride measurements are rarely of value in assessing disturbances of fluid balance.

Urine osmolality

Measurements of urine osmolality are of value in the investigation of:

1 *Polyuria*. In the differential diagnosis of polyuria, a relatively concentrated urine suggests that polyuria is due to an osmotic diuretic (e.g. glucose), whereas a dilute urine suggests that there is primary polydipsia or diabetes insipidus (p. 129).

Patients with chronic renal failure may also have polyuria, with a urine osmolality that is usually within 50 mmol/kg of the plasma value.

2   *Oliguria.* In oliguric patients with suspected acute renal failure (p. 135).

3   *SIADH.* In the investigation of patients thought to have SIADH (p. 42), the urine osmolality is not maximally dilute despite a dilutional hyponatraemia.

Urine sodium

The wide variability in Na^+ intake leads to a corresponding variability in urine Na^+ excretion, limiting the value of a random urine $[Na^+]$ measurement. Excretion of Na^+ measured on a 24-hour urine collection may be easier to interpret, but it is still important to take account of the patient's plasma $[Na^+]$ and ECF volume, whether the measurement is being used to help diagnose a disturbance in body Na^+ and water handling or to plan replacement fluid therapy.

Patients with natriuresis

In hyponatraemic patients *with evidence of ECF volume depletion*, continuing natriuresis (i.e. urine $[Na^+]$ greater than 20 mmol/L) suggests one of the following:

1   Volume depletion that is so severe as to have led to acute renal failure. The patient will be oliguric with a rising plasma [urea] and [creatinine]; diuresis fails to occur after volume repletion.

2   In the absence of acute renal failure, this occurs with over-zealous diuretic use, with salt-losing nephritis, and with defects in the hypothalamic–pituitary–adrenal axis, including Addison's disease.

Natriuresis may also occur in hyponatraemic states associated with SIADH or acute water intoxication. There is *no evidence of ECF volume depletion* in these patients. Indeed, there is some expansion of both ICF and ECF compartments, although interstitial oedema is usually absent.

Patients with low urine sodium

A low urine $[Na^+]$ is an appropriate response in patients who are volume-depleted with oliguria but normally functioning kidneys; urine $[Na^+]$ is usually less than 10 mmol/L, and urine flow increases after volume repletion. Excessive retention of Na^+ and low urine $[Na^+]$ occur in the secondary hyperaldosteronism associated with congestive cardiac failure, in liver disease and hypoproteinaemic states, as well as in Cushing's syndrome and Conn's syndrome.

Potassium balance

Potassium is the main intracellular cation. About 98% of total body K^+ is in cells; only 2% (about 50 mmol) is in the ECF. There is a large concentration gradient across cell membranes, the ICF $[K^+]$ being about 150 mmol/L compared with about 4.0 mmol/L in ECF.

External balance

This is mainly determined, in the absence of GI disease, by intake of K^+ and by its renal excretion. A typical 'Western' diet contains 20–100 mmol K^+ daily; this intake is normally closely matched by the urinary excretion. The control of renal K^+ excretion is not fully understood, but the following points have been established:

1 Nearly all the K^+ filtered at the glomerulus is reabsorbed in the proximal tubule. Less than 10% reaches the distal tubule, where the main regulation of K^+ excretion occurs. Secretion of K^+ in response to alterations in dietary intake occurs in the distal tubule, the cortical collecting tubule and the collecting duct.

2 The distal tubule is an important site of Na^+ reabsorption. When Na^+ is reabsorbed, the tubular lumen becomes electronegative in relation to the adjacent cell, and cations in the cell (e.g. K^+, H^+) move into the lumen to balance the charge. The rate of movement of K^+ into the lumen depends on there being sufficient delivery of Na^+ to the distal tubule, as well as on the rate of urine flow and on the concentration of K^+ in the tubular cell.

3 The concentration of K^+ in the tubular cell depends largely on ATPase-dependent Na^+/K^+ exchange with peritubular fluid (i.e. the ECF). This is affected by mineralocorticoids, by acid–base changes and by ECF $[K^+]$. The tubular cell $[K^+]$ tends to be increased by hyperkalaemia, by mineralocorticoid excess and by alkalosis, all of which tend to cause an increase in K^+ excretion.

Internal balance

This is determined by movements across the cell membrane. Factors causing K^+ to move out of cells include hypertonicity, acidosis, insulin lack, and severe cell damage or death. Potassium moves into cells if there is alkalosis or when insulin is given.

The alterations that occur when acid–base balance is disturbed are initiated by changes in plasma $[H^+]$. In acidosis, plasma $[H^+]$ is raised causing H^+ to move into cells and, to maintain electro-neutrality within cells, K^+ moves out. In alkalosis, the fall in ECF $[H^+]$ causes H^+ to move out of cells and K^+ moves in to maintain electro-neutrality. This explanation is over-simple since the responses may be modified by the effects that acid–base disturbances have on the external balance of K^+.

Abnormalities of plasma potassium concentration

The reference range for plasma $[K^+]$ is 3.3–4.7 mmol/L. The important, and often life-threatening, clinical manifestations of abnormalities of plasma $[K^+]$ are those relating to disturbances of neuromuscular excitability and of cardiac conduction. Any patient who has, or who is considered likely to have, an abnormal plasma $[K^+]$ and who also shows signs of muscle weakness or of a cardiac arrhythmia should have ECG cardiac monitoring. Steps should be taken to correct the abnormal plasma $[K^+]$, and this measurement should be repeated to assess the response to treatment.

Hypokalaemia must not be equated with K^+ depletion, and hyperkalaemia must not be equated with K^+ excess. Although most patients with K^+ depletion have hypokalaemia, and most patients with K^+ excess may have hyperkalaemia, acute changes in the distribution of K^+ in the body can offset any effects of

Table 4.7 Causes of hypokalaemia

Causes	Categories	Examples
Artefact		Specimen collected from an infusion site or near to one
Redistribution of K^+ between ECF and ICF		Alkalosis, familial periodic paralysis (hypokalaemic form), treatment of hyperglycaemia
Abnormal external balance	Inadequate intake	Anorexia nervosa, alcoholism (both rare)
	Abnormal losses from the GI tract	Vomiting and aspiration, diarrhoea and fistula, laxative abuse, villous papilloma of the colon
	Abnormal losses from the renal tract	Diuretics, osmotic diuresis, renal tubular acidosis, aldosteronism, Cushing's syndrome, Bartter's syndrome

depletion or excess. To generalize but at the same time to over-simplify the position, *acute* changes in plasma $[K^+]$ are usually caused by movement of K^+ across cell membranes, whereas *chronic* changes in plasma $[K^+]$ are usually manifestations of an abnormal external K^+ balance.

Hypokalaemia (Table 4.7)
The causes divide into those related to acute shifts of K^+ within the body, and those related to K^+ depletion or deficient K^+ intake.

Altered internal balance: shift of K^+ into cells
Acute shifts of K^+ into the cell may occur in *alkalosis*, but the hypokalaemia may be more closely related to the increased renal excretion of K^+. Patients with respiratory alkalosis caused by voluntary hyperventilation rarely show hypokalaemia, but patients on prolonged assisted ventilation may have low plasma $[K^+]$ if the alveolar P_{CO_2} is low for a relatively long period.

Insulin in high dosage, given intravenously, promotes the uptake of K^+ by liver and muscle. Acute shifts of K^+ into the cells may occur in diabetic ketoacidosis shortly after starting treatment.

Adrenaline and other β-adrenergic agonists stimulate the uptake of K^+ into cells. This may contribute to the hypokalaemia appearing in patients after myocardial infarction since catecholamine levels are likely to be increased in these patients. Hypokalaemic effects of salbutamol (a synthetic β-adrenergic agonist) have also been described.

Cellular incorporation of K^+ may be very rapid in states where cell mass rapidly increases. Examples include the treatment of severe megaloblastic anaemia with vitamin B_{12} or folate, and the parenteral refeeding of wasted patients (especially if insulin is also administered). It also occurs when there are rapidly proliferating leukaemic cells.

Hypokalaemic familial periodic paralysis. This is a rare, inherited disorder in which there are attacks of muscle weakness and hypokalaemia, associated with unexplained acute shifts of K^+ into the cells.

Altered external balance: deficient intake of K^+

Prolonged deficient intake of K^+ can lead to a decrease in total body K^+, eventually manifesting itself as hypokalaemia. This may occur in chronic and severe malnutrition in the Third World, in the elderly on deficient diets, in anorexia nervosa, and in patients receiving prolonged post-operative parenteral nutrition but with inadequate K^+ replacement.

Altered external balance: excessive losses of K^+

Hyperaldosteronism, both primary and secondary, and *Cushing's syndrome* cause excessive renal K^+ loss due to increased K^+ transfer into the distal tubule in response to increased reabsorption of Na^+ from the tubular lumen. In addition, mineralocorticoid excess favours transfer of K^+ into the tubular cell in exchange for Na^+ at the peritubular border of the cell. Urinary K^+ loss in hyperaldosteronism returns to normal if there is dietary Na^+ restriction, which limits distal tubular delivery of Na^+.

Diuretic therapy has a direct effect on renal K^+ excretion by causing increased delivery of Na^+ to the distal tubule and increased urine flow rate. Diuretics may also cause hypovolaemia with consequent secondary hyperaldosteronism.

Acidosis and alkalosis both affect renal K^+ excretion in ways that are not fully understood. Acute acidosis causes K^+ retention and acute alkalosis causes increased K^+ excretion. However, chronic acidosis and chronic alkalosis *both* cause increased K^+ excretion.

Gastrointestinal fluid losses often cause K^+ depletion. However, if gastric fluid is lost in large quantity, the resultant metabolic alkalosis is the main cause of the K^+ loss rather than the direct loss of K^+ in gastric juice; the alkalosis affects renal K^+ excretion. In diarrhoea or laxative abuse, the increased losses of K^+ in faeces may cause K^+ depletion.

Renal disease does not usually cause excessive K^+ loss. However, a few tubular abnormalities are associated with K^+ depletion, in the absence of diuretic therapy:

1 *Renal tubular acidosis*. The K^+ loss is caused both by the acidosis and, in patients with *proximal* renal tubular acidosis (p. 132), by increased delivery of Na^+ to the distal tubule. In *distal* renal tubular acidosis, the inability to excrete H^+ may cause a compensatory transfer of K^+ to the tubular fluid.

2 *Bartter's syndrome*. The syndrome consists of persistent hypokalaemia with secondary hyperaldosteronism in association with a metabolic alkalosis; patients are normotensive. There is increased delivery of Na^+ to the distal tubule caused by an abnormality of chloride reabsorption in the loop of Henle.

Other causes of hypokalaemia

Artefact. Collection of a blood sample from a vein near to a site of an intravenous infusion, where the fluid has a low $[K^+]$.

Excessive sweating. The K^+ content of sweat is normally greater than 5 mmol/L, but less than 20 mmol/L.

Hyperkalaemia (Table 4.8)

Increased plasma $[K^+]$ can arise from altered internal balance. It can also arise from abnormal external balance, which may be due to increased intake or decreased excretion.

Plasma $[K^+]$ in excess of 6.5 mmol/L requires urgent treatment. Intravenous calcium gluconate has a rapid but short-lived effect in countering the neuromuscular effects of hyperkalaemia. Treatment with glucose and insulin causes K^+ to pass into the ICF. However, treatment with ion-exchange resins or renal dialysis may be needed.

Altered internal balance of K^+

Acidosis. The effects of acidosis on internal K^+ balance are complicated. As a general rule, acidotic states are often accompanied by hyperkalaemia, as K^+ moves from the ICF into the ECF. Although this is the case for acute respiratory acidosis, and for both acute and chronic metabolic acidosis, it is more unusual to find hyperkalaemia in chronic respiratory acidosis. It is important to note that a high plasma $[K^+]$ may be accompanied by a reduced total body K^+ as a result of excessive urinary K^+ losses in both chronic respiratory acidosis and in metabolic acidosis.

Hypertonic states. In these, K^+ moves out of cells, possibly because of the increased intracellular $[K^+]$ caused by the reduction in ICF volume.

Table 4.8 Causes of hyperkalaemia

Causes	Categories	Examples
Artefact		Trauma during blood collection, delay in separating plasma/serum, freezing blood
Redistribution of K^+ between ECF and ICF		Acidosis, hypertonicity, tissue and tumour necrosis (e.g. burns, leukaemia), haemolytic disorders, hyperkalaemic familial periodic paralysis, insulin deficiency
Abnormal external balance	Increased intake	Excessive oral intake of K^+ (rare by itself)
	Decreased renal output*	
	Renal causes	1 Renal failure, oliguric (acute and chronic) inappropriate oral intake in chronic failure 2 Failure of renal tubular response, due to systemic lupus erythematosus, K^+-sparing diuretics, chronic interstitial nephritis
	Adrenal causes	Addison's disease, selective hypoaldosteronism

* With or without appropriate intake.

Uncontrolled diabetes mellitus. The lack of insulin prevents K^+ from entering cells. This results in hyperkalaemia despite the K^+ loss caused by the osmotic diuresis.

Cellular necrosis may lead to excessive release of K^+ and may result in hyperkalaemia. Extensive cell damage may be a feature of rhabdomyolysis (e.g. crush injury), haemolysis, burns, or tumour necrosis (e.g. in the treatment of leukaemias).

Digoxin poisoning prevents K^+ from entering into cells, but therapeutic doses do not have this effect.

Hyperkalaemic familial periodic paralysis. This is a rare disorder. Attacks of paralysis due to hyperkalaemia are induced by a variety of apparently unrelated stimuli.

Altered external balance: increased intake of K^+

Increased K^+ intake only rarely causes accumulation of K^+ in the body since the normal kidney can excrete a large K^+ load. However, if there is renal impairment, K^+ may accumulate if salt substitutes are administered, or excessive amounts of some fruit drinks are drunk, or if potassium replacement therapy accompanies diuretic administration.

Altered external balance: decreased excretion of K^+

Decreased K^+ excretion arises from intrinsic renal disease. It is also caused by mineralocorticoid deficiency, due to a defect in the endocrine (aldosterone) mechanism responsible for controlling K^+ secretion by the distal nephron.

Intrinsic renal disease is an important cause of hyperkalaemia. It may occur in acute renal failure and in the later stages of chronic renal failure. In patients with renal disease that largely affects the renal medulla, hyperkalaemia may occur earlier. This may be because increased K^+ secretion from the collecting duct, an important adaptive response in the damaged kidney, is lost earlier in patients with medullary disease.

Mineralocorticoid deficiency may occur in Addison's disease and in secondary adrenocortical hypofunction. In both, K^+ retention may sometimes occur, but not invariably, presumably because other mechanisms can facilitate K^+ excretion. Selective hypoaldosteronism, accompanied by normal glucocorticoid production, may occur in patients with diabetes mellitus in whom juxtaglomerular sclerosis probably interferes with renin production. ACE inhibitors, by reducing angiotensin II (and, therefore, aldosterone) levels (p. 39) may lead to increased plasma $[K^+]$, but severe problems are only likely to occur in the presence of renal failure.

Patients treated with K^+-sparing diuretics (e.g. spironolactone, amiloride) may fail to respond to aldosterone. If the K^+ intake is high in these patients, or if they have renal insufficiency or selective hypoaldosteronism, these can all lead to dangerous hyperkalaemia.

Other causes of hyperkalaemia

Artefact. This is the commonest cause of hyperkalaemia. When red cells or, occasionally, white cells and platelets are left in contact with plasma or serum for too long, K^+ leaks from the cells. In any blood specimen which does not have its plasma or serum separated from the cells within about 3 hours, plasma $[K^+]$ is likely to be spuriously high.

Blood specimens collected into potassium edetate (potassium EDTA), an anticoagulant widely used for haematological specimens, have greatly increased plasma $[K^+]$. Sometimes, doctors decant part of a blood specimen initially collected by mistake into potassium edetate into another container and send this for biochemical analysis. Laboratory staff readily detect this source of artefact, which may increase plasma $[K^+]$ to 'lethal' levels (e.g. over 8 mmol/L), because there is an accompanying very low plasma [calcium], due to chelation of Ca^{2+} with EDTA.

'*Pseudohyperkalaemia*'. This is a rare familial condition in which the red cells leak K^+ abnormally rapidly following blood collection. Its importance lies in its distinction from 'true' hyperkalaemia. Plasma separated carefully soon after collection of blood from these patients has a normal $[K^+]$; serum is particularly unsuitable for measurements of $[K^+]$ in these patients. Pseudohyperkalaemia can also occur in acute and chronic myeloproliferative disorders, chronic lymphocytic leukaemia, and severe thrombocytosis as a result of cell lysis during venepuncture or if there is any delay in the separation of plasma following specimen collection.

Other investigations in disordered K^+ metabolism

Urine K^+ measurements may be of help in determining the source of K^+ depletion in patients with unexplained hypokalaemia, but are otherwise of little value. A 24-hour urine collection should be made.

Case 4.3

A 64-year-old man was admitted on a Sunday for an elective operation on his nasal sinuses; his previous hospital notes were not available. He appeared to be fit for operation on clinical examination, and his pre-operative electrocardiogram (ECG) was normal, but the following results were obtained on a blood specimen analysed as part of the ward's routine pre-operative assessment:

Plasma analysis	Result	Reference range	Units
[Urea]	7.0	2.5–6.6	mmol/L
[Na$^+$]	135	132–144	mmol/L
[K$^+$]	8.8	3.3–4.7	mmol/L
[Total CO$_2$]	30	24–30	mmol/L

How would you interpret the hyperkalaemia in relation to the findings on clinical examination and the normal ECG recording? Would your comments be influenced by the information that became available later that day, when the patient's medical records were received, that he had chronic lymphocytic leukaemia? This patient is discussed on p. 56.

Plasma total [CO$_2$] (p. 65) may prove helpful in the investigation of disorders of K$^+$ balance since metabolic acidosis and metabolic alkalosis are commonly associated with abnormalities of K$^+$ homeostasis. Only rarely is it necessary to assess acid–base status fully when investigating disturbances of K$^+$ metabolism; measuring plasma [total CO$_2$] usually suffices.

Other investigations may be indicated by the history of the patient's illness and the findings on clinical examination, e.g. plasma [creatinine].

Fluid and electrolyte balance in surgical patients

Patients admitted for major elective surgery, and who might be liable to develop disturbances of water and electrolyte balance post-operatively, require pre-operative determination of baseline values for plasma urea, creatinine, Na$^+$, K$^+$ and total CO$_2$ concentrations (the 'electrolyte' group).

Patients who present for emergency surgery, with disturbances of water and electrolyte metabolism already developed, require to have the severity of the disturbances assessed and corrective measures instituted pre-operatively. This usually involves the measurement of plasma 'electrolytes' as an emergency. Ideally, fluid and electrolyte disturbances should be corrected before operation.

The nutritional support of patients, including surgical patients post-operatively, is considered on p. 239.

Metabolic response to trauma

Accidental and operative trauma produce several metabolic effects, including breakdown of protein, release of K$^+$ from cells and a consequential K$^+$ deficit due to urinary loss, temporary retention of water, utilization of glycogen reserves, gluconeogenesis, mobilization of fat reserves and a tendency to ketosis that sometimes progresses to a metabolic acidosis. Hormonal responses include increased secretion of adrenal corticosteroids, with temporary abolition of negative feedback control, and increased secretion of aldosterone and AVP.

The metabolic responses to trauma are physiological and appropriate. They are the reason why 'post-operative states' are such frequent causes of temporary disturbances in electrolyte metabolism. Most patients after major surgery have a temporarily impaired ability to excrete a water load or a Na$^+$ load; they also have a plasma [urea] that is often raised due to tissue catabolism. Injudicious fluid therapy, especially in the first 48 hours after operation, may 'correct' the chemical abnormalities, e.g. by lowering the plasma [urea], but only by causing dangerous retention of fluid and the possibility of acute water intoxication.

Post-operatively, any tendency for patients to develop disturbances of water and electrolyte balance can be minimized by regular follow-up clinical assessment. In addition to plasma 'electrolytes', fluid balance charts and measurement of 24-hour urinary losses of Na$^+$ and K$^+$ or losses from a fistula can provide information of value in calculating the approximate volume and composition of fluid needed to replace continuing losses. This is discussed more fully on p. 241.

Acute water intoxication is a severe and dangerous disorder associated with acute neurological symptoms (drowsiness, fits) and later with coma and often death. The symptoms are due to acute swelling of the brain cells caused by the entry of water from the ECF, which has become hypotonic relatively rapidly with respect to the ICF. There is controversy about the appropriate treatment. However, in most centres this would be instituted as a matter of urgency with the infusion of hypertonic saline; a diuretic would also be given to avoid causing fluid overload.

Comments on Case 4.1 (p. 44)

The absence of clinical evidence of either salt retention or depletion of ECF volume argues in favour of a dilutional hyponatraemia. The most likely diagnosis would be inappropriate secretion. In the absence of AVP measurements, the *low* plasma osmolality combined with the *high* urine osmolality is good evidence for inappropriate AVP secretion. Urine Na^+ excretion tends to be high in these patients as the retention of water leads to mild expansion of the ECF, reduced aldosterone secretion and increased renal Na^+ loss. Dilutional hyponatraemia is also supported by the low plasma [urea].

Before diagnosing the syndrome of inappropriate AVP or ADH (SIADH, p. 42) secretion, it is important to exclude adrenal, pituitary and renal disease. In this patient, possible explanations relate to the recurrent chest infections, or an underlying bronchogenic carcinoma, with 'ectopic' secretion of AVP.

Comments on Case 4.2 (p. 47)

The osmolality can be *calculated* from the data using the formulae given on p. 36. These yield results of (i) 289.5 and (ii) 280 mmol/L respectively. The difference between these figures and the value for the directly *measured* osmolality (465 mmol/L) could be explained if there were to be other low mol mass solutes present in plasma. From the patient's history, it seemed that ethanol might be contributing significantly to the plasma osmolality, and plasma [ethanol] was measured the following day, on the residue of the specimen collected at the time of emergency admission. The result was 170 mmol/L, very close to the difference between the measured and calculated osmolalities.

Comments on Case 4.3 (p. 54)

The ECG changes that are associated with hyperkalaemia are not correlated closely with the level of plasma $[K^+]$, but it would be most unlikely for the ECG to be normal in a patient whose plasma $[K^+]$ was 8.8 mmol/L. It is much more likely that the hyperkalaemia was an artefact.

Intracellular $[K^+]$ is much higher than plasma $[K^+]$ and potassium leaks out of erythrocytes on prolonged storage of an unseparated blood specimen or as a result of haemolysis. Less often, hyperkalaemia may be due to lysis of leucocytes or platelets, and this is liable to occur in chronic lymphocytic leukaemia (as in this patient), in acute and chronic myeloproliferative syndromes, and in severe thrombocytosis, unless plasma is separated from the cells with care and very soon after the blood specimen has been collected.

Chapter 5
Acid–base Balance and Oxygen Transport

The hydrogen ion concentration of ECF is normally maintained within very close limits. To achieve this, each day the body must dispose of:

1 About 20 000 mmol of CO_2 generated by tissue metabolism.

2 About 40–80 mmol of non-volatile acids, mainly sulphur-containing organic acids, which are excreted by the kidneys.

The CO_2 produced in tissue cells diffuses freely down a concentration gradient across cell membranes into the ECF and red cells. The following reactions then occur:

$$CO_2 + H_2O \rightleftharpoons H_2CO_3 \tag{5.1}$$

$$H_2CO_3 \rightleftharpoons H^+ + HCO_3^- \tag{5.2}$$

Reaction 5.1, the non-ionic hydration of CO_2 to form carbonic acid (H_2CO_3), is very slow and carbonic anhydrase is needed as catalyst to enable the rapid removal of CO_2 from the tissues to be effected; this limits the site of Reaction 5.1 mainly to the erythrocytes, where carbonic anhydrase is located. The ionization of carbonic acid, Reaction 5.2, then occurs rapidly and spontaneously; as a result, erythrocytes are the principal site of H^+ and HCO_3^- formation in the blood. The H^+ are mainly buffered inside the red cell by haemoglobin. Bicarbonate ions, however, pass from the erythrocytes into plasma in exchange for chloride ions.

In the pulmonary capillaries, the blood P_{CO_2} is higher than the P_{CO_2} in the alveoli, so the gradient is reversed. The above reaction sequence shifts to the left, carbonic anhydrase again catalysing Reaction 5.1; CO_2 then diffuses into the alveoli down the concentration gradient and is excreted by the lungs.

The lungs and the kidneys together maintain overall acid–base balance. However, the ECF requires to be protected against rapid changes in $[H^+]$. This is achieved by various buffer systems, the capacity of which to act as buffers of H^+ is related to their concentration and the pK_a values. Thus, haemoglobin and plasma proteins act as efficient buffers in blood since they have pK_a values in the region of pH 7.0, relatively close to the normal blood pH of 7.40, whereas the bicarbonate buffer system has a pK_a value that is far removed, at pH 6.1, and thus has much lower physiological buffering capacity.

All the blood buffer systems are in equilibrium and changes in $[H^+]$ that affect one system produce corresponding changes in the others. Any convenient buffer system can be used to investigate and define acid–base status, and the H_2CO_3/HCO_3^- buffer system has proved to be the most appropriate for this purpose.

The Henderson equation

Two ways of expressing the dissociation of carbonic acid are widely used. Of these, the Henderson equation simply applies the Law of Mass Action to give:

$$[H^+] = K \times \frac{[H_2CO_3]}{[HCO_3^-]} \tag{5.3}$$

In this equation, K is the first ionization constant of carbonic acid. The $[H_2CO_3]$ term can be replaced by $S.P_{CO_2}$, where S is the solubility coefficient of CO_2, since H_2CO_3 is in equilibrium with dissolved CO_2 (Reaction 5.1). At 37°C, S has the value 0.23 mmol/J if P_{CO_2} is expressed in kilopascals (kPa); the numerical value of K is 7.94×10^{-7}. Equation 5.3 becomes:

$$[H^+] = 7.94 \times \frac{0.23\, P_{CO_2}}{[HCO_3^-]} \times 10^{-7}\, \text{mol/L} \tag{5.4}$$

In Equation 5.4, P_{CO_2} is sometimes referred to as the respiratory component because, in arterial blood, it is directly related to alveolar P_{CO_2}, which, in turn, depends on respiratory function. The $[HCO_3^-]$ term is sometimes referred to as the metabolic (or non-respiratory) component. However, the term 'metabolic component' is potentially misleading since plasma HCO_3^- reflects changes in both metabolic *and* respiratory disorders (see later).

The changes discussed in the previous paragraph are caused by changes in the equilibria of *chemical* reactions, and must be distinguished from the acid–base changes which occur as a result of respiratory or renal *physiological* mechanisms operating to return plasma $[H^+]$ towards normal. For example, if there is a rise in P_{CO_2}, this will be *immediately* reflected by a rise in both plasma $[H^+]$ and $[HCO_3^-]$ due to a shift to the right in Reactions 5.1 and 5.2. Only after several hours, however, would the effect of physiological renal compensatory changes become evident (p. 61).

The Henderson–Hasselbalch equation

This equation is Equation 5.3 rearranged into the corresponding logarithmic form:

$$pH = pK + \log_{10} \frac{[HCO_3^-]}{[H_2CO_3]} \tag{5.5}$$

The $[HCO_3^-]$ term can again be replaced by $S.P_{CO_2}$; in this case, the numerical value of S is 0.03. The value of pK is 6.10. Equation 5.5 then becomes:

$$pH = 6.10 + \log_{10} \frac{[HCO_3^-]}{0.03\, P_{CO_2}} \tag{5.6}$$

Investigating acid–base balance

The acid–base status of a patient can be fully characterized by measuring pH (from which $[H^+]$ is directly derived) and P_{CO_2} in arterial or arterialized capillary blood specimens that have been collected with due care, as described below. When discussing these results, and their interpretation, it is a matter of individual preference whether the Henderson or the Henderson–Hasselbalch equation is adopted. Our preference is for the Henderson equation as its use avoids the confusion that some experience when trying to reconcile the fact than an acidosis, in which there is an *increase* in $[H^+]$, is reflected by a *fall* in pH, and the converse apparent anomaly occurs in an alkalosis.

Because of the relationships described in Equations 5.4 and 5.6, it is only necessary to measure two of the three variables; the third variable, arterial bicarbonate or plasma $[HCO_3^-]$, is then obtained by calculation. Plasma $[HCO_3^-]$ has largely replaced terms such as standard bicarbonate, base excess and base deficit, although these derived values are still sometimes reported. We do not think they are necessary for the understanding of acid–base disturbances; indeed, at times, they may be frankly misleading.

Collection and transport of specimens

Arterial blood specimens are the most appropriate for full assessment of acid–base status. However, unless an arterial cannula is *in situ*, these specimens may be difficult to obtain for repeated assessment of patients whose clinical condition is rapidly changing. Arterialized capillary blood specimens are also widely used, especially in infants and children; it is essential for the capillary blood to flow freely, and collection of satisfactory samples may be impossible if there is peripheral vasoconstriction or the blood flow is sluggish.

Patients must be relaxed, and their breathing pattern should have settled after any temporary disturbance (e.g. due to insertion of an arterial cannula), before specimens are collected; some patients may hyperventilate temporarily because they feel apprehensive.

Blood is collected into syringes or capillary tubes that contain sufficient heparin to act as anticoagulant; excess heparin must be avoided. Specimens must be free from air bubbles; air must be ejected from the syringe *before* blood is mixed with heparin.

Arrangements should be made for the *immediate* performance of acid–base measurements. Unless this can be done, the specimens *must* be chilled in iced water; otherwise, glycolysis occurs and the acid–base composition of the blood alters rapidly. Specimens chilled in iced water can have their analysis delayed as long as 4 hours. However, the clinical reasons that gave rise to the need for full acid–base studies usually demand much more rapid answers. Under no circumstances should specimens of blood for acid–base measurement be frozen as this causes haemolysis.

Temperature effects

Acid–base measurements are nearly always made at 37°C. However, some patients on whom these investigations are requested may have body temperatures that are much removed from 37°C (e.g. severely hypothermic patients). Equations have been defined that relate $[H^+]$, Pco_2 and Po_2, determined at 37°C, to the 'equivalent' values that correspond to the patient's body temperature. The question is, 'Should acid–base data obtained at 37°C be 'corrected' to the temperature of the patient before being reported?'

Reference ranges for acid–base data have only been established by most laboratories for measurements made at 37°C. We cannot, therefore, recommend 'correction' of analytical results to values that would have been obtained, according to the equations used, at the temperature of the patient (e.g. 28°C). It is not possible, ethically, to establish reference ranges for hypothermic patients. If treatment aimed at reducing an acid–base disturbance (e.g. $NaHCO_3$ infusion) is given to a severely hypothermic patient, the effects of the treatment should be monitored frequently by repeating the acid–base measurements (at 37°C).

Disturbances of acid–base status

Acid–base disorders fall into two main categories, respiratory and metabolic:

1 *Respiratory disorders*. A primary defect in ventilation affects the P_{CO_2}.

2 *Metabolic disorders*. The primary defect may be production of non-volatile acids, or ingestion of substances (e.g. NH_4Cl) that give rise to them in excess of the kidney's ability to excrete these substances. Alternatively, the primary defect may be the loss of H^+ from the body, or it may be loss or retention of HCO_3^-.

We shall base our discussion on the relationships represented by Reactions 5.1 and 5.2, and restrict it mainly to consideration of *simple* acid–base disturbances, in which there is a single primary disturbance, *normally* accompanied by *compensatory* physiological changes which usually tend to correct plasma $[H^+]$ towards normal. We shall not consider mixed disturbances, where two or more primary simple disturbances are present, in any detail.

Sets of illustrative acid–base results for patients with the four categories of simple disorders of acid–base status are given in Table 5.1. The mechanisms of each of these disorders will now be briefly discussed.

Table 5.1 Illustrative data for patients with simple disturbances of acid–base balance

Nature of disturbance	$[H^+]$ 36–44 nmol/L*	P_{CO_2} 4.4–6.1 kPa*	Plasma $[HCO_3^-]$ 21.0–27.5 mmol/L*	Plasma [total CO_2] 24–30 mmol/L*
Respiratory acidosis				
Uncompensated	58	9.3	29	32
Partially compensated	49	9.3	34	37
Respiratory alkalosis				
Uncompensated	29	3.2	20	22
Partially compensated	32	3.2	18	20
Metabolic acidosis				
Uncompensated	90	5.3	10	14
Partially compensated	72	3.2	8	11
Metabolic alkalosis				
Uncompensated	26	5.3	37	40
Partially compensated†	32	7.3	40	44

* Reference range.

† Respiratory compensation for the alkalosis (i.e. hypoventilation) is usually minimal.

Table 5.2 Respiratory acidosis

Mechanism	Examples of causes
Alveolar P_{CO_2} increased	Lung disease, respiratory muscle weakness, CNS disease, drug overdose

Respiratory acidosis (Table 5.2)

This is caused by CO_2 retention due to hypoventilation. It may accompany defects in the control of ventilation, or diseases affecting the nerve supply or muscles of the chest wall or diaphragm, or disorders affecting the respiratory cage or intrinsic lung disease.

Acute respiratory acidosis. In this, a sudden rise in P_{CO_2} causes the equilibria in Reactions 5.1 and 5.2 to shift to the right. As immediate and direct results, *plasma [H$^+$] and [HCO$_3^-$] both increase.*

Equilibration of body buffers achieves a steady state within a few minutes. Unless the cause of the acute episode of acidosis is treated quickly, and successfully, *renal compensation* causes HCO_3^- retention and H^+ excretion, thereby returning plasma [H$^+$] towards normal whereas [HCO$_3^-$] increases even further; these compensatory changes occur over 4–5 days, by which time a new steady state is achieved and the daily renal H^+ excretion and HCO_3^- retention return to normal. The patient then has the pattern of acid–base abnormalities of *chronic respiratory acidosis.*

Respiratory alkalosis (Table 5.3)

This is due to hyperventilation, caused by an *abnormality of control* of respiration. The stimulus may be cortical hypoxaemia or mechanical. The reduced P_{CO_2} that results from overventilation causes the equilibrium positions of Reactions 5.1 and 5.2 to move to the left. As an immediate and direct result, *plasma [H$^+$] and [HCO$_3^-$] both fall.*

If conditions giving rise to a low P_{CO_2} persist for more than a few hours, the kidneys increase HCO_3^- excretion and reduce H^+ and NH_4^+ excretion; plasma [H$^+$] returns towards normal whereas plasma [HCO$_3^-$] falls even further. A new steady state will be achieved in 3–4 days, if the respiratory disorder persists. It is unusual for chronic respiratory alkalosis to be severe, and plasma [HCO$_3^-$] rarely falls below 12 mmol/L.

Table 5.3 Respiratory alkalosis

Mechanism	Examples of causes
Alveolar P_{CO_2} lowered	Voluntary overbreathing, artificial ventilation, drug overdose (e.g. salicylates sometimes)

Table 5.4 Metabolic acidosis

Mechanism	Examples of causes
Addition of H^+ to body fluids in excess of body's excretory capacity	Starvation ketosis, diabetic ketoacidosis, lactic acidosis, poisoning (e.g. methanol, salicylate)
Failure to excrete H^+ at the normal rate	Acute and chronic renal failure, distal renal tubular acidosis
Loss of HCO_3^- from the GI tract or in the urine	Severe diarrhoea, fistula, ureterosigmoidostomy, proximal renal tubular acidosis, carbonic anhydrase inhibitors

Metabolic acidosis (Table 5.4)

This disturbance is most commonly due to poisoning, diabetic ketoacidosis, acute anoxia or renal failure. The addition of H^+ to the ECF, or the accumulation of H^+ within the ECF, tends to disturb the equilibrium in Reaction 5.2; the consequence is a shift to the left as the extra H^+ combine with HCO_3^- to form H_2CO_3. However, since there is no ventilatory abnormality, P_{CO_2} remains constant and any increase in plasma $[H_2CO_3]$ is only transient as the related slight increase in dissolved CO_2 is immediately excreted by the lungs. The net effect is that a new equilibrium rapidly establishes itself in which the product, $[H^+] \times [HCO_3^-]$, remains unchanged since $[H_2CO_3]$ is unchanged. In consequence, *plasma $[H^+]$ rises and $[HCO_3^-]$ falls*.

The rise in ECF $[H^+]$ stimulates the respiratory centre. This causes *compensatory hyperventilation*. As a result, due to the fall in P_{CO_2}, plasma $[H^+]$ falls back towards normal while *plasma $[HCO_3^-]$ falls even further*. It is quite common for patients with metabolic acidosis to have very low plasma $[HCO_3^-]$, often below 10 mmol/L.

Metabolic alkalosis (Table 5.5)

This is most often due to prolonged vomiting but may be due to other causes. The loss of H^+ upsets the equilibrium in Reaction 5.2, causing it to shift to the right as H_2CO_3 dissociates to form H^+ and HCO_3^-. However, because there is no disturbance of ventilation, plasma $[H_2CO_3]$ and P_{CO_2} remain constant, with the net effect that *plasma $[H^+]$ falls and $[HCO_3^-]$ rises*. Respiratory compensation (i.e. hypoventilation) for the alkalosis is usually minimal.

Table 5.5 Metabolic alkalosis

Mechanism	Examples of causes
Loss of H^+ from the body	Vomiting, severe K^+ depletion, thiazide diuretics, glucocorticoid or mineralocorticoid excess
Addition of base to the body in excess of its excretory capacity	Milk-alkali syndrome ($NaHCO_3$ intake excessive)

Interpretation of results of full acid–base assessment

Results of acid–base measurements must be considered in the light of clinical findings, and the results of other chemical tests (e.g. plasma creatinine, urea, Na^+ and K^+); other types of investigation (e.g. radiological) may also be important. With the exception of patients with metabolic alkalosis, a simple primary disturbance of a given severity will generate a predictable compensatory response. For example, in a patient with a simple metabolic acidosis causing an initial plasma $[H^+]$ of 90 nmol/L, the degree of hyperventilatory response would predictably lower the P_{CO_2} to about 3 kPa and the plasma $[HCO_3^-]$ to about 8 mmol/L.

We shall present the following discussion in relation to numerical findings and also base it on the equilibria represented by Reactions 5.1 and 5.2 and the related Henderson equation. *We suggest that, after reviewing the clinical findings, acid–base results should be considered in the following order*:

1 *Plasma $[H^+]$*. Reference range, 36–44 nmol/L.
2 *Plasma P_{CO_2}*. Reference range, 4.5–6.1 kPa.
3 *Plasma $[HCO_3^-]$*. Reference range, 21.0–27.5 mmol/L.

This procedure immediately identifies those patients in whom there is an acidosis and those in whom there is an alkalosis, and initiates the orderly consideration of their further classification.

Plasma $[H^+]$ is increased

The patient has an acidosis. The P_{CO_2} result is considered next, as follows:

1 *P_{CO_2} is decreased*. The patient has a *compensated metabolic acidosis*. The reduced P_{CO_2} is due to hyperventilation, the physiological compensatory response (e.g. the overbreathing in patients with diabetic ketoacidosis). Plasma $[HCO_3^-]$ is reduced in these patients, often to below 10 mmol/L.

2 *P_{CO_2} is normal*. The patient has an *uncompensated metabolic acidosis*. Plasma $[HCO_3^-]$ will be decreased. This is a rather unusual combination of results as the normal compensatory response should lower the P_{CO_2} in patients with a simple metabolic acidosis (see above).

3 *P_{CO_2} is increased*. The patient has a *respiratory acidosis*. If this is a simple disturbance, plasma $[HCO_3^-]$ will be increased. The pattern of results will tend to differ, however, depending on whether the respiratory acidosis is acute or chronic:

(a) *Acute*: The patient is likely to have a high plasma $[H^+]$ and high P_{CO_2}, with a moderately raised plasma $[HCO_3^-]$.

(b) *Chronic*: The patient is likely to have a normal or slightly raised plasma $[H^+]$, a high P_{CO_2}, and a markedly raised plasma $[HCO_3^-]$ that is usually over 32 mmol/L, due to renal retention of HCO_3^-.

Plasma $[H^+]$ is decreased

The patient has an alkalosis. The P_{CO_2} result should be assessed next:

1 *P_{CO_2} is decreased*. The patient has a *respiratory alkalosis*. If this is a simple disturbance, plasma $[HCO_3^-]$ will be decreased (not below about 12 mmol/L).

2 *P_{CO_2} is normal*. The patient has an *uncompensated metabolic alkalosis*, and the plasma $[HCO_3^-]$ will be increased, see Equation 5.4.

3 *P_{CO_2} is increased*. It is unlikely that this patient has a *simple* acid–base

disturbance, since significant hypoventilation is not a feature of the compensatory response to a metabolic alkalosis (see above). The more usual explanation for a low plasma [H^+] and an increased P_{CO_2} is that the patient probably has a *mixed acid–base disturbance*, consisting of a metabolic alkalosis and a respiratory acidosis; plasma [HCO_3^-] is also increased.

Plasma [H+] is normal

The patient either has no acid–base disturbance, or no net acid–base disturbance as a result of one of the mechanisms described below. Considering the P_{CO_2} result next:

1 *P_{CO_2} is decreased.* The patient most probably has a *mixed acid–base disturbance* consisting of a respiratory alkalosis and a metabolic acidosis. Both these types of acid–base disturbance cause a decreased plasma [HCO_3^-], and the distinction can usually be made on clinical grounds. A fully compensated respiratory alkalosis is unlikely.

2 *P_{CO_2} is normal.* There is no significant acid–base disturbance. Since both plasma [H^+] and P_{CO_2} are normal, plasma [HCO_3^-] must be normal, (see Equation 5.4).

3 *P_{CO_2} is increased.* The patient either has a fully compensated respiratory acidosis or there is a mixed acid–base disturbance consisting of a respiratory acidosis and a metabolic alkalosis. Both these possibilities give rise to increased plasma [HCO_3^-], to over 30 mmol/L. They can usually be distinguished on clinical

---

Case 5.1

A 70-year-old man was admitted to hospital as an emergency. He gave a long history of epigastric pain and dyspepsia, extending over several years. One week prior to admission, he had started to vomit, and had since vomited frequently, being unable to keep down any food. He was clinically dehydrated and had marked epigastric tenderness, but no sign of abdominal rigidity. Analysis of an arterial blood specimen gave the following results:

Blood or plasma analysis	Result	Reference range	Units
[Urea]	17.3	2.5–6.6	mmol/L
[Na^+]	117	132–144	mmol/L
[K^+]	2.2	3.3–4.7	mmol/L
[Creatinine]	250	55–120	µmol/L
[H^+]	26	36–44	nmol/L
P_{CO_2}	6.2	4.4–6.1	kPa
[HCO_3^-]	44	21.0–27.5	mmol/L
P_{O_2}	9.7	12–15	kPa

How would you describe this patient's acid–base status? What might have caused the various abnormalities revealed by these results? This patient is discussed on p. 70.

grounds, which must include consideration of any treatment that the patient may have received (e.g. $NaHCO_3$).

Mixed acid–base disturbances

It may not always be possible to differentiate some mixed acid–base disturbances from simple ones by the scheme described above. For instance, some patients with chronic renal failure (which causes a primary metabolic acidosis) may also have chronic obstructive airways disease (which causes a primary respiratory acidosis); plasma $[H^+]$ will be increased in these patients, but the results for plasma P_{CO_2} and $[HCO_3^-]$ cannot be predicted. The history and clinical findings must be taken into account.

Alternatives to full acid–base assessment

The full characterization of acid–base status requires arterial or arterialized capillary blood samples since venous blood P_{CO_2} (even if 'arterialized') bears no constant relationship to alveolar P_{CO_2}. However, full acid–base assessment of all patients with acid–base disturbances would present difficulties in the collection of specimens, and the numbers of such full assessments might create serious logistic problems for the laboratory.

Total CO_2 (reference range, 24–30 mmol/L)

This test, performed on venous plasma or serum, is part of the frequently requested 'electrolyte' group of tests routinely performed by most clinical biochemistry laboratories. It includes contributions from HCO_3^-, H_2CO_3, dissolved CO_2 and carbamino compounds; however, about 95% of 'total CO_2' is contributed by HCO_3^-.

Total CO_2 measurements have the advantages of ease of sample collection and suitability for measurement in large numbers, but they cannot define a patient's acid–base status since plasma $[H^+]$ and P_{CO_2} are both unknown. For example, an increased plasma [total CO_2] may be due to either a respiratory acidosis or a metabolic alkalosis. However, when interpreted in the light of the clinical findings, plasma [total CO_2] can often give an adequate assessment of whether an acid–base disturbance is present and, if one is present, provide an indication of its severity. This is particularly true when there is a *metabolic* disturbance. However, patients with *respiratory* disturbances are much more likely to require full assessment of acid–base status, both for their definition and for monitoring and controlling their treatment.

Anion gap (AG) (reference range, 10–20 mmol/L)

This term describes a calculation frequently performed by those laboratories that still measure plasma [chloride]. It serves as a pointer to the presence of certain types of acid–base disturbance, especially a metabolic acidosis. The anion gap (or *ion difference*) derives from plasma electrolyte results, as follows:

$$AG = ([Na^+] + [K^+]) - ([Cl^-] + [\text{total } CO_2])$$

The difference between the cations and the anions represents the unmeasured anions or anion gap. It includes proteins, phosphate, sulphate and lactate ions. The anion gap may be increased because of an increase in unmeasured anions or, less often, a decrease in unmeasured cations (Table 5.6). A reduction in the anion gap occurs much less frequently, and can usually be traced to laboratory error.

Table 5.6 Causes of an increased anion gap

Mechanism	Examples
Plasma [unmeasured anions] increased with or without changes in $[Na^+]$ and $[Cl^-]$	Metabolic acidosis: Uraemic acidosis, lactic acidosis, diabetic ketoacidosis, salicylate toxicity, methanol toxicity, ethylene glycol toxicity, paraldehyde toxicity
Increase in plasma $[Na^+]$	Treatment with sodium salts, e.g. salts of some high-dose antibiotics such as carbenicillin; this increases plasma [unmeasured anions]
Artefact	Improper handling of specimens after collection, causing loss of CO_2

The main value of the anion gap is that it draws the attention of the clinician, on the basis of these plasma electrolyte measurements, to the possibility that there is present in plasma a significant amount of an analyte that is much less frequently measured, such as lactate or a drug metabolite.

Plasma chloride (reference range, 95–107 mmol/L)

The causes of metabolic acidosis are sometimes divided into those with an increased anion gap (Table 5.6) and those with a normal anion gap. In the latter group, the fall in plasma [total CO_2], which accompanies the metabolic acidosis, is associated with an approximately equal rise in plasma $[Cl^-]$. Patients with a metabolic acidosis and a normal anion gap are sometimes described as having a *hyperchloraemic acidosis*. Chronic renal failure is the commonest cause of hyperchloraemic acidosis.

Increased plasma $[Cl^-]$, out of proportion to any accompanying increase in plasma $[Na^+]$, may occur in patients with chronic renal failure, ureteric transplants into the colon or renal tubular acidosis, or in patients treated with carbonic anhydrase inhibitors. Increased plasma $[Cl^-]$ may also occur in patients who develop respiratory alkalosis as a result of prolonged assisted ventilation. An iatrogenic cause of increased plasma $[Cl^-]$ is the intravenous administration of excessive amounts of isotonic or 'physiological' saline, which contains 150 mmol/L NaCl.

Decreased plasma $[Cl^-]$. The chloride content of gastric juice is normally approximately 150 mmol/L. Patients who lose large volumes of gastric secretion (e.g. due to pyloric stenosis) often show a disproportionately marked fall in plasma $[Cl^-]$ compared with any hyponatraemia that may develop. They develop a metabolic alkalosis, and are often dehydrated.

Oxygen transport

The full characterization of the oxygen composition of a blood sample requires measurement of Po_2, haemoglobin (Hb) concentration and per cent oxygen saturation.

Measurements of Po_2 in arterial blood (reference range, 12–15 kPa) are important, especially at levels of Po_2 above 10.5 kPa. The results are often valuable in assessing the efficiency of oxygen therapy, when high Po_2 values may be found. Above a Po_2 of 10.5 kPa, however, Hb is almost fully saturated with oxygen (Fig. 5.1) so the per cent oxygen saturation is not often required at high Po_2 levels. On the other hand, results of Po_2 measurements may be misleading in conditions where the oxygen-carrying capacity of blood is grossly impaired, as in severe anaemia, carbon monoxide poisoning and when abnormal Hb derivatives (e.g. methaemoglobin) are present. Measurement of both the blood [Hb] and the per cent oxygen saturation are required in addition to Po_2 under these circumstances.

Haemoglobin measurements are widely available and Po_2 is one of the measurements automatically performed by most blood gas analysers as part of the full acid–base assessment of patients. Per cent oxygen saturation is much less frequently measured.

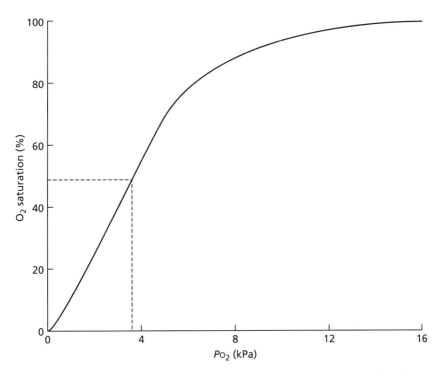

Fig. 5.1 The oxygen-dissociation curve of haemoglobin. It is important to note that, above a Po_2 of approximately 9 kPa, haemoglobin is over 95% saturated with O_2. Also shown in the figure is the value of the Po_2, 3.8 kPa, that corresponds to 50% saturation with O_2; this value is called the P_{50}.

Indications for full blood acid–base and oxygen measurements

The main indications for full acid–base assessment, coupled with Po_2 or per cent oxygen saturation measurements, are in the investigation and management of patients with pulmonary disorders, severely ill patients in intensive care units, and patients in the operative and peri-operative periods of major surgery who may often be on assisted ventilation. Other important applications include the investigation and management of patients with vascular abnormalities involving the shunting of blood.

Full acid–base assessment is much less often needed in patients with metabolic acidosis or alkalosis, for whom measurements of plasma [total CO_2] on venous blood usually give sufficient information. Full assessments are not often needed in patients with respiratory alkalosis, except for patients on assisted ventilation.

Respiratory insufficiency

This term is applied to two types of disorder in which lung function is impaired sufficiently to cause the Po_2 to become abnormally low, usually less than 8.0 kPa.

Type I: low Po_2 with normal or low Pco_2

Hypoxia without hypercapnia occurs in patients in whom there is a preponderance of alveoli that are adequately perfused with blood, but inadequately ventilated. It occurs, for example, in emphysema, pulmonary oedema, asthma or obesity; type II respiratory insufficiency can also occur in some of these conditions.

In type I respiratory insufficiency there is, in effect, a partial right-to-left 'shunt' bringing unoxygenated blood to the left side of the heart. Increased ventilation of the adequately perfused and ventilated alveoli is able to compensate for the tendency for the Pco_2 to rise. It cannot, however, restore the Po_2 to normal, since

---

Case 5.2

The junior doctor first on call for the accident and emergency (A & E) department examined a 22-year-old man who was having an acute attack of asthma. The patient was very distressed so the doctor treated him with nebulized terbutaline (10 mg) immediately and returned 10 minutes later to examine him when he was more settled and was breathing air. He decided to check the patient's arterial blood gases, the results of which were:

Analysis	Result	Reference range	Units
[H$^+$]	44	36–44	nmol/L
Pco_2	6.0	4.4–6.1	kPa
[HCO$_3^-$]	27.0	21.0–27.5	mmol/L
Po_2	10.2	12–15	kPa

The doctor asked the A & E consultant whether he could send the patient home. Would you consider that these results suggested that it would be safe to do so? This patient is discussed on p. 70.

the blood perfusing the normal alveoli conveys haemoglobin that is already nearly saturated with oxygen.

Type II: low P_{O_2} with high P_{CO_2}

This combination means that there is hypoventilation. The cause may be central in origin, or due to airways obstruction, or it may be neuromuscular. There may be altered ventilation/perfusion relationships, with an excessive number of alveoli being inadequately perfused; this causes 'wasted' ventilation and an increase in 'dead space'.

Chronic obstructive airways disease is an important cause of type II respiratory insufficiency. It also occurs with mechanical defects in ventilation (e.g. chest injuries, myasthenia gravis, polyneuritis). In status asthmaticus, if serial measurements show a rising P_{CO_2} and falling P_{O_2}, more intensive treatment is urgently needed.

Treatment of acid–base disturbances

The reliability of acid–base measurements and their value in the management of patients are critically dependent on the collection of satisfactory specimens and their proper subsequent handling, i.e. immediate presentation for analysis, or else immediate cooling in iced water if there is to be any delay before analysis. Also, the data *must* be interpreted in relation to clinical information, if they are to help provide a rational basis for treatment.

Having defined the nature of an acid–base disturbance, treatment should aim to correct the primary disorder and to assist the physiological compensatory mechanisms. In some cases, more active intervention may be necessary (e.g. treatment with $NaHCO_3$). It is often possible to correct an acid–base disturbance

---

Case 5.3

A 75-year-old widow, a known heavy smoker and chronic bronchitic, and a patient in a long-stay hospital, became very breathless and wheezy. The senior nurse called the doctor who was on duty but he was unable to come at once because he was treating another emergency. He asked the nurse to start the patient on 24% oxygen. One hour later, when the doctor arrived, he examined the patient and took an arterial specimen to determine her blood gases. The results were as follows:

Analysis	Result	Reference range	Units
$[H^+]$	97	36–44	nmol/L
P_{CO_2}	21.8	4.4–6.1	kPa
$[HCO_3^-]$	42	21.0–27.5	mmol/L
P_{O_2}	22.5	12–15	kPa

How would you describe this patient's acid–base status? Do you think that she was breathing 24% oxygen? This patient is discussed on p. 70.

by treatment aimed only at the causative condition (e.g. diabetic ketoacidosis is usually corrected without the administration of $NaHCO_3$). Where active treatment of the acid–base disturbance is necessary, this is usually needed for metabolic disturbances.

In *metabolic acidosis*, treatment with HCO_3^- is usually not indicated unless $[H^+]$ is very high (i.e. over 90 nmol/L), except for patients with proximal renal tubular acidosis, who lose HCO_3^- because of the primary defect.

In *metabolic alkalosis* many patients have lost Cl^-, either in the urine or from the stomach. The kidney responds by retaining HCO_3^- and it is necessary to provide Cl^- as part of the active treatment of the alkalosis; otherwise, the kidney continues to retain HCO_3^-. The majority of patients with metabolic alkalosis respond to administration of isotonic saline (150 mmol/L NaCl), but there are some who do not respond. These patients have mineralocorticoid excess, due to primary adrenal hyperfunction or to those causes of secondary adrenal hyperfunction that are not due to hypovolaemia and ECF depletion. These latter include renal artery stenosis, magnesium deficiency and Bartter's syndrome; treatment of these must in each case be directed at the primary disorder.

Comments on Case 5.1 (p. 64)

The patient had a metabolic alkalosis. This was caused by his persistent vomiting, the vomit being likely to consist almost entirely of gastric contents. In this age-group, the cause could be carcinoma of the stomach or chronic peptic ulceration with associated fibrosis, leading to obstruction of gastric outflow.

Gastric juice $[K^+]$ is about 10 mmol/L. Also, in the presence of an alkalosis, K^+ shifts from the ECF into cells. Furthermore, dehydration causes secondary hyperaldosteronism in order to maintain ECF volume, and Na^+ is avidly retained by the kidneys in exchange for H^+ and K^+. Patients such as this man, despite having an alkalosis and despite being hypokalaemic, often excrete an acid urine containing large amounts of K^+.

Comments on Case 5.2 (p. 68)

It would not be safe to send this patient home. In a moderately severe asthmatic attack, the ventilatory drive from hypoxia and from mechanical receptors in the chest normally results in a P_{CO_2} at or below the lower end of the reference range. A P_{CO_2} greater than this is a serious prognostic sign, indicative either of extensive 'shunting' of blood through areas of the lung that are underventilated because of bronchoconstriction or plugging with mucus, or of the patient becoming increasingly tired. A rising P_{CO_2} in an asthmatic attack is an indication for ventilating these patients.

Comments on Case 5.3 (p. 69)

This patient had a respiratory acidosis. Although she gave a long history of chest complaints, the history of the recent illness was short and it was most unlikely that renal compensation could have accounted in that short time for the very high arterial plasma $[HCO_3^-]$.

From the arterial P_{O_2} result, it was apparent that the patient was breathing a much higher concentration of oxygen than 24%. Atmospheric pressure is approximately 100 kPa, and the P_{O_2} of inspired air (in kPa) is numerically equal, approximately, to the percentage of oxygen inspired. Further, it is approximately true that:

Inspired P_{O_2} = alveolar P_{O_2} + alveolar P_{CO_2}

Since alveolar P_{CO_2} equals arterial P_{CO_2}, this equation can be rewritten as:

Alveolar P_{O_2} = inspired P_{O_2} – arterial P_{CO_2}

It was thus possible to conclude that the patient must have been breathing oxygen at a concentration of at least 40%. On checking, it was found that the wrong mask had been fitted, and that oxygen was being delivered at 60%.

It was concluded that the patient had an underlying chronic (compensated) respiratory acidosis with carbon dioxide retention (type II respiratory failure), and that the administration of oxygen had removed the hypoxic drive to ventilation, thereby superimposing an acute respiratory acidosis on the underlying chronic acid–base disturbance.

Chapter 6
Plasma Enzyme Tests in Diagnosis

Most of the enzyme tests required for diagnostic purposes determine activities of enzymes released into plasma as a result of cell death or damage caused by normal 'wear and tear' or by disease. In general, these enzymes have no known function in blood. The activities of most enzymes normally detectable in plasma remain fairly constant in health, although some may show temporary increases after severe muscular exercise (e.g. creatine kinase), or after a meal (e.g. intestinal isoenzyme of alkaline phosphatase).

The observed activities are governed by the *rate of release* of enzymes from cells, their *volume of distribution* in the ECF, and their *rates of removal* from plasma, by catabolism or excretion. Purely analytical factors, such as the presence in plasma of inhibitors or activators of enzyme activity, may also be relevant. Changes in plasma enzyme activity can nearly always be attributed to increases in the *rate of release* of enzymes into the circulation. *Increased release is most commonly caused by*:

1 *Necrosis or severe damage to cells.* This is usually caused by ischaemia or by toxic substances. The enzymes released are principally those present in the cytoplasm.

2 *Increased rate of cell turnover.* This occurs normally during periods of active growth (e.g. alkaline phosphatase in the first year of life, and at puberty), or tissue repair (e.g. alkaline phosphatase in patients recovering from multiple fractures), or in association with several forms of malignant disease.

3 *Increased concentrations of enzymes within cells.* Synthesis of some enzymes is *induced* by disease or drugs, e.g. gamma-glutamyl transferase (GGT) synthesis in the liver is induced by ethanol.

4 *Duct obstruction.* Enzymes normally present in exocrine secretions (e.g. amylase) may be regurgitated into the blood, if the normal route of outflow is obstructed.

There is considerable variation in the rate of removal of enzymes from the circulation, mainly by uptake into the cells of the lymphoreticular system but partly by excretion in the urine. The plasma half-lives of enzymes most often measured for diagnostic purposes vary from about 10 hours to more than 5 days.

Selecting plasma enzyme tests

Organ damage releases increased amounts of many enzymes into the bloodstream. *The most important diagnostic questions are*:

1 *Has tissue damage occurred and, if so, what is its extent?* This will determine the *sensitivity* of the test which will largely depend on the tissue : plasma ratio of enzyme activity (Table 6.1).

2 *Which tissues have been damaged?* This is often a major problem since most enzymes are widely distributed and may be released following damage to several different organs, leading to *lack of specificity*. This may be overcome, at least in part, either by measuring more than one enzyme or by isoenzyme measurements.

3 *How does plasma enzyme activity change during the course of the disease?* The interpretation of enzyme activities depends on the stage of the disease when the sample was taken, e.g. after a myocardial infarction (p. 82).

Enzyme units

Plasma enzyme measurements are usually made in terms of *activity*, since these determinations are relatively easy to perform and are sensitive. In a few instances, enzyme *concentrations* are now measured, by immunoassay. Enzyme concentrations and activities are usually proportional to one another, but catalytic activity is sometimes lost before loss of immunoreactivity.

Catalytic activity is measured in terms of reaction rates. The *international unit (IU) of enzyme activity* is defined as 'that amount of enzyme which, under given assay conditions, will catalyse the conversion of 1 μmol of substrate per minute'. Although international units were introduced in order to achieve a greater degree of standardization of enzyme measurements between laboratories, the numerical values of results are still liable to variation, depending on the *nature and concentration of substrate, reaction temperature, pH, type of buffer*, nature and concentration of co-factors, etc.

International recommendations specifying these various conditions have been made for several of the commonly performed enzyme activity measurements, but it will still be several years before most laboratories adopt these recommendations in full. Meanwhile, reference ranges for plasma enzyme activity measurements and results for the related analyses continue, in many cases, to show considerable differences between laboratories. Therefore, for simplicity, we have adopted a pragmatic approach and usually express enzyme activity (and concentration) as the ratio between the result observed and the upper reference value for the method of measurement.

Table 6.1 Tissue : plasma ratios of activities of four frequently measured enzymes (the activity of each enzyme in plasma is taken as unity)

Tissue	AST	ALT	LD	CK
Heart	8 000	400	1 000	10 000
Liver	7 000	3 000	1 500	< 10
Skeletal muscle	5 000	300	700	50 000
Erythrocytes	15	7	300	< 1

ALT, alanine aminotransferase; AST, aspartate aminotransferase; CK, creatine kinase; LD, lactate dehydrogenase.

Examples of clinically important plasma enzymes

Several commonly measured enzymes will be described here, and the subject of isoenzymes (and isoforms) introduced. Detailed consideration of specific clinical applications for these tests will mostly be deferred until later chapters.

Isoenzymes are proteins that possess similar catalytic activity, but which show genetically determined differences in their structure and in certain other properties (e.g. electrophoretic mobility, stability to heat). When an enzyme is released from damaged tissue, the isoenzyme pattern of the organ may be reflected by a corresponding change in the pattern detectable in plasma. Isoenzyme studies may thus help to localize the tissue of origin of an increased plasma enzyme activity.

Lactate dehydrogenase (LD)

Human tissues contain five major proteins, all designated lactate dehydrogenase; an additional, minor, LD isoenzyme is present in testes.

Each of the major LD isoenzymes (M_r, 135 kDa) is a tetramer consisting of four polypeptide chains; each chain may be one of two types, H or M. Combinations of these two types of subunit give rise to its five major isoenzymes; these have subunit structures H_4, H_3M, H_2M_2, HM_3 and M_4. These can be distinguished on the basis of their electrophoretic mobilities; the isoenzyme that migrates most rapidly towards the anode (H_4) is termed LD_1, and the slowest moving isoenzyme (M_4) is called LD_5. Isoenzyme patterns of LD within various tissues fall into three main groups:

1 Predominant LD_1 and LD_2 (anodal isoenzymes), as in heart and red cells.
2 Predominant LD_5 and LD_4 (cathodal isoenzymes), as in liver and some skeletal muscles.
3 No one isoenzyme component of LD predominates, as in lung and spleen.

Total LD activity (i.e. the combined activity of the five isoenzymes of LD) is often measured and may be increased in patients with myocardial infarction, hepatocellular damage, haemolytic anaemia, skeletal muscle disease, various malignant diseases, etc. In addition, LD isoenzyme studies are frequently performed. All five isoenzymes can normally be detected in serum, although LD_1 and LD_2 are normally present in considerably larger amounts than LD_3 and usually there are only small amounts of LD_4 and LD_5 (Fig. 6.1).

Isoenzymes of LD differ in their biological, chemical and physical properties and show a gradation of these properties, with LD_1 and LD_5 representing the extremes (e.g. the half-life of LD_1 in plasma is about 100 hours and the half-life of LD_5 is about 10 hours). Some of the biochemical and physical differences between the isoenzymes may be used as the basis for methods to distinguish LD isoenzymes (Table 6.2).

Isoenzyme studies of LD are most often used in the investigation of myocardial infarction (discussed later, p. 82) in which LD_1 and LD_2 are raised and the normal $LD_1 : LD_2$ ratio of less than 1.0 is reversed (sometimes called a 'flipped' LD isoenzyme ratio). Since LD_1 and LD_2, however measured, are raised most commonly in plasma from patients with myocardial damage, they are often called 'heart-specific LD'. However, this term is a misnomer and can be misleading, as

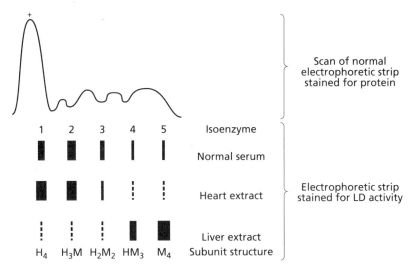

Fig. 6.1 Approximate relative proportions of the five principal LD isoenzymes in normal serum and in extracts of heart and liver tissue, after electrophoretic separation on cellulose acetate. Also shown is the corresponding normal densitometric scan of the serum proteins, following their separation and staining. The direction of flow of the electric current is from right to left, with the anodal isoenzymes of LD moving most rapidly towards the anode (+). Reading from left to right, the peaks in the serum pattern correspond, respectively, to albumin, α_1-globulin, α_2-globulin, β-globulin and γ-globulin. The serum was applied to the cellulose acetate at a point corresponding to the trough between the β-globulin and γ-globulin peaks. Thus, LD_4 stays at or very close to the origin, and LD_5 migrates towards the cathode.

Table 6.2 Examples of differences between the isoenzymes of lactate dehydrogenase

Methods used to differentiate isoenzymes	LD_1 (H_4)	LD_5 (M_4)	Measurement's name*
Physical methods			
Electrophoretic mobility	α_1-Globulin region	γ-Globulin region	Individual activities of LD_1–LD_5 isoenzymes
Heat at 60°C for 30 min before assay	Unaffected	Destroyed	**Heat-stable LD activity**
Selective inhibitors			
(a) Urea (2.0 mol/L)	Slight inhibition	Complete inhibition	**Urea-stable LD activity**
(b) Anti-M subunit antibody	No effect	Complete inhibition	LD-H activity
Selective substrate			
2-Oxobutyrate substrate instead of lactate	High activity relatively	Low activity relatively	**'Hydroxybutyrate dehydrogenase'**

* 'Heart-specific' LD isoenzyme measurements widely performed routinely are in bold.

such rises may also be due to release from other tissues, especially from red or white blood cells or blood cell precursors. This may occur either *in vivo* (megaloblastic and haemolytic anaemia, leukaemia) or *in vitro* due to lack of care in the collection, transport or storage of blood specimens, leading to haemolysis.

Creatine kinase (CK)

There are three principal CK isoenzymes, each composed of two polypeptide chains, denoted B and M; these give the dimers BB, MB and MM. Skeletal muscle has a very high total CK content; over 98% of this is normally CK-MM, the rest being CK-MB. Cardiac muscle also has a high CK content consisting of 70–80% CK-MM and 20–30% CK-MB. In most other tissues which contain CK (e.g. brain, thyroid), the BB isoenzyme predominates.

The most important point to note about the distribution of CK isoenzymes is that the myocardium is normally the only tissue which contains more than about 5% CK-MB. There are occasional exceptions to this. For example, in patients with muscle disease, the proportion of CK-MB in skeletal muscles may rise to 5–15%. Also, in athletes in training, skeletal muscle CK-MB rises slightly.

Immunological and electrophoretic methods can be used to quantitate the CK isoenzymes. Normally, 95% or more of plasma CK activity is due to CK-MM and less than 5% to CK-MB; CK-BB is normally undetectable in plasma.

Total plasma CK activity is frequently measured in patients who are suspected of having had a myocardial infarction (p. 82), and in patients with diseases of the skeletal muscles. Very large increases occur in muscle disease (see below). Increases are more variable, but may sometimes be large, after accidental trauma, surgical operations or even intramuscular injections, in comatose patients, diabetic ketoacidosis, acute renal failure and hypothyroidism. Increased plasma total CK activity is also found after prolonged muscular exercise, especially in unfit individuals.

Raised plasma CK-BB activity is unusual. It may occur in patients with carcinoma, especially of the prostate, and after acute brain damage. The measurement has not been found to be of much diagnostic value.

Creatine kinase isoforms

After the release of CK into plasma, a carboxypeptidase normally present in plasma splits the terminal lysine residue off the CK-M polypeptide chains without affecting enzyme activity. However, their charge is changed as a result of the loss of lysine residues and, hence, their electrophoretic mobility is altered.

In the case of CK-MM, the enzyme which is released from tissue contains two intact polypeptide chains and is termed CK-MM3. The removal of lysine from one of the chains causes the formation of CK-MM2 (a hybrid) and the subsequent removal of lysine from the other chain leads to the formation of CK-MM1. The different forms produced in this way are called *isoforms* of CK-MM. Generally, the presence of different isoforms in plasma is of no diagnostic significance, as the subtle differences in structure are usually difficult to detect. However, it has been suggested that increases in the CK-MM3 : CK-MM1 ratio, which occur very soon after myocardial infarction, may be of diagnostic value (p. 82).

Creatine kinase and muscle disease

Several plasma enzyme activities can be measured in order to detect muscle damage. However, plasma total CK is usually the measurement of choice, irrespective of the aetiology of the disorder; it is increased in the greatest number of cases and shows the largest changes. Plasma AST, LD and ALT activities may be increased also. The enzyme tests will be considered under several disease categories:

1 *Muscular dystrophy.* This group of disorders includes the Duchenne, limb girdle and facioscapulohumeral types. Duchenne dystrophy is usually transmitted as a sex-linked recessive disorder and predominantly affects males. High levels of plasma CK activity are present from birth, before the onset of clinical signs. During the early clinical stages of the disease, very high activities are usually present, but these tend to fall as the terminal stages of the disease are reached.

About 75% of female carriers of the Duchenne dystrophy gene have raised plasma CK activities, but the increases are usually relatively small. The incidence of raised activities in more benign forms of muscular dystrophy is about 70%; the increases tend to be much smaller than in the Duchenne type.

2 *Malignant hyperpyrexia.* This is a rare but serious disorder characterized by raised body temperature, convulsions and shock following general anaesthesia. Many of the patients show evidence of myopathy. Extremely high plasma CK activities are seen in the acute, post-anaesthetic stage, but smaller increases often persist and can also be detected in relatives of affected patients.

Measurements of plasma CK activity pre-operatively are not a reliable way of detecting patients liable to develop malignant hyperpyrexia, even if such screening were practicable logistically. Pre-operative screening for susceptibility to malignant hyperpyrexia should be limited to those patients with a family history of anaesthetic deaths or of malignant hyperpyrexia.

3 *Other myopathies and myotonias.* There is a large group of rare, genetically determined myopathies and myotonias. Plasma CK activity is raised in most of these and in patients with alcoholic myopathy.

4 *Polymyositis.* This may be due to infective agents or collagen disease or other less well-defined causes. Plasma CK activity is often raised, the amount of the increase reflecting the activity of the disease.

5 *Neurogenic muscle disease.* Plasma CK activity is usually normal in peripheral neuritis, poliomyelitis and motor neurone disease.

The aminotransferases

Aspartate aminotransferase (AST), previously known as glutamic oxaloacetic transaminase (GOT), is present in most tissues, but especially in skeletal and cardiac muscle, liver and kidney (Table 6.1). There are two major isoenzymes of AST, one cytoplasmic and the other mitochondrial. Both have been demonstrated in plasma following tissue damage, but their differentiation has not been shown to be of much diagnostic value. On the other hand, total AST activity is one of the most widely and frequently performed plasma enzyme activity measurements. Its principal applications are in the investigation of patients with suspected myocardial infarction (p. 82) and liver disease (p. 114).

Alanine aminotransferase (ALT), previously called glutamic pyruvic transaminase (GPT), is also widely distributed. Its concentration in most tissues is considerably less than AST, but in liver the activities of the two enzymes are of the same order of magnitude (Table 6.1). ALT activity is most often measured as one of a group of 'liver function tests', as a measure of hepatocellular damage (p. 107); it is more liver-specific than AST (Table 6.1).

The rises of both AST and ALT when there is hepatocellular damage, such as in infectious hepatitis, are often of the same order of magnitude although some forms of liver disease tend to affect one enzyme more than the other (p. 115). Small increases in plasma ALT activity occur in uncomplicated myocardial infarction; larger increases may occur when there is cardiac failure, presumably as a result of hepatic venous congestion.

Both AST and ALT are widely distributed, and increased plasma activity of both enzymes may be observed in many other conditions associated with tissue injury such as acute pancreatitis, acute renal disease, muscle disease and disseminated carcinoma. These findings are not specific enough to be much help in diagnosis.

Alkaline phosphatase

This is the generic name for a group of enzymes that display maximum activity in the pH range 9.0–10.5. They are widely distributed, different tissues possessing one (occasionally more) characteristic and analytically distinguishable form. Liver, bone, placenta and intestine are clinically important sources of plasma alkaline phosphatase activity.

It is possible to determine the tissue of origin of increased alkaline phosphatase activity in serum by electrophoresis. Simpler methods of differentiation, for example using inhibitors or heat-stability, have been described and are occasionally used in routine laboratories. However, the most important clinical distinction, between the liver and bone forms, is still most often made by electrophoretic methods.

The precise biochemical role of alkaline phosphatase is not known. In many tissues it is attached to cell membranes, suggesting an association between alkaline phosphatase activity and membrane transport. In the liver, for example, activity is localized on the cell membrane that adjoins the biliary canaliculus and on the sinusoidal border of the parenchymal cell. Although alkaline phosphatase is present in bile, this has not come from the plasma but has rather been produced in the liver, by cells lining the biliary canaliculi. Alkaline phosphatase is removed from plasma by cells of the lymphoreticular system, like other intracellular enzymes released into the circulation.

Physiological changes in activity

Plasma alkaline phosphatase activity may be significantly increased (compared with adult reference values) for entirely physiological reasons. It is important to consider these possibilities before regarding as pathological what at first sight might seem to be an abnormal result. They are:

1 *Normal pregnancy.* Release of alkaline phosphatase from the placenta may

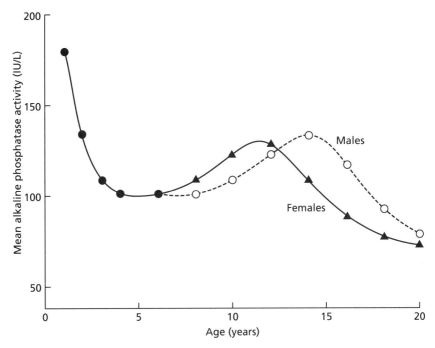

Fig. 6.2 The data presented illustrate the considerable variation in *mean* plasma alkaline phosphatase activity with age and sex that is normally found in healthy individuals between 1 and 20 years old. The reference ranges at each age are wide, and are subject to considerable variation depending on the analytical method used, but the overall pattern of variation in activity with age remains the same no matter what method is used. With the method used here, the combined reference range for adults (both sexes) is 40–125 IU/L (mean value 80 IU/L). Reference ranges for plasma alkaline phosphatase activity in neonates, infants and childhood are given in Table 21.1 (p. 322).

cause its total activity in plasma to rise in the second and third trimesters to about twice the normal adult levels.

2 *Infancy and childhood.* The upper reference value is as much as three or four times the adult value (Fig. 6.2). This increase is a direct result of the intensive osteoblastic activity associated with normal bone growth (e.g. at puberty) since osteoblasts secrete alkaline phosphatase.

3 *Meals containing fat.* These may cause transient small increases in plasma intestinal alkaline phosphatase activity. Blood for alkaline phosphatase measurements should preferably be collected from patients who have not eaten recently.

Changes in activity due to disease

Alkaline phosphatase activity is one of the most frequently requested plasma enzyme measurements. Its principal uses are in the investigation of patients with liver and bone disease. Most laboratories include alkaline phosphatase in their standard grouping of 'liver function tests' (p. 107); its activity is often greatly increased whenever there is cholestasis, but hepatocellular damage causes relatively little increase.

In bone disease, plasma alkaline phosphatase activity is raised when there is increased osteoblastic activity, as in Paget's disease, hyperparathyroidism, rickets and osteomalacia (Chapter 13). The uses of these measurements as a tumour marker are discussed on p. 102.

Gamma-glutamyl transferase (GGT)

This enzyme, sometimes called gamma-glutamyl transpeptidase, is found mainly in kidney, liver, biliary tract and pancreas. The kidney contains by far the largest amount of GGT of any of these tissues. However, renal GGT is not released into plasma and is of little diagnostic importance. Much of the GGT activity in liver, as with alkaline phosphatase, is associated with the cell membrane adjoining the biliary canaliculus.

In liver disease, plasma GGT activity generally increases in parallel with alkaline phosphatase, i.e. it rises most when there is cholestasis. However, it tends to be raised more than alkaline phosphatase in other disorders affecting the liver, such as hepatocellular damage. Hepatic synthesis of the enzyme is also induced by alcohol and by several drugs (e.g. the anti-epileptics) thereby causing plasma GGT to rise. Its activity is not raised in bone disease so plasma GGT measurements can help to identify the tissue of origin of a raised plasma alkaline phosphatase activity; the activity of both enzymes is increased if there is hepatic disease.

Plasma GGT activity is sometimes increased after myocardial infarction, and occasionally in other diseases that do not primarily involve the liver, biliary tract or pancreas. In all these cases, the increased GGT activity can usually be attributed to secondary hepatic involvement, e.g. due to venous congestion.

Acid phosphatase

The prostate contains high concentrations of acid phosphatase. Non-prostatic tissues (e.g. liver, spleen, red cells, platelets) contain relatively small amounts of other acid phosphatases. The prostatic and non-prostatic isoenzymes can be differentiated by using a substrate that is preferentially hydrolysed by one of the isoenzymes, or by measuring activity in the presence of a selective inhibitor (e.g. L(+)-tartrate) or by specific immunoassay procedures.

The prostatic isoenzyme is the component of principal diagnostic interest. Acid phosphatase measurements are used mainly for the diagnosis of metastatic or invasive prostatic carcinoma, and for monitoring the course of the disease and its response to treatment (p. 101).

Increased plasma acid phosphatase activity occurs in several other disorders. A tartrate-stable (i.e. non-prostatic) isoenzyme is often increased in patients with bone disease, especially Paget's disease, but also in patients with hyperparathyroidism and metastatic breast carcinoma. Plasma total acid phosphatase may be increased in liver disease and Gaucher's disease, and in thrombocytopenia (due to an increased rate of platelet lysis).

α-Amylase (amylase)

Large amounts of amylase are present in the pancreas and salivary glands, and smaller amounts in other tissues. Salivary and pancreatic isoenzymes (both have

M_r, 45 kDa) are partially filtered from plasma at the glomerulus. These iso-enzymes can be differentiated by immunological or electrophoretic methods, or by using an inhibitor (a wheat protein) that preferentially inhibits non-pancreatic isoenzymes of amylase.

Plasma amylase measurements are mostly used to help distinguish acute pancreatitis, in which surgery is not indicated, from other acute abdominal disorders many of which require immediate operation. Although plasma amylase activity is nearly always greatly increased in acute pancreatitis, it is also often considerably raised in other acute intra-abdominal conditions (p. 149). However, in general, the magnitude of the rise is greatest in acute pancreatitis.

Cholinesterase (ChE)

There are two principal ChE: (i) the enzyme which is synthesized in the liver and which is present in plasma (formerly known as pseudocholinesterase); and (ii) acetyl cholinesterase, which is present at nerve endings and in the erythrocytes, but not in plasma (formerly known as 'true' cholinesterase).

Plasma ChE is of particular value in the diagnosis of patients with scoline apnoea and organophosphorus insecticide poisoning (p. 375), but changes also occur in other conditions (Table 6.3).

Scoline apnoea

Some patients exhibit prolonged apnoea, lasting several hours, after succinyl dicholine (scoline) administration. This drug is normally hydrolysed by plasma ChE. Over 50% of patients sensitive to scoline have genetically determined abnormalities in the ChE enzyme protein. At least four allelic genes are involved: E_1^u codes for the usual form of ChE, present in over 95% of the UK population. E_1^a codes for an atypical ChE that is resistant to inhibition by dibucaine. E_1^f codes for an atypical ChE that is resistant to inhibition by fluoride. E_1^s codes for a protein that has little or no ChE activity.

Most individuals with abnormal variants have low plasma ChE activity, but the only reliable way of demonstrating the variants is by means of inhibitor studies. The abnormal enzymes are less affected by some inhibitors than is the normal enzyme. Dibucaine and fluoride are the two most widely used inhibitors.

Plasma ChE activity is measured in the absence of inhibitor and again in the

Table 6.3 Causes of low plasma cholinesterase activity

Category of cause	Examples
Physiological reasons	Infancy, third trimester of pregnancy
Inherited abnormality	Scoline sensitivity (ChE variants)
Acquired abnormality	
(a) Liver disease	Whenever synthesis of the plasma proteins impaired due to hepatocellular dysfunction
(b) Industrial poisoning	Organophosphorus insecticides (p. 375)
(c) Drug effects	Oral contraceptives, monoamine oxidase inhibitors, cytotoxic drugs

presence of (i) dibucaine and (ii) fluoride. For example, individuals who possess the $E_1^a E_1^a$ genotype, which shows great sensitivity to scoline, are usually found to have low plasma ChE activity, but this low activity is only inhibited to a small extent by dibucaine (8–28%) and by fluoride (10–28%). This contrasts with the $E_1^u E_1^u$ genotype, which is not sensitive to scoline, and which has normal plasma ChE activity, that is, however, strongly inhibited by dibucaine (77–83%) and by fluoride (50–68%). The percentage inhibition values are known as *dibucaine numbers* and *fluoride numbers*, respectively.

Detection of individuals liable to scoline apnoea and identification of heterozygotes are important. Affected relatives can then be traced, and anaesthetists warned not to use certain muscle relaxants, especially scoline.

Plasma enzyme tests in myocardial infarction

Activities of many enzymes may become raised in plasma after an infarct, but only four enzyme tests are used with any frequency. These are CK, the MB isoenzyme of CK (CK-MB), AST and LD. Total LD activity is not used much because it is not tissue-specific, but measurement of its anodal isoenzymes (LD_1 and LD_2), which are more cardio-specific, is more common, using either electrophoresis or simpler tests such as heat-stable LD (Table 6.2, p. 75). It should be remembered that the anodal LD isoenzymes are not truly heart-specific since they also occur, for example, in red cells and red cell precursors.

Time-course of enzyme changes

After a myocardial infarction, the time-course of plasma enzyme changes always follows the same general pattern (Fig. 6.3). After an initial 'lag' phase of at least 3 hours, during which activities remain normal, they rise rapidly to a peak. Activities then return to normal at rates that depend on the half-life of each enzyme in plasma.

The rapid rise and fall of CK-MB activity should be particularly noted and the fact that LD activity remains raised for considerably longer than the other enzymes. It has also been shown that changes in the ratio of CK-MM3, the CK-MM isoform released from tissue (p. 76), to CK-MM1 is the *earliest detectable enzyme change* in plasma; increases in this ratio can usually be detected between 2 and 5 hours after the onset of chest pain. However, the methods for measuring CK-MM isoforms are not straightforward and the place of such measurements in routine diagnosis is not yet clear.

Thrombolytic therapy

In patients treated with thrombolytic agents, the general pattern of plasma enzyme activity changes shown in Fig. 6.3 is slightly modified. Following successful thrombolytic therapy (e.g. with streptokinase), plasma enzyme activities rise rapidly to reach an early peak, at 10–18 hours. This peak is higher than the peak that is usually observed in the absence of thrombolytic therapy; plasma enzyme activities then return to normal at the usual rate. These findings are probably due to 'wash out' of enzymes from the infarcted area immediately after reperfusion occurs. It is possible, using serial CK-MB measurements during and immediately

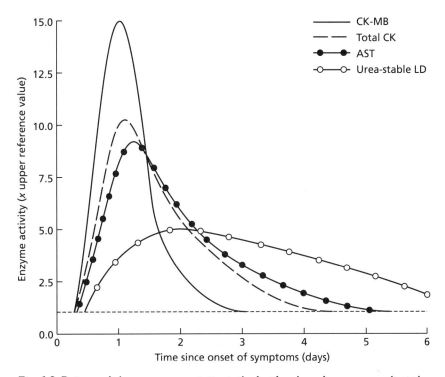

Fig. 6.3 Patterns of plasma enzyme activities in the first few days after an uncomplicated myocardial infarction. The time-relationships of these patterns are liable to modification as a result of treatment with thrombolytic agents, but their inter-relationships are otherwise generally maintained. Urea-stable LD is an example of so-called 'heart-specific' LD. Note the delay of a few hours before any of the activities become abnormal after an infarction.

after thrombolytic therapy, to detect whether or not therapy has been successful from the rate of rise of plasma enzyme activity.

Optimal times for blood sampling

The first priority is to obtain a sample with the optimal chance of being abnormal if indeed infarction has occurred. This should be between 18 and 30 hours after the onset of symptoms for CK and AST measurements (Table 6.4), slightly earlier

Table 6.4 Time-course of plasma enzyme activity changes after myocardial infarction

Enzyme	Abnormal activity detectable (hours)	Peak value of abnormality (hours)	Duration of abnormality (days)
CK-MB isoenzyme	3–10	12–24	1.5–3
Total CK	5–12	18–30	2–5
AST	6–12	20–30	2–6
'Heart-specific' LD	8–16	30–48	5–14

AST, aspartate aminotransferase; CK, creatine kinase; LD, lactate dehydrogenase.

for CK-MB (especially if thrombolytic therapy has been given), and somewhat later for LD. It is also useful to have an earlier sample, taken on admission, to provide a 'baseline'. Except for the occasional patient seen for the first time 2 days or more after the episode, in whom LD measurements might still be useful, it is *very rarely of any value to take samples for plasma enzyme studies after 48 hours from the onset of symptoms that suggest a diagnosis of myocardial infarction.*

Selection of tests

Enzyme activity measurements, especially plasma CK-MB, are very sensitive tests of myocardial damage. Probably over 95% of patients with myocardial infarction show detectable increases in plasma enzyme activity, provided that specimens are taken at the optimal times.

The magnitude of the rise in enzyme activity is strongly correlated with infarct size. Patients with large increases, for example plasma CK activity rising to more than 10 times the upper reference value, have a much poorer prognosis than those with small increases in activity.

Plasma total CK measurements and measures of LD_1 and LD_2 activities are the enzyme tests that are requested most often to help confirm a clinical diagnosis of myocardial infarction. Because these enzymes have different tissue specificities, we consider it advisable to request more than one test as a matter of routine. The pattern of release of AST after myocardial infarction is very similar to that of CK; AST measurements may, therefore, be preferred in place of CK in some laboratories. The specificities of the two enzymes (AST and CK) do differ, however, since AST (but not CK) is released in hepatocellular disease or damage, whereas CK is released from damaged skeletal muscle much more readily than AST.

CK-MB isoenzyme

There is little doubt that CK-MB is the most sensitive and specific test for myocardial damage currently available. However, the test has certain drawbacks which have precluded its general introduction as the 'first-line' test for myocardial infarction in all laboratories. The rise in plasma CK-MB is relatively transient. Also, CK-MB methods are often less reliable or more expensive, or both, than other enzyme tests. In the following circumstances, however, *plasma CK-MB measurements are strongly indicated*:

1 When *very early confirmation* of the diagnosis of myocardial infarction is required, i.e. within 6 hours of the incident.

2 When investigating *post-operative patients* for suspected myocardial infarction. In these patients, plasma CK-MB remains normal in the absence of myocardial damage, whereas AST, total CK and LD activities are often increased in plasma for non-cardiac causes.

3 In patients suspected of having had a *second infarct* within a few days of the first. It is easier to show that a second rise in plasma enzyme activity has occurred if the activity of the enzyme that is being measured rises and falls rapidly after the previous incident involving myocardial damage (Fig. 6.3).

4 When it is suspected that an increased plasma total CK activity may be due to release of the enzyme from skeletal muscle (e.g. after an intramuscular injection).

Trauma and operations

The activities of several enzymes are increased in plasma shortly after major operations, or as a result of severe trauma (e.g. road traffic accident). The changes are similar to those observed after myocardial infarction except that plasma CK-MB activity is not increased.

Enzyme tests and the ECG

In many patients with suspected myocardial infarction it might seem unnecessary to measure plasma enzymes, since the ECG often provides unequivocal evidence of infarction. However, it is possible to misinterpret ECG traces, especially in the presence of arrhythmias, and the ECG is by no means always abnormal in patients who have recently had a myocardial infarction.

Plasma enzyme activity measurements can provide confirmation of the diagnosis of myocardial infarction, independent of the ECG findings. They can also provide information about the size of an infarct and give an indication of prognosis. Therefore, we recommend that plasma enzyme tests, normally CK (or AST) and a method that measures LD_1 and LD_2, should be requested on all patients suspected of having had a myocardial infarction within the previous 48 hours.

Plasma enzyme activity measurements should be treated as complementary to ECG recordings, in the investigation of patients with suspected myocardial infarction. Assuming that the correct combination of enzyme tests has been performed at the appropriate time, and that the ECG was recorded under optimal conditions, the sensitivities and specificities of the two methods of investigation are approximately:

	Sensitivity	Specificity
ECG	70%	100%
Plasma enzymes	95%	90%

By performing both types of investigation correctly, few wrong diagnoses of myocardial infarction should be made.

Chapter 7
Abnormalities of Proteins in Plasma

Plasma proteins are mostly synthesized in the hepatocytes. They form a diverse group of substances that, between them, carry out a wide range of functions. Their principal functions are concerned with:

1 *Maintenance of colloid osmotic pressure*, mainly a function of albumin.
2 *Transport functions, by various carrier proteins* (Table 7.1).
3 *Defence reactions*, a function which depends on:
   (a) *Immunoglobulins*, synthesized in the lymphoreticular system.
   (b) *The complement system.*
4 *Coagulation and fibrinolysis.* This involves some of the proteins circulating in plasma, and others liberated from damaged cells or tissues (e.g. platelets).

We shall not consider the complement system in this book, nor the proteins concerned in coagulation and fibrinolysis (except for prothrombin, p. 113), as their investigation is normally all or mostly carried out in haematology or blood transfusion laboratories.

Some diseases may affect virtually all the plasma proteins, e.g. if there is malnutrition or loss of blood. In other diseases, only certain specific proteins are affected. In this chapter, we shall consider both general disorders of plasma protein metabolism and more specific disorders affecting individual proteins. We shall also discuss proteins that may be released from tumours into plasma and there serve as tumour markers.

Table 7.1 Examples of the transport functions of plasma proteins

Carrier proteins	Carrier functions
Pre-albumin	Retinol (vitamin A), T4 and T3
Albumin	Inorganic constituents of plasma (e.g. calcium) Hormones (e.g. T4 and T3) Excretory products (e.g. unconjugated bilirubin) Drugs and other toxic substances
Hormone-binding proteins	Corticosteroids and thyroid hormones each have their own specific binding proteins
Metal-binding proteins	Copper (by ceruloplasmin); iron (by transferrin)
Lipoproteins	Lipids (transport of essential metabolites)

Methods of investigating plasma proteins

Techniques for measuring the concentrations of proteins in plasma include:

1 *Direct chemical measurement.* The biuret method is one example of methods that measure the total concentration in a specimen, whether there be one protein present or a mixture containing several proteins. Total protein measurements may be carried out on plasma or serum. At best, this is a screening investigation.

2 *Direct physical measurement.* Relatively specific dye-binding methods are available for albumin.

3 *Measurement after separation.* Serum protein electrophoresis separates the proteins into five fractions—albumin, α_1-globulins, α_2-globulins, β-globulins and γ-globulins; each of the globulin fractions consists of a mixture of several proteins (Table 7.2). Serum protein electrophoresis has limited diagnostic value, but

Table 7.2 Examples of plasma proteins commonly measured for the diagnosis and monitoring of disease

Proteins and (in italics) their *electrophoretic mobility*	Principal function(s)	Used in the detection or investigation of disease
Pre-albumin	Unknown (has some transport functions)	Malnutrition, liver disease, effects of trauma
Albumin	Colloid oncotic pressure, transport functions	Diseases of liver, kidney and gastrointestinal tract etc., malignancy, malnutrition
α_1-Globulins		
α_1-Fetoprotein	Unknown	Neural tube defects, also as a tumour marker
α_1-Protease inhibitor (API)	Antiprotease	API deficiency
Prothrombin	Blood clotting	Coagulation screen; also as a 'liver function test'
α_2-Globulins		
Ceruloplasmin	Copper transport	Wilson's disease
Haptoglobin	Haemoglobin binding	Haemolytic disorders
α_2-Macroglobulin	Antiprotease, transport functions	Proteinuria (e.g. selectivity investigations)
Thyroxine-binding globulin	T4 and T3 transport	Thyroid disease
β-Globulins		
C-Reactive protein	Body's defence mechanisms	Non-specific test that may be used instead of the ESR
β_2-Microglobulin	Body's defence mechanisms	Monitoring myeloma, renal failure
Transferrin	Iron transport	Iron deficiency
γ-Globulins		
Immunoglobulins (IgG, IgA, IgM, etc.)	Body's defence mechanisms	Liver disease, infections, auto-immune disease, paraproteinaemias, etc.

another (less widely available) separation technique, isoelectric focusing, is more powerful.

4 *Immunological methods.* These include radioimmunoassay and immunoprecipitation. These are very sensitive and specific methods and can be used to measure individual plasma proteins even when they are present in very low concentration.

5 *Measurements of enzymic activity.* These methods are both sensitive and specific. They provide the basis for clinical enzymology (Chapter 6).

Plasma proteins and disease

A summary of the proteins commonly measured in clinical practice is given in Table 7.2. Most diseases that alter plasma protein concentrations do so by affecting their volume of distribution or their rates of synthesis, catabolism or excretion. In some patients, more than one of these factors may be operating.

Total protein (reference range for plasma, 63–83 g/L)

Many laboratories have stopped measuring plasma or serum [total protein], as a fall in the concentration of one protein or group of proteins may be masked by a coincident or compensatory increase in another, e.g. a fall in plasma [albumin] masked by an increase in plasma [immunoglobulins]. Others continue to perform it as a preliminary to more specific measurements of individual proteins. Causes of changes in plasma [total protein] include:

1 *Increased [total protein].* This may be an artefact due to excessive stasis at the time of venepuncture. *Pathological causes include:*

  (a) *Dehydration.*

  (b) *Increased [Ig]*, which may be monoclonal or polyclonal (p. 96).

2 *Decreased [total protein].* This may be physiological, as in pregnancy when there is increased plasma volume (p. 315), or due to artefact caused by collecting a blood specimen from close to the site of an intravenous infusion. *Pathological causes include:*

  (a) *Impaired synthesis*, as in severe malnutrition, chronic liver disease and in intestinal malabsorptive disease.

  (b) *Excessive loss*, via the kidneys, GI tract or skin.

  (c) *Overhydration*, which is usually iatrogenic.

Albumin (reference range, 36–47 g/L)

Albumin (M_r, 66 kDa) is quantitatively the most important contributor towards maintaining the colloid oncotic pressure of plasma, and hypoalbuminaemia may lead to the development of oedema. Albumin also acts as a non-specific transport vehicle (Table 7.1) for many endogenous and exogenous substances, the latter sometimes displacing endogenous substances from their binding to albumin (e.g. unconjugated bilirubin can be displaced by salicylates or sulphonamides).

Over 20 structural variants of albumin have been described, none of which is associated with disease. Albumin normally appears as a single, fairly discrete band on serum protein electrophoresis. Heterozygotes for some variant albumins may show two bands, usually staining with equal intensity; this condition (bisalbuminaemia) represents the product of two genes.

Hypoalbuminaemia occurs whenever there is increased plasma volume (e.g. in pregnancy). It may also be due to many different *pathological causes*:

1   *Reduced synthesis*, due to liver disease (p. 113), both acute and chronic, although there may be no reduction observed in acute liver disease because of the long half-life of albumin of about 20 days; malnutrition and intestinal malabsorptive disease, if this is severe and prolonged.

2   *Altered distribution*, due to increased capillary permeability, which enables plasma to leak into the extravascular fluid (e.g. severe burns), or to overhydration or to serous effusion (e.g. ascites), when there is sequestration of proteins.

3   *Increased catabolism*, as a result of injury (e.g. major surgery or trauma), infection or malignant disease.

4   *Abnormal losses*. The liver can normally replace albumin losses of up to 5 g/day. Greater losses (which may involve losses of other proteins besides albumin) may occur in:

   (a) *Renal disease*, in the nephrotic syndrome (p. 139).

   (b) *Gastrointestinal tract disease*, in the relatively rare protein-losing gastroenteropathies especially; smaller losses also occur in some other disorders (e.g. ulcerative colitis, Crohn's disease).

   (c) *Skin disease*, e.g. exfoliative dermatitis, extensive burns.

Hereditary abnormalities

Analbuminaemia is a rare disorder in which plasma [albumin] is usually less than 1.0 g/L. However, there may be no symptoms or signs, not even oedema, due to there being compensatory increases in plasma [globulins]. Bisalbuminaemia has no pathological significance.

The haptoglobins

This is a group of proteins, all α_2-globulins, that bind haemoglobin to form haptoglobin–haemoglobin complexes; the complexes are then rapidly broken down in the lymphoreticular system. Only a small proportion of red cell destruction occurs inside the vascular system, and it seems likely that only this component leads to the formation of these complexes. This small amount may, cumulatively, fulfil a useful function by helping to conserve the body's iron stores. Uncomplexed haemoglobin (M_r, 68 kDa) can pass the glomerular filter, with consequent loss of its iron from the body. By combining with haptoglobin, the small amount of haemoglobin normally released into the circulation is conserved and its iron is not lost.

   Plasma [haptoglobin] falls whenever intravascular haemolysis is increased (e.g. in haemolytic anaemia) and free haptoglobin may then be undetectable. Decreased plasma [haptoglobin] is found also in liver disease, and rarely as a congenital abnormality.

   Plasma [haptoglobin] increases in acute infections and following trauma: haptoglobin is one of the acute phase reactants (p. 92). It is also increased in the nephrotic syndrome.

Genetic polymorphism

The structure of haptoglobin varies between individuals. The basic molecule comprises two types of chain, α and β, giving rise to the structure $\alpha_2\beta_2$. The β

Table 7.3 The haptoglobin phenotypes

Phenotype	Subunit structure	Molecular mass (daltons)	Electrophoretic appearance
Hp1-1	$\alpha^{1F}\alpha^{1F}\beta_2$ $\alpha^{1F}\alpha^{1S}\beta_2$ $\alpha^{1S}\alpha^{1S}\beta_2$	100 000	Single band
Hp 2-1	$\alpha^{1S}\alpha^2\beta_2$ $\alpha^{1F}\alpha^2\beta_2$	105 000 210 000 315 000 etc.	Multiple bands
Hp 2-2	$\alpha_n^2\beta_n$, where n = 3-8	220 000 300 000 370 000 etc.	Multiple bands

chains (M_r, 40 kDa) are the same in all haptoglobins, but the α chain may be of three types — α^{1S} (9 kDa), α^{1F} (9 kDa) and α^2 (17 kDa); the α^{1S} and α^{1F} polypeptide chains differ by only a single amino acid. Three allelic genes (HP^{1F}, HP^{1S} and HP^2) code for the chains in each $\alpha\beta$ pair, so several phenotypes are possible (Table 7.3).

Individuals inherit a characteristic genotype, which determines the nature of their plasma haptoglobin; this is an example of the phenomenon known as genetic polymorphism. Several other plasma proteins show similar inherited variations (e.g. IgG, apolipoprotein E, α_1-protease inhibitor). With the haptoglobins these are of considerable genetic interest but are of no pathological significance.

α_1-Protease inhibitor (API)

This is a glycoprotein (M_r, 54 kDa), previously called α_1-antitrypsin. Present at a mean concentration of about 3.0 g/L, API comprises approximately 90% of the α_1-globulin band seen on serum protein electrophoresis. It inhibits proteases, particularly elastase, probably having the function thereby of limiting and localizing proteolytic activity at sites of inflammation. Interest principally relates to the association between certain diseases of the lung and liver and API deficiency.

Reduced plasma API levels

API deficiency is usually first recognized by finding a greatly reduced α_1-globulin band on serum protein electrophoresis. Specific immunological or enzymic methods can then be used to measure plasma [API] or API activity, respectively.

α_1-Protease inhibitor is another example of a protein that exhibits genetic polymorphism. Several allelic genes code for API, the alleles being given the general designation Pi (protease inhibitor). The normal allele is Pi^M and the normal homozygote Pi^{MM} (the MM type). Individuals who are homozygous for the Pi^Z allele, (i.e. who are Pi^{ZZ}, the ZZ type) make up one in 3000 of the UK population. Individuals of the ZZ type produce about 15% of the normal amount of plasma API, and have a relatively high incidence of lung or liver disease:

1 *Pulmonary emphysema.* About 1% of patients with emphysema have API deficiency, but this percentage is much higher in young patients. When associated

with API deficiency, emphysema tends to manifest itself in the 20–40 age-group. Smoking seems to be a strong predisposing factor for the development of the disease in these patients.

2 *Hepatic disorders.* Neonatal jaundice, usually presenting a predominantly cholestatic picture, is common in type ZZ individuals. Although the jaundice may resolve, there is usually progression to hepatic cirrhosis. In about 20% of children with cirrhosis, the hepatic disorder can probably be attributed to API deficiency. In adults, cirrhosis and hepatoma are associated with the Pi^Z phenotype.

Phenotyping of API can be best performed by isoelectric focusing, and is desirable in all cases where plasma API levels are low or borderline: the results are required before appropriate genetic counselling can be given to affected individuals or to their parents. Molecular biology techniques (e.g. Southern blotting) can be used to investigate relatives of patients with API deficiency (p. 354, 361).

Increased plasma API levels

These occur in pregnancy, in acute infections and following trauma; API is one of the acute phase reactants. Increases in plasma API are not important in themselves. However, individuals who are deficient in API also show increases in plasma API in pregnancy, in acute infections and after trauma. These increases may be sufficient to bring the levels for an individual with API deficiency into the lower part of the API reference range, and delay in diagnosis of API deficiency may occur as a result.

Other plasma proteins

The concentrations of many other plasma proteins may be altered either in diseases that primarily affect their metabolism or as a result of dehydration, overhydration or malnutrition. In the rest of this section, we shall consider briefly some of the other proteins listed in Table 7.2, most of which are able to be measured in most clinical biochemistry laboratories, but there are many other proteins present in plasma that are not considered here.

Pre-albumin (M_r, 55 kDa)

This protein, normally present in plasma in small amounts, is synthesized by the hepatocytes. It acts as one of the transport proteins for vitamin A and thyroxine. Plasma [pre-albumin] falls in states of malnutrition. It also falls rapidly in response to injury and is decreased in acute as well as in chronic liver disease, because its half-life is much shorter than that of albumin.

α_1-Fetoprotein (M_r, 69 kDa)

This protein is present in the tissues and plasma of the fetus. Its concentration falls very rapidly after birth, but minute amounts (up to 15 μg/L) can still be detected in plasma from adults, if sensitive immunoassay methods are used. The functions of α_1-fetoprotein (AFP) are unclear but it may play an immunoregulatory role during pregnancy. Measurements of AFP have two important applications:

1 *Pregnancy.* Women carrying fetuses with open neural tube defects have increased plasma [AFP]. Screening programmes involving measurement of maternal serum [AFP] at 16–18 weeks' gestation are now widely practised (p. 316).

2 *Tumour marker.* This application is considered on p. 103.

Ceruloplasmin (M$_r$, 132 kDa)

This is a copper-containing protein, an α_2-globulin with a mean concentration in plasma of 0.35 g/L. It has oxidase properties. It normally binds about 90% of the copper present in plasma. However, it is not known whether ceruloplasmin is primarily concerned with plasma copper transport, or whether its enzymic properties as an oxidase are of physiological importance.

Plasma [ceruloplasmin] is reduced in Wilson's disease (p. 121), in patients with malnutrition, and in the nephrotic syndrome.

Plasma [ceruloplasmin] is increased in pregnancy and in women taking oestrogen-containing oral contraceptives. It is also raised in acute infections, in some types of chronic liver disease and in neoplastic disease.

α_2-Macroglobulin (M$_r$, 820 kDa)

This is the major α_2-globulin; it has a mean concentration of about 2.5 g/L in plasma. It binds endopeptidases such as trypsin and chymotrypsin; the resulting complexes have no endopeptidase activity. It is not known whether this antiprotease activity represents the major biological function of α_2-macroglobulin. It also has transport functions.

Plasma [α_2-macroglobulin] is increased greatly in the nephrotic syndrome, in some patients with cirrhosis, and in some of the collagen disorders.

β_2-Microglobulin (M$_r$, 11.8 kDa)

This protein forms part of the HLA system and is a surface constituent of most cells. The β_2-microglobulin in plasma is mainly derived from myeloid and lymphoid cells and is normally synthesized at a fairly constant rate. Plasma levels (mean concentration, normally about 1.5 mg/L) are increased whenever there is lymphoid or myeloid proliferation.

The rate of removal of β_2-microglobulin from plasma depends on the GFR, and *plasma [β_2-microglobulin] is increased* in the presence of renal failure. It may also rise in some malignant and immunological disorders. Its measurement is of value in monitoring patients with renal failure, and in following the progress of patients with multiple myeloma (p. 99, 141).

C-reactive protein (M$_r$, 105 kDa)

This protein is a β-globulin, originally named after a property of serum that had been obtained from acutely ill patients and which caused the precipitation of a polysaccharide (fraction C) from pneumococcal extracts. C-reactive protein (CRP) binds strongly to certain lipids, particularly phospholipids. It seems that CRP is somehow concerned with the body's response to foreign materials.

The acute phase response

Several proteins are synthesized in increased amounts as a response to 'injury'. They include CRP, API, fibrinogen and the haptoglobins, and are collectively known as acute phase reactants. 'Injury' is used here as a general term to include acute tissue damage due to trauma, myocardial infarction, burns, acute infections, etc. as well as chronic inflammation (e.g. rheumatoid arthritis, Crohn's disease) and malignant disease.

Most acute phase reactants increase two- to threefold after 'injury', but plasma [CRP] may be increased much more, often 10-fold to 100-fold. Measurements of plasma [CRP] can be used as a screening test for organic disease, as an alternative to the erythrocyte sedimentation rate, and to monitor the progress of conditions such as rheumatoid arthritis. However, the CRP response may be modest or absent in some chronic inflammatory conditions.

The concentrations of albumin, pre-albumin, transferrin and some other plasma proteins may fall during the acute phase response to 'injury'.

The immunoglobulins

These are a group of structurally related proteins that function as antibodies; they are synthesized by the cells of the lymphoreticular system. Although predominantly moving with the γ-globulins on serum protein electrophoresis, some may migrate with the β- or with the α_2-globulins.

The basic immunoglobulin (Ig) molecule is made up of four polypeptide chains consisting of a pair of heavy chains (M_r, 50–75 kDa each) and a pair of light chains (M_r, 22 kDa each). There are five principal types of heavy chain (γ, α, μ, δ and ε) and two types of light chain (κ and λ). Every immunoglobulin can be assigned a formula that indicates its composition, according to its types of chain (e.g. $\alpha_2 \lambda_2$, $\gamma_2 \kappa_2$, etc.). The antigen-combining sites are between the adjacent light and heavy chains (Fig. 7.1).

The immunoglobulin classes

Three major (IgG, IgA and IgM) and two minor (IgD and IgE) classes of immunoglobulin have been recognized; the type of heavy chain determines the

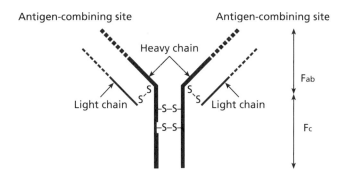

Fig. 7.1 The immunoglobulin molecule, which consists of two identical pairs of heavy and light chains, held together by disulphide bonds (shown as –S–S–). The molecule can be split by papain into three components; these are the two antigen-binding fragments (Fab), each of which has one binding site, and the crystallizable fragment (Fc). The variable regions of the Ig molecule are shown as interrupted lines. The heavy chains are one of five types (α, δ, ε, γ, or μ) and the light chains are one of two types (κ or λ).

Table 7.4 Some features of the major classes of the immunoglobulins

Feature	IgG	IgA	IgM
Average mol mass	146 000 Da	160 000 Da	875 000 Da
Plasma concentration	5.0–13.0 g/L	0.5–4.0 g/L	0.3–2.5 g/L
Light chain type	κ or λ	κ or λ	κ or λ
Heavy chain type	γ	α	μ
Structure of protein	$\gamma_2\kappa_2$ or $\gamma_2\lambda_2$	$\alpha_2\kappa_2$ or $\alpha_2\lambda_2$	$(\mu_2\kappa_2)_5$ or $(\mu_2\lambda_2)_5$
Plasma half-life	21 days	6 days	5 days
Amount in the circulation	50%	70%	80%
Immune response	Secondary	Local, secretory	Primary
Present in secretions	Trace	Yes	Trace
Transplacental passage	Yes	No	No

class. Table 7.4 lists several features of the major classes. Both light and heavy chains have 'constant' and 'variable' sections. The 'constant' portion varies little within each particular chain type, whereas the variable portion (which is associated with the antigen-combining site) is different for each immunoglobulin even within a single chain type. The variable portion is responsible for the specificity of the antibody.

IgG immunoglobulins are formed particularly in response to soluble antigens such as toxins and the products of bacterial lysis. They are widely distributed in the ECF and cross the fetoplacental barrier.

IgM immunoglobulins in plasma are pentamers of the basic immunoglobulin structure. They tend to be formed especially in response to particulate antigens, such as those on the surface of bacteria. In the presence of complement, IgM are very effective in producing lysis of these cells. Following an antigenic stimulus, IgM formation usually precedes IgG formation, and IgM are thought to provide an early defence mechanism against intravascular spread of infecting organisms.

IgA immunoglobulins, as they occur in plasma, are monomers. However, over 50% of IgA synthesis occurs in lymphoreticular cells under the mucosa of the respiratory and alimentary tracts. The IgA molecules are taken up here by the mucosal epithelial cells with the formation of an IgA dimer, e.g. $(\alpha_2\lambda_2)_2$; a secretory piece is also added, which protects the molecule from proteolysis. The resulting protein, called secretory IgA, is secreted into the alimentary or the respiratory tract, and may form part of the defence mechanism against local viral and bacterial infections.

IgD immunoglobulins are present in minute amounts in plasma. They are also often present, with monomer IgM, on the surface of B lymphocytes. Their function in plasma is unknown. However, on lymphocytes they are probably concerned with antigen recognition and with the development of tolerance.

IgE immunoglobulins include the reagins, which bind to cells such as the mast cells of the nasopharynx. In the presence of antigen (allergen), one result of the antigen–antibody reaction is the release of histamine and other amines and polypeptides from the cell, giving rise to a local hypersensitivity reaction.

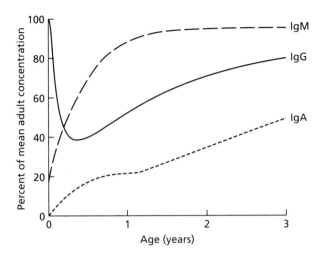

Fig. 7.2 The *average* concentrations of the three major immunoglobulin classes in the first 3 years of life, expressed as percentages of the mean concentrations of these classes in healthy adults. Adult reference ranges are given in Table 7.4.

Immunoglobulins in children

In neonates, IgG is present in plasma in relatively high concentration, having been transferred across the placenta; its concentration falls soon after birth. IgM is present in plasma at birth in very small quantities, having been synthesized by the fetus *in utero*. In the healthy neonate, IgA is undetectable in plasma.

During infancy and childhood, plasma [total Ig] rises towards the values observed in healthy adults, plasma [IgM] increasing fairly rapidly but plasma [IgG] and [IgA] more slowly (Fig. 7.2). In some children, Ig development may be delayed.

Disorders of immunoglobulin synthesis

There are two broad categories of disorder. In one, plasma [Ig] is decreased; in the other, their concentration is increased (Table 7.5). The two categories are not

Table 7.5 Disorders of immunoglobulin synthesis

Hypogammaglobulinaemia	Hypergammaglobulinaemia
Inherited (all rare conditions)	*Diffuse*
Agammaglobulinaemia	Infections
Hypogammaglobulinaemia	Chronic liver disease
Dysgammaglobulinaemia	Auto-immune disease
Acquired (or secondary)	*Discrete*
Prematurity and delayed maturity	Multiple myeloma
Protein-losing syndromes	Macroglobulinaemia
Lymphoid neoplasia	Heavy chain disease
Drug treatment	Benign paraproteinaemia

mutually exclusive; reductions in one Ig class may be accompanied by increases in another.

Inherited deficiencies of immunoglobulin synthesis

Hypogammaglobulinaemia and, rarely, agammaglobulinaemia are conditions in which there is defective production of IgG, IgA and IgM. Children begin to develop severe, recurrent bacterial infections when over the age of 1 year.

Dysgammaglobulinaemias comprise a group of very rare conditions in which there is a deficiency of one or more of the immunoglobulin classes. Nearly all the possible combinations of deficiencies of IgG, IgA and IgM have been described. These disorders may be associated with defective cell-mediated immunity. Affected children are prone to viral infections and normally minor viral illnesses may prove fatal.

Acquired deficiencies of immunoglobulin synthesis

These are usually secondary to some other disease, but occasionally Ig deficiency may occur in adult life with no apparent precipitating cause.

Secondary hypogammaglobulinaemia is much commoner than the inherited deficiencies. It may occur in lymphoid neoplasia (e.g. chronic lymphatic leukaemia, Hodgkin's disease, multiple myelomatosis), in 'toxic' disorders or certain types of drug therapy, in protein-losing syndromes (e.g. nephrotic syndrome), and in prematurity and delayed maturity.

In the lymphoid disorders, the cause of the suppression of synthesis is not known but there is a consequent increased tendency to infection. Severe infections, or treatment with cytotoxic drugs, may adversely affect Ig synthesis and exacerbate the deficiency.

Diffuse hypergammaglobulinaemia

Serum protein electrophoresis reveals a broad band, due to increased amounts of γ-globulin. The increase may affect all the Ig classes or it may affect predominantly one class. The antibodies produced are heterogeneous. Quantitation of the separate Ig classes is occasionally helpful in diagnosis. In most cases, however, the cause of the diffuse increase in plasma [total Ig] is apparent. The causes include:

1 *Infections.* In both acute and chronic infections, the increases are a part of the body's physiological response to infection, larger increases generally being seen in chronic infection. All three major Ig classes are commonly affected, but sometimes one class tends to be associated with certain diseases (e.g. IgA is often increased in diseases of the skin and lungs, IgM in tropical diseases).

2 *Liver disease.* Most patients with cirrhosis show a diffuse increase in γ-globulin on serum protein electrophoresis, the major Ig classes all being affected, with plasma [IgA] characteristically showing the greatest increase. However, in primary biliary cirrhosis there is a predominant increase in plasma [IgM] in over 90% of patients, and in chronic active hepatitis [IgG] tends to be most increased.

3 *Auto-immune disease.* In systemic lupus erythematosus, Sjögren's syndrome

and chronic thyroiditis, for example, patients tend to show an increase in plasma [IgG], although other Ig classes are also affected.

Discrete hypergammaglobulinaemia (paraproteinaemia)

Discrete immunoglobulin bands, visible on electrophoresis of serum, are known as paraproteins or 'M' (monoclonal) components. They are due to production of a single immunoglobulin or immunoglobulin fragment (e.g. light chain) by a single clone of B cells. The detection of a paraprotein in blood or urine requires further investigation, to determine whether the paraproteinaemia is malignant or benign. Malignant paraproteinaemias include multiple myeloma, macroglobulinaemia and some lymphomas (Table 7.6).

Multiple myeloma is a disease in which there is proliferation of plasma cells and plasma cell precursors. Most myelomas produce complete Ig molecules, usually either IgG or IgA, together with excessive amounts of Ig fragments; these may be light chains or parts of heavy chains or other fragments. About 10–20% of myelomas, usually the less differentiated, secrete insignificant amounts of complete immunoglobulins. Instead, they produce large quantities of Ig fragments consisting mainly of dimers of light chains (M_r, 44 kDa), when the disease is called Bence Jones myeloma or light chain disease.

Waldenström's macroglobulinaemia usually follows a more prolonged course than multiple myeloma. There is proliferation of cells that resemble lymphocytes rather than plasma cells. They produce complete IgM molecules and often an excess of light chains. Increased plasma [IgM] causes increased plasma viscosity, which tends to make the circulation sluggish and thromboses are common.

Table 7.6 Features of the malignant paraproteinaemias

Disease	Incidence (%)	Serum 'M' component		Urine protein	
		Nature	Frequency (%)	Nature	Frequency (%)
IgG myeloma	50	IgG	> 95	Bence Jones	50–90
IgA myeloma	25	IgA	> 95	Bence Jones	50–90
IgD myeloma	1–3	IgD	> 50	Bence Jones	> 90
Light chain disease	10–25	κ or λ chains	Variable	Bence Jones	100
Macroglobulinaemia	5–10	IgM	> 95	Bence Jones	10–60
Heavy chain disease	Very rare	α,γ,μ chain fragments	Variable	Heavy chain fragments	Variable

Notes
1 The figures for the incidence are the approximate percentages that each disease contributes to the whole group of conditions that together comprise the malignant paraproteinaemias.
2 The frequency of occurrence is the approximate percentage of patients with a particular condition that exhibits the related feature (serum 'M' component, urinary paraprotein).
3 The urine protein data refer to urine protein electrophoresis carried out after concentration of the specimen. In variable percentages of cases, urine also contains albumin and other proteins.
4 The table does not contain data for IgE myeloma or IgM monomer disease, both very rare.

Heavy chain disease (Franklin's disease) comprises a group of rare conditions in which heavy chain fragments corresponding to the Fc portion of the immuno-globulins are synthesized and excreted in urine. Abnormal production of α and γ heavy chains are the most common derangements.

Benign paraproteinaemia may be transient or persistent. Paraproteins may occur transiently during acute infection and in auto-immune disease due to antigen stimulation. Stable or persistent benign paraproteinaemia may be due to a benign tumour of the B cells, but this can only be determined on follow-up (see below).

Cryoglobulins

These are immunoglobulins that precipitate when cooled to 4 °C and redissolve when warmed to 37 °C; sometimes they precipitate at temperatures intermediate between 37 °C and 4 °C. They occur in a number of diseases associated with hypergammaglobulinaemia, both the diffuse and the discrete forms. Their detection is of little value in determining the aetiology of the conditions in which they are formed. However, their importance lies in the fact that they may be associated with Raynaud's phenomenon.

If cryoglobulin determinations are to be performed, blood needs to be collected into a warmed syringe, no anticoagulant, and maintained at 37 °C until the serum for cryoglobulin investigation has been separated from the cells.

Investigation of paraproteinaemia

Chemical, haematological and radiological investigations and lymph node biopsy are all of value when investigating cases of suspected paraproteinaemia. The chemical tests are used to detect the paraprotein, to determine its concentration and type, and to follow the progress of the disease. Serum protein and urine protein electrophoresis should be carried out in all cases of suspected parapro-teinaemia. However, immunochemical methods for measuring serum [immuno-globulins] may be unreliable in the presence of paraproteins.

Initial investigations

Serum protein electrophoresis shows a single discrete band, usually in the γ-globulin region but occasionally in the β- or α_2-globulin region, in over 90% of patients in whom there is overproduction of complete immunoglobulin molecules (Table 7.5); the concentrations of the other immunoglobulins may be reduced. Occasionally, a band due to the presence of light chains may be observed. Electrophoresis is the most sensitive widely available test for paraproteins; plasma must *not* be used as the fibrinogen band may obscure or mimic paraproteins.

Urine protein electrophoresis is usually needed to demonstrate Bence Jones protein; its small size (M_r, 44 kDa) means that it is cleared rapidly by the kidney. If Bence Jones protein is detected, the monoclonal nature of the light chains can be confirmed by immunofixation. In multiple myeloma the light chains are nearly always dimers of type κ or type λ, but not a mixture of the two. Protein electrophoresis is much more sensitive than 'side-room' tests (p. 14) as a means of detecting Bence Jones protein in urine. Most cases of myeloma and many cases of macroglobulinaemia have Bence Jones proteinuria. In light chain disease, there is Bence Jones proteinuria but usually no serum paraprotein or 'M' component. The principal protein findings in myeloma and macroglobulinaemia are summarized in Table 7.4.

On finding a paraprotein, *the most important diagnostic decision is whether the condition is benign or malignant*. Chemical features that point to the condition being benign are: (i) other immunoglobulin classes are normal; (ii) Bence Jones proteinuria is absent; (iii) the serum [paraprotein] is less than 10 g/L; and (iv) the serum [paraprotein] does not increase with time.

Further investigations

If a paraprotein is found, further chemical measurements should usually be performed, as follows:

1 *The concentration and type of paraprotein* (IgG, IgA, etc.) should be determined.

2 *'Normal' (i.e. non-paraprotein) Ig*. The serum concentrations of these immunoglobulins should be measured, to assess the likelihood of intercurrent infection.

3 *Plasma [β_2-microglobulin]*. This provides a good index of prognosis, presumably because this determination depends both on the turnover of tumour cells and on renal function. High levels indicate a poor prognosis.

4 *Plasma [creatinine]*, to assess renal (glomerular) function. Myeloma is commonly associated with both glomerular and tubular dysfunction.

5 *Plasma [calcium]*. This is often raised due to increased release of calcium from bone. Plasma alkaline phosphatase activity is usually normal or only slightly raised as osteoblastic activity is not increased in multiple myeloma.

6 *Plasma [urate]*. This may be raised due to increased cell breakdown, especially after cytotoxic therapy. Urate deposition may cause renal damage in myeloma.

Many of the results of these tests will be abnormal not only in multiple myeloma but in the other paraproteinaemias, particularly in Waldenström's macroglobulinaemia.

Progress of paraproteinaemia

Both malignant and benign paraproteinaemias can be followed up by measuring serum [paraprotein], serum ['normal' immunoglobulins], and plasma [β_2-microglobulin]. These investigations may need to be repeated several times before it becomes clear whether the paraproteinaemia is benign or malignant. Monitoring the progress of benign paraproteinaemias indicates that they only rarely become malignant.

The efficacy of treatment for the malignant paraproteinaemias can be assessed by measuring serum [paraprotein], and plasma [β_2-microglobulin], [calcium] and [creatinine]. Potentially adverse effects of treatment may require periodical reassessment of plasma [urate], 'liver function tests', etc., depending on the nature of the treatment.

Tumour markers

Many tumour markers have been described, but so far their measurement has been of little value in the detection of asymptomatic cancer. Some have proved useful

---

Case 7.1

A 70-year-old man complained to his doctor of back pain, which he had had for several months, and of feeling generally unwell. He appeared pale and he was tender over the lumbar spine. His urine contained protein (1 g/L) on 'side-room' testing and his erythrocyte sedimentation rate (ESR) was very high (90 mm in the first hour). The following abnormalities were reported for chemical analyses on a blood specimen:

Analysis	Result	Reference range	Units
[Albumin]	32	36–47	g/L
[Calcium]	2.72	2.12–2.62	mmol/L
[Creatinine]	180	55–120	µmol/L
[Protein, total]	84	63–83	g/L
[IgA]	< 0.4	0.5–4.0	g/L
[IgG]	37	5.0–13	g/L
[IgM]	< 0.2	0.3–2.5	g/L

How would you interpret these results and what further chemical investigations would you request on this patient? He is discussed on p. 104.

---

in the early detection of recurrence of malignant disease *after* treatment, or in indicating the development of metastases. The markers that are most commonly measured at present to detect and monitor malignant tumours and premalignant conditions are listed in Table 7.7.

Hormones as tumour markers

The secretion of hormones by tumours of the endocrine glands is discussed later in

Table 7.7 Examples of tumour markers

Marker	Condition to be monitored*
Well-established tumour markers	
α₁-Fetoprotein (AFP)	Hepatoma, teratoma of the testis
Calcitonin	Medullary carcinoma of the thyroid
Carcinoembryonic antigen (CEA)	Carcinoma of the colon
Heat-stable alkaline phosphatase isoenzymes (e.g. Regan, Nagao)	Tumours of the ovary, testis
Human chorionic gonadotrophin (hCG)	Hydatidiform mole, choriocarcinoma
Prostatic acid phosphatase and prostate-specific antigen	Carcinoma of the prostate
Less well-established tumour markers	
CA 125	Carcinoma of the ovary
CA 15-3	Carcinoma of the breast
CA 19-9	Gastrointestinal cancers
Neurone-specific enolase	Small cell carcinoma of the lung

* Tumour markers are only rarely or very occasionally used for *detection* of tumours.

the appropriate chapters. Various of these hormones are also sometimes secreted by tumours originating elsewhere, from 'non-endocrine' tissue. Their secretion is then described as 'inappropriate' or 'ectopic'.

'Ectopic' hormone production is a misleading description since it implies that the hormone's synthesis is inappropriate for the tissue and its release merely that of a chance by-product. It is now known that many tissues previously regarded as 'non-endocrine', including brain and lung, contain several peptide hormones that may be important for their local effects on cell growth and differentiation. The hormones and hormone-like substances produced by tumours derived from these 'non-endocrine' tissues may be important autocrine growth factors; receptors for many hormones have been found associated with some tumours.

The production of hormones by 'non-endocrine' tumours is generally not subject to normal physiological negative feedback mechanisms of control. This lack of control allows high levels of the hormone to be produced unchecked and the clinical syndrome then becomes apparent by the action of the hormone on its target organ.

Many hormones may be secreted by 'non-endocrine' tumours but few are now used as tumour markers (Table 7.7). Some tumours are particularly associated with 'ectopic' hormone production, e.g. small cell carcinoma of the lung may produce them in 25–30% of patients; ACTH and AVP are the hormones most often released by these tumours.

Enzymes as tumour markers

Alterations in the activities or concentrations of many enzymes in plasma have been described in association with neoplastic disease, but few specific associations have been identified. The best example is the association between increased plasma acid phosphatase activity and the presence of metastatic carcinoma of the prostate in bone.

Prostatic acid phosphatase (PAP)

The main value of this measurement is in confirming the presence and spread of prostatic carcinoma, and in assessing the response to treatment. While carcinoma is confined within the prostate, plasma PAP activity is raised in only about 20% of patients. However, local or distant spread of the neoplasm causes increased activity, often to high levels, in up to 80% of patients. Enzyme activity falls rapidly after successful oestrogen therapy, but quickly rises again if relapse occurs. When investigating patients with prostatic disease by measuring plasma acid phosphatase activity, the following points should be noted:

1 *The prostatic isoenzyme* is unstable and specimens should be sent to the laboratory for assay, or for storage under correct conditions, as soon as possible after collection.

2 *Rectal examination.* Where possible, blood samples should be collected before a rectal examination since temporary (and occasionally large) increases in plasma PAP activity have been reported after this procedure. However, most recent reports have stated that rectal examination has no effect on plasma PAP activity.

Measurement of PAP by radioimmunoassay (RIA) offers few diagnostic advantages over methods based on enzyme activity measurements. The RIA methods are no better at detecting intracapsular prostatic carcinoma, nor are they much better at detecting and following the course of more extensive disease. It seems likely that measurement of prostate-specific antigen (see below) will be increasingly adopted in place of PAP in view of its greater sensitivity as a marker of prostatic cancer.

Alkaline phosphatase

The causes of an increased plasma alkaline phosphatase activity in patients with malignant disease can be grouped as follows:

1 *Bone alkaline phosphatase.* Its activity is increased in osteoblastic bone tumours, primary or secondary, e.g. in osteogenic sarcoma. It is not raised as a rule when the lesions are primarily osteolytic, as in multiple myeloma.

2 *Liver alkaline phosphatase.* Its activity is increased in a high proportion of patients with primary or secondary neoplasms in the liver. The increase is usually associated with areas of obstruction to biliary flow caused by these tumours. Other membrane-associated hepatic enzymes (e.g. GGT) may be similarly affected.

3 *'Tumour-specific' isoenzymes.* Several malignant tumours express isoenzymes of alkaline phosphatase that are not normally associated with the tissue of origin of the tumour; these are then released into the circulation. Plasma activities of these isoenzymes are often low and insufficient to cause significant increases in plasma total alkaline phosphatase activity, but specific monoclonal antibodies enable the detection and quantitation of these isoenzymes.

The commonest 'tumour-specific' alkaline phosphatases are the Regan (so called after the patient in whom it was first described) and the Nagao isoenzymes. These are, respectively, placental and placental-like isoenzymes and both are found particularly in specimens from patients with malignant disease of the reproductive system. Less often, an alkaline phosphatase similar to the fetal form of the intestinal isoenzyme can be detected in patients with GI and liver cancers (Kasahara isoenzyme).

Serum placental and placental-like alkaline phosphatase isoenzyme measurements are useful in monitoring patients treated for seminoma or dysgerminoma. In the common malignancies (e.g. breast, lung, stomach), however, their prevalence is usually less than 20%.

Neurone-specific enolase (NSE)

This is an isoenzyme of enolase present in large amounts in nerve cells and in cells with neuroendocrine properties. The main use of plasma NSE measurements is in monitoring small cell lung cancer since approximately 70% of patients with untreated disease have elevated levels.

Tumour antigens as markers

Many tumour antigens have been described as potential markers for the presence of malignant disease. The two that have been most fully evaluated are CEA and AFP. The extent of their usefulness and their limitations as diagnostic tests or as aids to the management of patients who have been treated for cancer are now reasonably well defined. Both CEA and AFP are normally detectable in small amounts in plasma. They may be increased in the presence of non-neoplastic conditions as well as in the presence of malignant disease, but the largest increases are nearly always due to malignancy.

Carcinoembryonic antigen (CEA)

Measurements of plasma [CEA] do not have the sensitivity or the specificity required for use as a screening test, and should never be used in isolation to establish a diagnosis of cancer. There is considerable overlap between plasma [CEA] in patients with inflammatory diseases and in patients with benign and malignant tumours. Smoking may also increase plasma [CEA]. However, in patients with symptoms suggesting a diagnosis of malignant disease, if plasma [CEA] is increased to more than five times the upper reference value (i.e. to over 25 µg/L), this is strong evidence pointing to the presence of cancer.

Plasma [CEA] should be measured pre-operatively in patients with colorectal or bronchial carcinoma. However, a low plasma [CEA] does not necessarily imply a good prognosis, as about 20% of patients in whom malignant disease is later proved never have raised plasma [CEA]. Also, poorly differentiated colorectal carcinomas do not seem, in general, to synthesize CEA to the same extent, or to release as much CEA, as better differentiated tumours.

The main indication for measuring plasma [CEA] is in the post-operative monitoring of colorectal carcinoma; it should be measured at follow-up assessments. If the concentration was increased pre-operatively, it should return to normal within 6 weeks following successful operation. Thereafter, if plasma [CEA] starts to rise slowly, this may indicate local recurrence; rapidly increasing plasma [CEA] is usually associated with the presence of metastases.

a_1-Fetoprotein (AFP)

Plasma [AFP] is increased in association with malignant tumours arising in many organs. It may also be raised in several non-neoplastic conditions but, in these, the increase may be temporary, associated with the tissue's response to injury, and usually the increase is smaller.

The main value of plasma [AFP] measurements in neoplastic disease is in the diagnosis and management of hepatocellular carcinoma where greatly increased amounts are detectable in 50–90% of patients. With malignant teratoma, 50–70% of patients show marked increases. Raised plasma [AFP] also occurs in about 20% of patients with gastric, pancreatic and biliary tract neoplasms.

Measurements of plasma [AFP] are used to monitor the course of malignant teratoma and its response to treatment. Serial measurements of plasma [AFP] may also be of value in monitoring for recurrence of hepatoma after treatment by local resection or liver transplantation.

Prostate-specific antigen (PSA)

This is an enzyme (a serine protease) that is normally confined to the epithelial tissue of the prostate. Measurement of serum [PSA] provides a very sensitive index of prostatic cancer, it being increased in over 90% of cases when first diagnosed whereas only about 50% of cases have increased serum prostatic acid phosphatase activity at this stage. However, serum [PSA] is also increased in most patients with benign prostatic hypertrophy, so the measurement lacks specificity as a test for prostatic cancer. Periodic measurements of serum [PSA] may prove valuable in monitoring the response of prostatic cancer to treatment.

Carbohydrate and glycoprotein antigens

Monoclonal antibodies have been raised to several carbohydrate or glycoprotein antigenic determinants found in several specific types of tumour. These include:

1 An antibody that reacts with a carbohydrate antigen (designated CA 19-9). Measurement of serum [CA 19-9] appears to be of value in the diagnosis and monitoring of patients with pancreatic, hepatobiliary and gastric carcinomas.

2 An antibody that reacts with a glycoprotein antigen (designated CA 125). Measurement of serum [CA 125] appears to be of value in monitoring the progress of patients with ovarian carcinoma. Raised serum [CA 125] has also been observed in patients with cirrhosis and with hepatoma.

3 Two monoclonal antibodies have been produced that, in conjunction, can be used to measure another cancer antigen (designated CA 15-3). These measurements have been advocated for monitoring patients with carcinoma of the breast.

Comments on Case 7.1 (p. 100)

Serum and urine protein electrophoresis would both be indicated. The serum pattern showed a discrete band in the γ-globulin region, with marked reduction of the other immunoglobulins, and urine electrophoresis revealed the presence of Bence Jones protein, subsequently identified as of the λ type. The diagnosis of multiple myeloma was confirmed on X-ray examination (which demonstrated osteolytic lesions in the skull, vertebral column, ribs and pelvis) and by the finding of plasma cells in the bone marrow.

Hypercalcaemia is present in about 30% of patients with multiple myeloma, and about 50% show some evidence of impaired renal function at the time of presentation; this is associated with a poor prognosis. Plasma [albumin] is often reduced, whereas [total protein] is often increased due to the high [paraprotein]; these abnormalities in plasma proteins account for the high ESR.

Chapter 8
Liver Disease

The liver plays a key role in many of the processes of intermediary metabolism. Its functions include the synthesis of carbohydrates, lipids and a wide range of proteins. It exchanges substances with the plasma, adding some for distribution in the body and removing others, often with subsequent metabolism. Bile is formed by the liver, and it is the organ mainly responsible for the detoxication of many drugs and carcinogens. The liver excretes a wide range of compounds into bile.

Structure of the liver

It is a common fallacy to think of the liver as being composed almost exclusively of a single type of cell, the hepatocyte or parenchymal cell. Only about 60% of the cells are hepatocytes, subdivided on the basis of their zonal location; zone 1 cells are those closest to the portal tract, zone 2 cells are between zones 1 and 3, and zone 3 cells are those closest to the hepatic vein. Endothelial (Kupffer) cells line the hepatic sinusoids and comprise 30% of the liver cells; the remaining 10% consists of vascular and supporting tissue and bile ducts.

The functional unit of each liver acinus consists of the portal tract surrounded by radiating cords of hepatocytes. Blood enters the acinus via the portal tract and passes along the sinusoids towards the central vein. Hepatocytes in zone 1 receive relatively well oxygenated blood, whereas the hepatocytes in zone 3 receive blood that has lost much of its oxygen and exchanged other substances with the cells of zones 1 and 2. Cells in zone 3 are the most susceptible to anoxia, and to injury by a wide range of toxic substances.

There is some degree of enzymic localization that relates to differences in oxygenation of the three zones (Fig. 8.1). Cells in zone 1, for instance, have relatively high concentrations of alkaline phosphatase and the aminotransferases. Differences in localization of enzymes help to explain why some patients with liver damage may have normal levels of some enzyme activities in plasma. For instance, ethanol, which mainly damages cells in zone 3, causes the release of relatively less of the aminotransferases than damage by viral hepatitis, which predominantly affects cells of zones 1 and 2.

The hepatocytes

Hepatocytes are arranged in sheets which are effectively one cell thick. Their membranes are raised into microvilli at the surface related to the sinusoidal cells and within the biliary canaliculi. They thus have a direct relationship with plasma across a large surface area, and a rapid, two-way exchange between hepatocytes and plasma probably occurs through pores in the lining of the sinusoids.

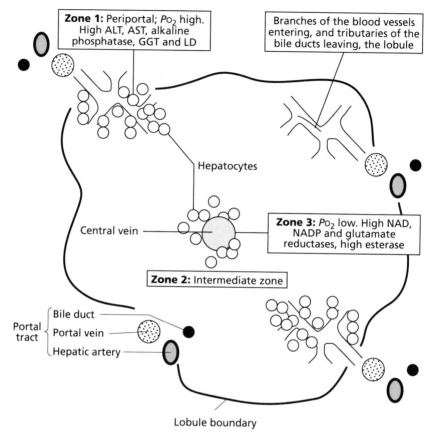

Fig. 8.1 A hepatic lobule, showing examples of the relative localization in the lobule of several enzymes. Hepatocytes are shown as small open circles; they are well oxygenated in zone 1, and relatively poorly oxygenated in zone 3. Cells in zone 2, the intermediate zone, are not shown.

Hepatocytes have many receptors on their plasma membrane; these are involved in the uptake and removal of many substances from the blood. They include receptors for LDL, glycoproteins and various organic anions (e.g. bilirubin, bile acids). Substances taken up by the liver may be metabolized or conjugated; some are excreted into bile.

Hepatocytes produce canalicular (hepatic) bile. The smallest radicles of the biliary tree are formed by fusion of the membranes of adjacent liver cells. There is a rapid one-way exchange between hepatocytes and newly secreted canalicular bile. Several substances undergo an enterohepatic circulation following biliary excretion (e.g. bile acids, urobilinogen, cholesterol). The hepatic transport systems for organic anions are very important. There are at least two systems, for the excretion of (i) bile acids and (ii) bilirubin, drugs, dyes (e.g. bromsulphthalein) and other anions.

Various substances, including bilirubin, many drugs, some hormones and carcinogens, are inactivated or detoxicated by the liver. For example, most steroid hormones are metabolized to inactive, water-soluble substances, and some carcinogens are conjugated. These products are excreted in the bile or in the urine.

'Liver function tests'

The history of a patient's illness and the findings on clinical examination, including the results of 'side-room' urine tests (p. 12), provide the essential basis on which to select chemical investigations for suspected liver disease and, more especially, the basis on which to interpret their results.

Many tests for assessing 'liver function' have been described but most laboratories perform a standard group consisting of plasma bilirubin, albumin and certain enzyme activity measurements (Table 8.1). This group of investigations does not assess genuine liver function but the tests are useful in detecting the presence of active hepatobiliary disease. Single tests, by themselves, are relatively non-specific and each may be abnormal in conditions other than liver disease. It is only when the results of *two or more biologically and physiologically independent tests* become abnormal that patterns begin to emerge which, taken together with clinical information and the results of 'side-room' tests, point with increasing certainty to the presence of liver disease.

Attempts have been made to develop chemical tests that genuinely assess liver function (e.g. plasma [bile acids]), but these are not widely used due to the wide availability of ultrasound, CT scanning and endoscopy. The chemical tests of 'liver function' described in this chapter are particularly valuable for:

1 Detecting the presence of liver disease.
2 Placing the liver disease into the appropriate broad diagnostic category.
3 Following the progress of liver disease.

Table 8.1 Routine groups of 'liver function tests' (examples of widely performed groups of plasma measurements)

Standard group of tests	Alternative or additional tests	Function or property being assessed
Plasma [albumin]		Protein synthesis
Plasma [bilirubin (total)]		Hepatic anion transport
Plasma enzyme activities		
ALT	AST	Hepatocellular integrity
Alkaline phosphatase	GGT	Presence of cholestasis

ALT, alanine aminotransferase; AST, aspartate aminotransferase; GGT, gamma-glutamyl transferase.

Notes
1 Many laboratories measure plasma alkaline phosphatase *and* GGT activities routinely as part of their group of 'liver function tests'. Some measure both plasma ALT and AST, and then calculate the ratio of the activities of these two enzymes in the specimen (this is sometimes called the de Ritis ratio).
2 In patients with symptoms or signs of hepatic dysfunction, liver-related tests additional to those routinely performed by the laboratory as 'liver function tests' may be indicated. Examples of extra tests are considered in the text.

Chemical investigations have their limitations, however, and are only rarely instrumental in pinpointing the diagnosis. 'Liver function tests' will be discussed under the following headings:

1   Hepatic anion transport, mainly concerned with bilirubin excretion.
2   Plasma protein abnormalities.
3   Plasma enzyme tests.
4   Miscellaneous chemical tests.

Hepatic anion transport: bilirubin excretion

About 80% of bilirubin formed from haem each day (400–500 µmol, 240–300 mg) arises from red cells; 1 g of haemoglobin gives rise to approximately 35 mg of bilirubin. The remaining 20% comes from red cell precursors destroyed in the bone marrow ('ineffective erythropoiesis'), and from other haem proteins such as myoglobin, the cytochromes and peroxidase. Iron is removed from the haem molecule and the porphyrin ring opened to form bilirubin. Bilirubin is soluble in lipid solvents but almost insoluble in water. These characteristics enable it to cross cell membranes readily, but special mechanisms are needed to make it water-soluble for carriage in plasma and excretion in bile.

Transport in plasma and hepatic uptake

Bilirubin is rendered soluble in plasma by protein-binding, mainly to albumin. In this form it does not readily enter most tissues, nor is it filtered at the glomerulus unless there is glomerular proteinuria. The bilirubin–albumin complex appears to be dissociated by the receptors on the plasma membrane of the hepatocytes; bilirubin is at the same time taken up, probably by a specific carrier mechanism, leaving albumin in the plasma. Liver cells contain several relatively non-specific anion-binding proteins. Of these, one family of proteins, the glutathione S-transferases, is thought to be particularly important.

Conjugation of bilirubin and secretion into bile

Conjugation of bilirubin within the hepatocyte makes it water-soluble. Three glucuronides (glucosiduronates) are formed by the action of bilirubin-UDP-glucuronyltransferase in the endoplasmic reticulum, two isomeric bilirubin mono-glucuronides and one diglucuronide. Secretion of bilirubin glucuronides into bile occurs against a high concentration gradient; a carrier-mediated energy-dependent process is probably involved. About 75% of bilirubin in bile consists of its diglucuronide, the rest being a mixture of the two monoglucuronides.

Further metabolism of bilirubin in the gut

After secretion into the intestine, bilirubin glucuronides are degraded by bacterial action, mainly in the colon, being deconjugated and then converted into a mixture of compounds collectively termed urobilinogen (alternatively, sometimes called stercobilinogen).

Urobilinogen (M_r, about 600 Da) is water-soluble. It is mostly excreted in the faeces but a small percentage is reabsorbed and then mostly re-excreted by the liver, one example of an enterohepatic circulation. After excretion, urobilinogen (which is colourless) oxidizes spontaneously to urobilin, which is brown. Some of the reabsorbed urobilinogen passes through the liver into the systemic circulation and is then excreted in the urine, where it can be detected by 'side-room' tests on *fresh* specimens of urine.

Measurements of plasma bilirubin (reference range, 2–17 μmol/L)

Plasma contains unconjugated lipid-soluble bilirubin which is being transported, bound to albumin, from the lymphoreticular system to the liver. It also contains a little conjugated water-soluble bilirubin, regurgitated from the liver into the plasma. Normally, more than 95% of bilirubin in plasma is unconjugated.

The chemical measurement most often performed is plasma or serum [total bilirubin], the sum of the unconjugated and conjugated forms. It is technically more difficult and time-consuming to measure plasma [conjugated bilirubin] and plasma [unconjugated bilirubin] separately. For most purposes, plasma [total bilirubin] is sufficient, especially when results are interpreted in relation to the patient's history and findings on clinical examination, and the results of 'side-room' tests on urine specimens for urobilinogen and bilirubin.

Table 8.2 summarizes the findings for bilirubin and urobilinogen measurements in the jaundiced patient.

Abnormalities of bilirubin metabolism

Clinical jaundice is nearly always attributable to hyperbilirubinaemia. It becomes apparent when the plasma [bilirubin] exceeds 50 μmol/L, but smaller degrees of hyperbilirubinaemia may be of diagnostic significance. Disorders of bilirubin metabolism can occur at several sites and it is convenient to consider them under three headings (Fig. 8.2).

Pre-hepatic hyperbilirubinaemia

Overproduction of bilirubin occurs in all forms of haemolytic anaemia and, less commonly, in conditions where there is much ineffective erythropoiesis (e.g.

Table 8.2 Bilirubin and urobilinogen measurements (examples of results in various conditions)

| | Urine tests ('side-room') | | Plasma [bilirubin] | |
Condition	Urobilinogen	Bilirubin	Total* (μmol/L)	Conjugated
Healthy individuals	Trace	Nil	2–17	About 5%
Gilbert's syndrome	Trace	Nil	< 50	Below 5%
Haemolytic diseases	Increased	Nil	< 60	Below 5%
Hepatitis				
Prodromal	Increased	Detectable	< 35	Raised
Icteric stage	Undetectable	Present	< 250	Much raised
Recovery stage	Detectable	Falling	Falling	Falling
Biliary obstruction	Undetectable	Present	< 400	Much raised

* Values for plasma [total bilirubin] are included so as to give indications of the order of severity of the hyperbilirubinaemia that may be observed in the various conditions listed.

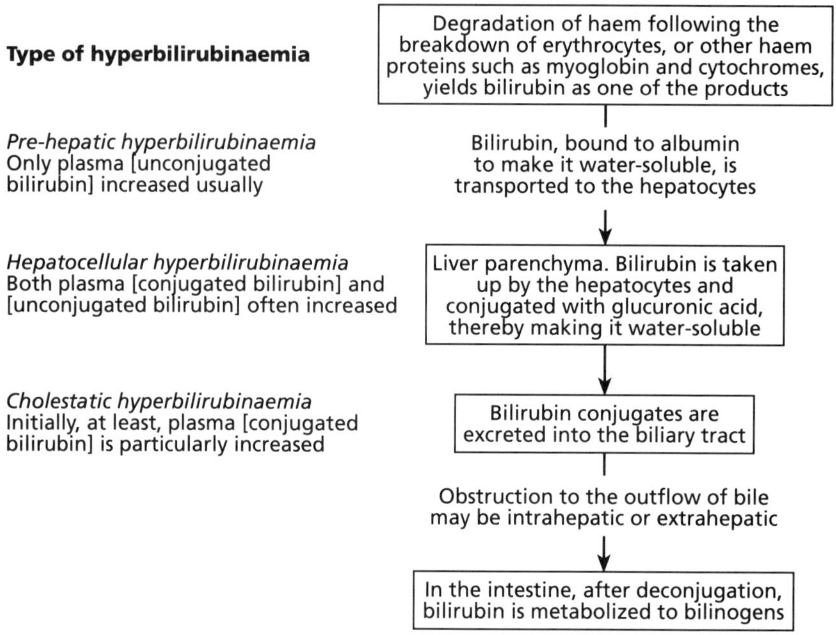

Type of hyperbilirubinaemia	

Degradation of haem following the breakdown of erythrocytes, or other haem proteins such as myoglobin and cytochromes, yields bilirubin as one of the products

Pre-hepatic hyperbilirubinaemia
Only plasma [unconjugated bilirubin] increased usually

Bilirubin, bound to albumin to make it water-soluble, is transported to the hepatocytes

Hepatocellular hyperbilirubinaemia
Both plasma [conjugated bilirubin] and [unconjugated bilirubin] often increased

Liver parenchyma. Bilirubin is taken up by the hepatocytes and conjugated with glucuronic acid, thereby making it water-soluble

Cholestatic hyperbilirubinaemia
Initially, at least, plasma [conjugated bilirubin] is particularly increased

Bilirubin conjugates are excreted into the biliary tract

Obstruction to the outflow of bile may be intrahepatic or extrahepatic

In the intestine, after deconjugation, bilirubin is metabolized to bilinogens

Fig. 8.2 The formation and metabolism of bilirubin, and its excretion into the intestine. A small percentage of the intestinal bilinogens is normally absorbed from the intestine.

pernicious anaemia). In haemolytic disease of the newborn due to rhesus incompatibility, if untreated, the concentration of lipid-soluble unconjugated bilirubin may reach sufficiently high levels in plasma for appreciable amounts to cross the blood–brain barrier, with resulting kernicterus (p. 333). However, for kernicterus to occur, there may also need to be damage to the blood–brain barrier. Pre-hepatic hyperbilirubinaemia is also sometimes due to bleeding into the tissues (e.g. sports injuries), and sometimes occurs in patients with rhabdomyolysis.

Hepatocellular hyperbilirubinaemia

Hepatic uptake of bilirubin may be abnormal in Gilbert's syndrome (see below). Uptake may also be abnormal in patients with hepatitis or cirrhosis. Plasma [unconjugated bilirubin] is increased.

Conjugation of bilirubin may be impaired in the newborn, especially in premature infants since bilirubin-UDP-glucuronyltransferase normally develops at about full term. Plasma [unconjugated bilirubin] is increased. Conjugation of bilirubin may also be abnormal in generalized hepatocellular damage (e.g. due to viral hepatitis, cirrhosis), in congenital deficiency of the conjugating enzyme (Gilbert's and Crigler–Najjar syndromes), and as a result of competitive inhibition of the conjugating enzyme (e.g. due to novobiocin).

Secretion of conjugated bilirubin into bile is abnormal in the Rotor and Dubin–Johnson syndromes (see below), and in generalized hepatocellular damage.

Hepatocellular damage (e.g. due to viral hepatitis, cirrhosis) may thus interfere with the uptake of bilirubin by the liver, or with its conjugation in the hepatocyte, or with the secretion of conjugated bilirubin into bile, or with all three processes.

Cholestatic hyperbilirubinaemia

General impairment of bilirubin metabolism is often associated with cholestasis. Cholestasis may be intrahepatic or extrahepatic; in both, there is conjugated hyperbilirubinaemia and bilirubinuria.

Intrahepatic cholestasis commonly occurs in acute hepatocellular damage (e.g. due to infectious hepatitis), cirrhosis and intrahepatic carcinoma. It may also be due to drugs (e.g. methyltestosterone, phenothiazines), or to primary biliary cirrhosis.

Extrahepatic cholestasis is most often due to gallstones or carcinoma of the head of the pancreas or of the biliary tree.

The congenital hyperbilirubinaemias

These are all due to inherited defects in the mechanism of bilirubin transport.

Gilbert's syndrome

This familial condition is inherited as an autosomal dominant trait and is probably present in 2–3% of men; it is two to seven times more common in men than in women. Usually there is an asymptomatic, mild, unconjugated hyperbilirubinaemia but a variety of non-specific symptoms (e.g. abdominal discomfort, fatigue, malaise) may be present. The plasma [bilirubin] fluctuates, higher levels tending to occur during intercurrent illness. Most patients have a plasma [bilirubin] less than 50 μmol/L but higher levels are not uncommon. Other commonly performed tests of 'liver function' are normal and there is no bilirubinuria.

The defect is complex and has not been defined precisely, but in many cases there is both an abnormality of hepatic uptake of bilirubin and a mild deficiency of bilirubin-UDP-glucuronyltransferase; the uptake defect is probably secondary to the enzyme deficiency. Patients with Gilbert's syndrome are unable to metabolize some drugs normally. Their plasma [bile acids], however, are normal and this measurement (not often available) is the best test for differentiating Gilbert's syndrome from hyperbilirubinaemia due to hepatic disease.

Gilbert's syndrome can be differentiated from the mild degree of hyperbilirubinaemia in haemolytic anaemia, and from the mild jaundice of some patients with hepatic disease, by haematological investigations or by observing the effects on plasma [unconjugated bilirubin] of (i) a reduced energy intake or (ii) an injection of nicotinic acid:

1 *Reduced energy intake* (1.67 MJ/day; 400 cal/day), particularly a reduction in the intake of lipids, for 72 hours results in at least a doubling of plasma [unconjugated bilirubin] in patients with Gilbert's syndrome. In normal individuals, it does not rise above 25 μmol/L. Usually no increase is seen in patients with haemolytic anaemia. However, in hepatitis there is an increase similar to the rise seen in Gilbert's syndrome.

2 *Nicotinic acid test.* After intravenous injection of nicotinic acid (50 mg), plasma [unconjugated bilirubin] normally rises to a maximum value within 90 minutes. In patients with Gilbert's syndrome, it rises to more than twice the basal level; the peak occurs after 2–3 hours.

Crigler–Najjar syndrome

This rare condition gives rise to severe hyperbilirubinaemia in neonates, leading to kernicterus and often to early death. The unconjugated hyperbilirubinaemia is due to very low activity of bilirubin-UDP-glucuronyltransferase.

Dubin–Johnson syndrome and Rotor syndrome

These are characterized by a benign conjugated hyperbilirubinaemia, accompanied by bilirubinuria. In both, there is a defect in the transfer of conjugated bilirubin into the biliary canaliculus. The mechanisms of these defects are not known.

Urinary coproporphyrins are normal in patients with the Dubin–Johnson syndrome, but increased in Rotor syndrome. The response to bromsulphthalein injection is different in the two syndromes (see below).

Other tests of hepatic anion transport function

Plasma bile acids are secreted as their conjugates into bile. They are normally

---

Case 8.1

A 13-year-old was taken by his mother to see their general practitioner because he had been running a temperature (38°C) and for the past 2 days had been complaining that his muscles ached. On examination, the doctor found that the boy was pyrexial (38.4°C) and that he appeared to be jaundiced. There was no abdominal pain or tenderness, no lymphadenopathy or enlargement of either liver or spleen, and no obvious signs of muscle tenderness. 'Side-room' tests on urine showed that the urobilinogen content was normal, and there was no bilirubin detectable in the specimen. The doctor requested 'liver function tests', the results of which were:

Plasma analysis	Result	Reference range	Units
[Albumin]	45	36–47	g/L
Alkaline phosphatase activity	180	40–125	IU/L
ALT activity	30	10–40	IU/L
[Bilirubin, total]	60	2–17	μmol/L
GGT activity	35	10–55	IU/L

Five days later, the boy had recovered. He no longer had pyrexia and his jaundice had gone (plasma [bilirubin], 30 μmol/L); his alkaline phosphatase activity was still 175 IU/L. The reticulocyte count and other haematology investigations had all been normal on both occasions. What is the most likely diagnosis, and how would you explain the abnormal results among the 'liver function tests'? This patient is discussed on p. 123.

mainly absorbed from the terminal ileum into the portal bloodstream from which they are rapidly cleared by the liver. Bile acids undergo an enterohepatic circulation round which approximately 60 mmol (30 g) bile acids circulate each day. If available, measurement of fasting or post-prandial plasma [bile acids], particularly conjugated cholate, is a very sensitive test of hepatic anion transport function. Increased plasma [bile acids] occur in patients with liver disease.

Bromsulphthalein (BSP) is an anionic dye still occasionally used to test hepatic anion transport function in unjaundiced or selected, mildly jaundiced, patients (e.g. Dubin–Johnson, Rotor syndromes). After intravenous injection, BSP is bound to albumin and is normally cleared rapidly by the liver. In patients with the Dubin–Johnson syndrome, the rate of clearance of BSP is impaired. Also, instead of plasma [BSP] falling progressively, a secondary rise in plasma [BSP] occurs about 90 minutes after the injection. In patients with the Rotor syndrome, the rate of clearance is also impaired but there is no secondary rise in plasma [BSP]. The test is not entirely free from risk, and many hospitals no longer perform it.

Plasma protein abnormalities

Albumin

The capacity of the hepatocyte to synthesize albumin is impaired in many patients with liver disease. In chronic hepatocellular damage, plasma [albumin] falls and, in the later stages, provides a fairly good index of the progress of the disease. In acute liver disease, however, there may be little or no reduction in plasma [albumin] as the biological half-life of albumin is about 20 days and the fractional clearance rate is therefore low. Factors other than impaired hepatic synthesis may lead to a decreased plasma [albumin], including loss of albumin into the extravascular compartment and ascites, increased degradation and poor nutritional status (p. 89).

Increased portal venous pressure combined with a low plasma colloid oncotic pressure, together with Na^+ retention due to secondary hyperaldosteronism, leads to the formation of ascites in cirrhotic patients. Ascites (p. 122) usually develops in patients with portal hypertension, when plasma [albumin] falls below 30 g/L.

Coagulation factors

Multiple defects occur in liver disease. In patients with hepatocellular damage, plasma [prothrombin] is often decreased. It is, however, unusual to measure coagulation factors individually in these patients. Instead, measurements of the *prothrombin time* (usually performed in haematology departments) often suffice. This may be prolonged due to:

1   Deficiency of fat-soluble vitamin K due to failure of absorption of lipids, caused by cholestasis (p. 236).

2   Failure to synthesize one or more of the coagulation factors collectively measured by the prothrombin time, due to hepatocellular damage.

In vitamin K deficiency the coagulation defect can often be corrected by parenteral administration of vitamin K, but this has no effect in hepatocellular damage. The prothrombin time becomes prolonged relatively late in hepatic disease. However, it then alters rapidly as the fractional turnover rates of the coagulation factors are short. The prothrombin time can be used to assess progress and prognosis in patients with acute hepatocellular failure.

Other plasma proteins

Plasma immunoglobulin (Ig) measurements are of little value in liver disease because the changes are of low specificity. In acute liver disease abnormalities are inconstant, but in chronic liver disease there is usually an overall increase in plasma [Ig]. In most types of cirrhosis, plasma [IgA] is moderately increased and there are usually smaller increases in plasma [IgG] and [IgM]. In primary biliary cirrhosis, however, plasma [IgM] increases greatly but the increases in plasma [IgG] and [IgA] are much smaller, and in chronic active hepatitis plasma [IgG] tends to be most increased.

Ceruloplasmin, α_1-protease inhibitor (API) and cholinesterase provide other examples of proteins synthesized in the liver that are all able to be measured specifically. Their concentrations fall when there is hepatocellular dysfunction. As tests of the liver's ability to synthesize proteins, however, their measurement offers no advantage over plasma albumin.

Serum protein electrophoresis

Abnormal patterns often occur in liver disease reflecting the composite effect of changes in the concentrations of individual serum proteins. In cirrhosis, for example, serum [albumin] is reduced and there is a polyclonal increase in serum [γ-globulin]; there is also filling of the trough between the β- and the γ-globulins, due to an increase in the electrophoretically fast-moving IgA fraction. In cholestasis, increases in serum [γ-globulin] are smaller, but there are increases in the concentrations of α- and β-globulins, due in part to increased concentrations of the serum lipoproteins.

It is doubtful whether much diagnostic information derives from serum protein electrophoresis in patients with liver disease, except in API deficiency (p. 90) where there is often a reduced α_1-globulin band. However, specific measurement of plasma [API] is preferable.

Plasma enzyme tests in liver disease

Three patterns of altered plasma enzyme activity may be seen in patients with liver disease, due to the following derangements:

1 Release of soluble cytoplasmic enzymes and, to a lesser extent, mitochondrial enzymes. This occurs in hepatocellular damage.

2 Release of membrane-associated enzymes. This occurs in cholestasis.

3 Impaired synthesis of certain enzymes (e.g. cholinesterase), when hepatocellular function is greatly impaired. This group of measurements is rarely used for assessing the severity of liver disease.

Soluble cytoplasmic and mitochondrial enzymes

Aminotransferase (either ALT or AST) activity measurements are included in the standard group of 'liver function tests' performed in most hospital laboratories.

They are sensitive tests of hepatocellular damage, and continue to be widely used even though some other plasma enzymes (e.g. alpha-class glutathione S-transferase) have been shown to be more specific and, in some reports, more sensitive indices of liver damage. Aminotransferases continue to be measured because of their analytical convenience and simplicity but, since they are mainly located in the periportal hepatocytes, they do not give a reliable indication of centrilobular liver damage.

Plasma ALT measurements are more liver-specific than AST (Table 6.1, p. 73) and increases in ALT activity are usually greater than AST in early hepatocellular disease. Aspartate aminotransferase has both cytoplasmic and mitochondrial isoenzymes and tends to be released more than ALT in chronic hepatocellular disease (e.g. cirrhosis).

Membrane-associated enzymes

Many enzymes are 'anchored' to cell membranes. Those anchored to the biliary canaliculus include alkaline phosphatase and gamma-glutamyl transferase (GGT). 'Anchorages' take the form of hydrophobic domains in the enzyme's polypeptide chain, inserted into the lipid membrane. Circumstances facilitating release from the membrane vary from enzyme to enzyme and are not fully understood. However, it seems that detergent action (e.g. bile acids) and pro-teolytic action (e.g. intracellular proteases removing the 'anchor peptide') may both play a part.

Because they are firmly anchored to the membrane, alkaline phosphatase and GGT tend to be released into plasma only in small amounts following hepatocel-lular damage. However, they are released in much greater amounts when there is cholestasis, since their synthesis is induced in these circumstances and they are rendered soluble prior to regurgitation. Plasma activities of both these enzymes may be greatly increased if the bile duct draining a lobe or lobule of the liver is obstructed (p. 119).

Alkaline phosphatase is included in a standard group of 'liver function tests' by almost all hospital laboratories. Changes in the activities of most of the other membrane-associated enzymes usually accompany the changes in plasma alkaline phosphatase in cholestatic liver disease. Plasma GGT activity, however, provides a more sensitive index of cholestasis than alkaline phosphatase, and has the advantage of being more liver-specific as plasma alkaline phosphatase may also be increased if there is bone disease; some laboratories include both alkaline phos-phatase and GGT in their routine group of 'liver function tests'.

Miscellaneous chemical tests

Tests of metabolic capacity

The clearance of certain substances from the blood is dependent on the metabolic capacity of the liver. Tests which have been developed to assess metabolic capacity include the galactose or caffeine clearance tests and the aminopyrine breath test. None of these tests is widely used but each provides a good index of functional liver volume.

Tests for the presence of hepatic fibrosis

Chronic liver disease is usually accompanied by increased collagen deposition in the space of Disse and the formation of basement membranes beneath the endothelial cell layer. These events, coupled with excessive production of other proteins such as fibronectin and proteoglycans, lead to the development of fibrosis and impairment of the metabolic functions of the liver together with alterations in blood flow.

At least 10 types of collagen occur in the body, but types I and III comprise approximately one-third of the total hepatic collagen. Type I and type III collagens are synthesized as 'procollagens' that contain additional C-terminal and N-terminal peptides which are removed by specific proteases and released into the circulation when procollagen is converted to collagen.

Measurement of the N-terminal peptide of procollagen type III in plasma by radioimmunoassay provides a non-invasive method of monitoring the extent of fibrotic change. However, the test is not specific as increased plasma [N-terminal peptide] occurs in many other diseases including rheumatoid arthritis, myelofibrosis, Paget's disease and various malignancies.

Desialated transferrin

In patients with alcohol-induced liver disease, transferrin in plasma has a reduced sialic acid content. Plasma [desialated transferrin] is increased in about 90% of patients who drink more than 60 g alcohol per day, according to some reports.

Disordered nitrogen metabolism

There is ineffective conversion of amino acids and ammonia to urea in patients with severe liver disease. As a result, plasma [amino acids] may be increased and there may then be generalized (overflow) amino aciduria (p. 132). However, these tests do not have sufficient diagnostic or prognostic value to justify their performance as 'liver function tests' in these patients.

Plasma [ammonia] increases in patients with acute hepatocellular failure and with portal-systemic encephalopathy complicating hepatic cirrhosis. Reliable measurement of plasma [NH_3] is difficult and this has limited the use of this test; results tend to correlate poorly with other indices of acute hepatic decompensation.

Significant decreases in plasma [urea] may occur late in hepatic disease, due to failure of the liver to convert amino acids and NH_3 to urea. There are, however, other causes of a low plasma [urea] (Table 9.2, p. 127); patients with liver disease are sometimes maintained for long periods on diets low in protein and high in carbohydrate, so a falling plasma [urea] in a patient with liver disease may not be a sign of deteriorating hepatic function.

Disordered carbohydrate metabolism

Hypoglycaemia may occur in severe liver disease due to impaired gluconeogenesis or glycogen breakdown, or both. However, measurements of plasma [glucose] are of little value in the diagnosis of liver disease.

Disordered lipid metabolism

In cholestatic syndromes the concentrations of all the plasma lipid fractions are frequently raised. In contrast to most other causes of hyperlipidaemia, plasma [phospholipids] are increased at least as much as plasma [cholesterol] and [triglycerides].

An abnormal lipoprotein, *lipoprotein X*, is present in plasma in nearly all cases of cholestasis. Its mechanism of production is poorly understood. It is not found in healthy people and is rarely present in patients with hepatocellular damage unless there is cholestasis also.

Serological tests

Anti-mitochondrial antibodies are present in over 95% of patients with primary biliary cirrhosis, and anti-smooth muscle antibodies are found in about 50% of patients with chronic active hepatitis.

The place of chemical tests in the diagnosis of liver disease

The jaundiced patient (Fig. 8.3)

'Side-room' tests (p. 15) on fresh urine specimens, for bilirubin and urobilinogen, can be a great help in the investigation of patients suspected of having liver disease, especially if the patient is jaundiced. They should always be performed as

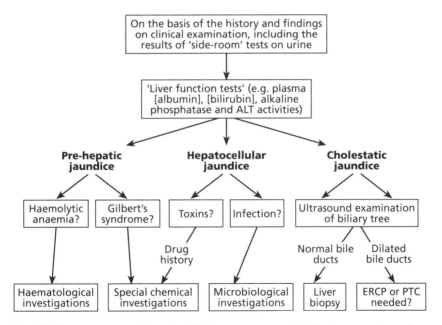

Fig. 8.3 The investigation of jaundice. Endoscopic retrograde cholangiopancreatography (ERCP) or percutaneous trans-hepatic cholangiography (PTC) may be needed whenever the cause of dilated bile ducts is uncertain.

Table 8.3 Hepatocellular damage and cholestasis (plasma or serum measurements that may help to differentiate between these conditions)

| Investigation | Hepatocellular damage | | Cholestasis |
	Acute	Chronic	
Albumin	N or ↓	N, ↓ or ↓↓	N or ↓
Bilirubin (total)	N, ↑ or ↑↑	N or ↑	N* ↑ or ↑↑
Aminotransferases	↑↑ or ↑↑↑	N or ↑	↑
Alkaline phosphatase	N or ↑	N or ↑	↑↑
GGT	N or ↑	N or ↑	↑↑
Immunoglobulins	N or ↑	↑ (Note 1)	↑ (Note 2)
Lipoprotein X	Not present unless there is cholestasis		Present
Prothrombin time (PT)	N or ↑	N or ↑	N or ↑
Effect of parenteral vitamin K on PT	None	None	May correct PT

N, normal; ↑, increased; ↑↑ and ↑↑↑, much increased and very much increased, respectively; ↓, decreased; ↓↓, much decreased. N* indicates that plasma [bilirubin] is often normal when cholestasis is localized, as it often is with secondary deposits in the liver.

Notes
1 Plasma [IgA] is particularly increased in cirrhosis, and plasma [IgG] in chronic active hepatitis.
2 Plasma [IgM] is increased in primary biliary cirrhosis.

early in the illness as possible, and their results interpreted in relation to the history of the illness and the findings on clinical examination. Where jaundice is present, these tests help to categorize the hyperbilirubinaemia into pre-hepatic, hepatocellular, and cholestatic (post-hepatic) jaundice.

Measurements of plasma [bilirubin] give a quantitative index of its severity. There are many causes of jaundice and it is important to differentiate between them; plasma enzyme activity measurements are very important in this respect (Table 8.3).

Acute hepatitis

In the pre-icteric phase of infectious hepatitis and serum hepatitis, plasma ALT and AST activities are increased and may be the only abnormal chemical findings, developing before increased amounts of urobilinogen are present and before bilirubin becomes detectable in the urine. By the time clinical jaundice appears, plasma ALT and AST activities are usually more than six times, and occasionally more than 100 times, the upper reference value; plasma ALT activity is usually increased to a relatively greater extent than AST. The stools may be very pale, due to impaired biliary excretion of bilirubin, and urobilinogen then disappears more or less completely from the urine. Alkaline phosphatase activity is usually only slightly increased, up to about twice the upper reference value, but it may be considerably raised in those cases (relatively uncommon) where there is a marked cholestatic element, as often occurs in acute alcoholic hepatitis.

Acute viral hepatitis usually resolves quickly, and chemical indices of abnormality revert to normal within a few weeks. However, chronic persistent hepatitis occurs in a few patients, in whom plasma aminotransferase activities and plasma [bile acids] may remain high for months.

Findings similar to those in acute viral hepatitis are observed in patients with hepatocellular toxicity due to drugs (e.g. paracetamol overdosage, halothane jaundice, carbon tetrachloride poisoning).

Cholestasis

This is most often due to extrahepatic obstruction. Intrahepatic cholestatis may be prolonged and severe, especially when due to primary biliary cirrhosis or drugs such as the phenothiazines. Relatively benign and short-lasting intrahepatic cholestasis sometimes occurs in pregnancy.

Plasma [bilirubin] is often greatly increased and there is marked bilirubinuria; urobilinogen often becomes undetectable in urine. Plasma alkaline phosphatase activity is considerably increased, often to more than three times the upper reference value, but plasma ALT and AST activities are usually only moderately raised. In long-standing cholestatic jaundice, hepatic protein synthesis may be impaired and plasma alkaline phosphatase activity may start to fall as a result, and even return to normal; this emphasizes the importance of performing a baseline set of investigations as early as possible in patients with liver disease.

Alkaline phosphatase and GGT activities may be markedly increased in plasma in the presence of only minor degrees of cholestasis. For instance, in patients with *partial biliary obstruction* due to obstruction to one of the smaller biliary ducts, such as often occurs in both primary and secondary carcinoma of the liver, higher concentrations of alkaline phosphatase and GGT occur in the part of the liver normally drained by the obstructed bile duct, due to induction of enzyme synthesis. Partial biliary obstruction may have little or no effect on the capacity of the liver to excrete bilirubin, so there may be no evidence of jaundice in these patients, at least initially; bilirubin excretion in the other parts of the liver may be able to compensate fully for the sector affected by the local biliary obstruction.

Plasma protein concentrations do not show characteristic changes in cholestasis except for the increase in plasma [IgM] seen in primary biliary cirrhosis. Plasma [albumin] tends to fall, especially if cholestasis is prolonged. Plasma lipids show a variable increase in cholesterol, triglyceride and phospholipid concentrations. Lipoprotein X is usually demonstrable.

Chemical features that may help to distinguish cholestasis from hepatocellular damage are summarized in Table 8.3. It should be emphasized that these are 'typical' findings. Many cases do not follow these patterns exactly. The distinction between intrahepatic and extrahepatic cholestasis can rarely be made by chemical tests; it is usually made by radiological investigations or by liver biopsy.

Infiltrations of the liver

The liver parenchyma may be progressively disorganized and destroyed by a wide variety of pathological conditions that can loosely be described as 'infiltrations'. These include multiple deposits of secondary carcinoma (e.g. lung, stomach), amyloidosis, the reticuloses, tuberculosis, sarcoidosis and abscesses.

'Infiltrations' are often characterized, in terms of their effects on the liver, by finding considerably increased plasma alkaline phosphatase (hepatic isoenzyme) and GGT activities in the presence of normal or only slightly increased plasma [bilirubin]. This is due to enzyme induction as a result of cholestasis locally in parts of the liver where the infiltration has prevented excretion of bile. Plasma ALT and AST activities may be normal or slightly increased. Measurement of plasma [AFP] is of value if hepatoma is suspected; it is often greatly increased with hepatoma.

Cirrhosis of the liver

Alcoholism, viral hepatitis and prolonged cholestasis are thought to be the most frequent known causes of cirrhosis in Britain, but in half the cases no obvious cause is found. Less often, cirrhosis is associated with metabolic disorders such as Wilson's disease (see below), cystic fibrosis (p. 335), API deficiency (p. 90), haemochromatosis (p. 220), or galactosaemia (p. 179).

It is convenient to divide cirrhosis into mild and severe cases. In mild cases no clinical abnormalities may be apparent due to the reserve functional capacity of the liver; in these cases the term 'compensated cirrhosis' is sometimes used. In severe cases, haematemesis may occur and various clinical features including ascites may be present; acute hepatic decompensation may arise and often proves fatal.

Mild or latent cirrhosis. Plasma [bile acids] are likely to be abnormal more frequently than other tests. However, these measurements are not often available; instead, plasma GGT activity measurements are widely used. Although GGT measurements provide a sensitive means of detecting mild cirrhosis, most heavy drinkers (many of whom do *not* have cirrhosis of the liver) have raised plasma GGT activities; these mostly fall within 2 months of stopping drinking. Plasma aminotransferase and alkaline phosphatase activities are less often increased at this stage, while plasma [bilirubin] is usually below 25 µmol/L. Alterations in plasma [albumin] and [Ig] are rarely present when cirrhosis is mild or latent.

More severe cirrhosis. Jaundice may develop and plasma [albumin] falls, the prothrombin time becomes abnormal and plasma [Ig] increases. Clinical deterioration accompanied by prolonged prothrombin time, a generalized amino aciduria, increased plasma [NH_3] and reduced plasma [urea] may herald the development of acute hepatic failure.

Copper in liver disease

The liver is the principal organ involved in copper metabolism. The amount it contains is maintained at normal levels by excretion of copper in bile and by incorporation into ceruloplasmin (p. 92). The liver's copper content is increased in Wilson's disease, primary biliary cirrhosis, prolonged extrahepatic cholestasis, and intrahepatic bile duct atresia in the neonate. Increased liver [copper] may be a factor in the continuing hepatic damage that occurs in primary biliary cirrhosis.

Wilson's disease (hepatolenticular degeneration) is a rare, hereditary, autosomal recessive disorder with a prevalence of about one in 30 000. Copper is deposited in many tissues including the liver, brain and kidney. Symptoms are mainly due to liver disease and to degenerative changes in the basal ganglia. The

Case 8.2

A 40-year-old housewife complained to her general practitioner of generalized severe itching for the previous 9 months. She had no other symptoms and she said that her consumption of alcohol was small (2–3 units/week). On clinical examination she was found to be slightly jaundiced, and bilirubin was detected in the urine on 'side-room' testing. 'Liver function tests' were requested, and gave the following results:

Plasma analysis	Result	Reference range	Units
[Albumin]	38	36–47	g/L
Alkaline phosphatase activity	450	40–125	IU/L
ALT activity	60	10–40	IU/L
[Bilirubin, total]	60	2–17	μmol/L
GGT activity	150	5–35	IU/L

How would you interpret these results? This patient is discussed on p. 123.

biochemical defect has not been precisely defined but the liver is unable to excrete copper in normal amounts into the bile. Plasma [ceruloplasmin] is nearly always low but it is not clear how this relates to the aetiology of Wilson's disease.

The diagnosis may be suspected from the family history or on clinical grounds, such as liver disease in patients less than 20 years old, or characteristic neurological disease. Kayser–Fleischer rings, due to the deposition of copper in the cornea, can be detected in most patients. The following chemical tests may be valuable:

1 *Plasma [ceruloplasmin]*. This is usually less than 200 mg/L, and often below 100 mg/L (reference range, 250–450 mg/L).

2 *Plasma [copper]*. This is usually less than 12 μmol/L (reference range, 12–26 μmol/L).

3 *Urinary copper output*. This is always more than 1.0 μmol/24 hours (normally below 0.5 μmol/24 hours).

4 *Liver [copper]* is always raised. This is the most sensitive test, but it involves liver biopsy and may only be required when investigating patients with a positive family history.

These tests are not 100% specific for Wilson's disease. For example, plasma [ceruloplasmin] may occasionally be low in severe cirrhosis and urinary copper output and liver [copper] may be raised in biliary cirrhosis. However, urinary copper output is valuable for case-finding among relatives since a normal result virtually excludes Wilson's disease.

Abnormalities of other chemical tests are often present in Wilson's disease, e.g. increased plasma [bilirubin] and aminotransferase activities. There is usually evidence of renal tubular damage, with a generalized (overflow) amino aciduria. There may also be glucosuria and phosphaturia and, in advanced cases, renal tubular acidosis.

Alcoholic liver disease

Chronic over-indulgence in ethanol is a common cause of hepatic cirrhosis. Ethanol is metabolized by alcohol dehydrogenase, catalase and an NADP-dependent microsomal enzyme oxidizing system (MEOS). The relative importance of these enzymes varies, depending on the blood [ethanol] and on the length of any period of chronic over-indulgence.

Blood [ethanol] is worth measuring in patients in whom the differential diagnosis includes alcohol abuse. Ethanol is not normally present in blood (except in trace amounts) unless some has been drunk recently, but a negative result does not exclude the diagnosis. For the diagnosis of alcoholism, the American National Council on Alcoholism has proposed as criteria the finding of blood [ethanol] greater than 65 mmol/L (300 mg/100 mL) at any time, or greater than 33 mmol/L in the absence of symptoms.

Plasma enzyme activity measurements have been widely used as pointers to the diagnosis of chronic alcohol abuse, notably plasma GGT; alcohol induces the synthesis of GGT by the liver. As a single test for the recognition of chronic alcohol abuse, plasma GGT lacks sensitivity, but its diagnostic value can be increased by measuring the mean cell volume of erythrocytes (MCV) also. The finding of both a slight macrocytosis and an increased plasma GGT activity provides probably the best routinely available combination of measurements for detecting alcohol abuse. These tests are better at ruling out alcohol abuse, but only have moderate sensitivity (30–40%) for detecting it. As neither test is specific for this latter purpose, a diagnosis of alcohol abuse should not be made hastily even when both tests yield abnormal results.

Measurement of plasma [desialated transferrin] may prove to be a useful indicator of alcoholic liver disease. Chronic ethanol abuse is one of the commonest causes of increased fasting plasma [triglycerides], and plasma [urate] may also be increased.

Chronic over-indulgence in ethanol may produce these and other chemical abnormalities, but the diagnosis is likely to depend greatly on the history and clinical examination, unless blood [ethanol] is measured and found to be abnormal.

Disulfiram (antabuse) is sometimes prescribed as treatment for alcoholism. In these patients, the laboratory may be called upon to check the patient's compliance, by measuring blood [ethanol] and examining the urine for disulfiram metabolites.

Drugs and the liver

Drug therapy with potentially hepatotoxic agents may cause increased plasma enzyme activities before any other abnormalities are apparent. This applies to drugs, such as iproniazid which causes raised plasma ALT and AST activities. It also applies to drugs that may cause cholestasis, such as chlorpromazine; in this case, the activities of alkaline phosphatase and GGT in plasma are particularly increased. Plasma GGT is also increased in patients treated with phenytoin, phenobarbitone and other barbiturates, and certain other drugs; as with chronic alcoholics, these increases are all due, at least partly, to liver enzyme induction.

Ascites

Several measurements, including plasma [albumin], [bilirubin], aminotransferase and GGT activities tend to be performed routinely in any patient who develops ascites, as liver disease is the commonest cause. If a diagnostic paracentesis is performed, the appearance of the fluid (blood-stained, bile-stained, milky, etc.) should be noted and fluid [total protein] determined.

Ascites with a fluid [protein] less than 30 g/L is called a *transudate*. It is usually associated with non-infective causes such as uncomplicated cirrhosis, in which there is a combination of back-pressure effects and low plasma [albumin]. However, fluid [protein] may be greater in some of these patients, and 30 g/L is not a reliable diagnostic cut-off point.

Ascites with a fluid [protein] much in excess of 30 g/L is called an *exudate*. It usually indicates the presence of infective conditions such as tuberculous peritonitis, or malignant disease or pancreatic disease. If pancreatic disease is thought to be the cause, fluid amylase activity should be measured; a sero-sanguinous fluid with a high amylase activity will help to confirm the diagnosis. If hepatoma is suspected, plasma and ascitic fluid [AFP] may both be considerably increased.

Chemical investigations are generally relatively non-specific and of minor importance in the examination of ascitic fluid. Bacteriological and cytological examinations are likely to be much more informative. This generalization is also true for pleural fluid, where again the most frequently performed chemical measurement is the determination of fluid [total protein], to help differentiate between a transudate and an exudate.

Comments on Case 8.1 (p. 112)

This patient has Gilbert's syndrome. This was revealed when he developed a flu-like illness and went off his food. Caloric restriction in these patients can be used as a test to unmask the latent mild hyperbilirubinaemia. The absence of bilirubin in the urine showed that the hyperbilirubinaemia was due to increased plasma [unconjugated billirubin], and the normal reticulocyte count excluded haemolytic anaemia as the cause. The alkaline phosphatase activity, which was elevated in relation to the reference range quoted by the laboratory that performed the analyses (a range applicable to adults), is normal for a child of this age (Table 21.1, p. 322) and in keeping with this stage in the patient's development; the plasma GGT activity was normal, which helped to confirm this explanation.

Comments on Case 8.2 (p. 121)

This patient had cholestatic jaundice. Her pruritus was caused by the retention of bile salts. The presence of serum anti-mitochondrial antibodies in high titre indicated that the diagnosis was primary biliary cirrhosis, one of the causes of intrahepatic cholestasis. Retention of bile salts within the liver is liable to cause hepatocellular damage, which could account in this patient for the increased plasma ALT activity.

Chapter 9
Renal Disease

Many diseases affect renal function. In some, several functions are affected; in others, there is selective impairment of glomerular function or of one or more tubular functions. Most types of renal disease cause destruction of complete nephrons; this is particularly true for chronic renal disease. It has been suggested, therefore, that alterations in renal function can be most readily explained on the basis of the remaining nephrons being functionally normal but overloaded. This 'intact nephron hypothesis' is almost certainly an over-simplification.

Chemical investigations, including 'side-room' tests (p. 14), are mainly of value in detecting the presence of renal disease by its effects on renal function, and in assessing its progress. They are of less value in determining the causes of disease.

Glomerular function

The glomerular filtration rate (GFR) depends on the net pressure across the glomerular membrane, the physical nature of the membrane and its surface area, which reflects the numbers of functioning glomeruli. All three factors may be modified by disease but, in the absence of large changes in blood pressure or in the structure of the glomerular membrane, the GFR provides a useful index of the numbers of functioning glomeruli. It gives an estimate of the degree of renal impairment by disease. Until recently, GFR was most often assessed by determining urinary creatinine clearance; latterly, measurements of plasma [creatinine] have largely replaced creatinine clearance measurements.

Plasma creatinine (reference range, 55–120 μmol/L, in adults)

Creatine is synthesized in the liver, kidneys and pancreas. It is transported to its sites of usage, principally muscle and brain. About 1–2% of the total muscle creatine pool is converted daily to creatinine through the spontaneous, non-enzymic loss of water. Creatinine is an end-product of nitrogen metabolism.

Creatinine in the plasma is filtered unchanged freely at the glomerulus. A small amount undergoes tubular reabsorption whilst a larger amount, up to 10% of urinary creatinine, results from tubular secretion. Although endogenous production of urea may rise sharply following a protein-containing meal, under normal circumstances plasma [creatinine] remains fairly constant unless renal glomerular function changes.

Low plasma creatinine (Table 9.1)

Creatinine production is determined by the size of the creatine pool. Hence, a

Table 9.1 Causes of an abnormal plasma [creatinine]

Reduced plasma [creatinine]	
Physiological	Pregnancy
Pathological	Reduced muscle bulk (e.g. starvation, wasting diseases, steroid therapy)
Increased plasma [creatinine]	
No pathological significance	High meat intake, strenuous exercise
	Drug effects (e.g. salicylates)
	Analytical interference (e.g. due to cephalosporin antibiotics)
Pathological	Renal causes, i.e. any cause (acute or chronic) of a reduced GFR

smaller muscle mass leads to lower daily creatinine production, and vice versa. A low plasma [creatinine] may therefore be found in children and values are, on average, normally lower in women than in men. Abnormally low values may be found in wasting diseases and starvation, and in patients treated with corticosteroids due to their protein catabolic effect.

Creatinine production is increased in pregnancy, but this is more than offset by the combined effects of the retention of fluid and the physiological rise in GFR that occur in pregnancy, so plasma [creatinine] is usually low.

High plasma creatinine (Table 9.1)

Increased muscle bulk elevates plasma [creatinine]. Other *non-renal causes* of increased plasma [creatinine] include:

1 *High meat intake*: this can cause a temporary increase.

2 *Exercise*: transient, small increases may occur after vigorous exercise.

3 *Analytical overestimation*: some analytical methods are not specific for creatinine; they also measure endogenous and exogenous interfering substances. For example, if plasma [acetoacetate] or [pyruvate] is increased, or if certain cephalosporin antibiotics are administered, with some methods plasma [creatinine] will be overestimated.

4 *Drugs*: some drugs (e.g. salicylates, cimetidine) compete with creatinine for the tubular transport mechanism, thereby reducing tubular secretion of creatinine and elevating plasma [creatinine].

If non-renal causes can be excluded, the finding of an increased plasma [creatinine] indicates a fall in GFR. The *renal causes* of this include:

1 Any disease in which there is impaired renal perfusion (e.g. reduced blood pressure, fluid depletion, renal artery stenosis).

2 Most diseases in which there is loss of functioning nephrons (e.g. acute and chronic glomerulonephritis).

3 Diseases where pressure is increased on the tubular side of the nephron (e.g. urinary tract obstruction due to prostatic enlargement).

Creatinine clearance or plasma creatinine?

Accurate measurement of the GFR by clearance tests requires determination of the concentrations, in plasma and urine, of a substance that is filtered at the glomerulus, but which is neither reabsorbed nor secreted by the tubules; its concentration in plasma needs to remain constant throughout the period of urine collection. It is convenient if the substance is present endogenously, and important for it to be readily measured.

Creatinine only meets some of these criteria. Its concentration may not remain constant over the period of urine collection, it is secreted by the tubules and its measurement is subject to analytical overestimation. In practice, the effects of tubular secretion and analytical overestimation tend to cancel one another out at normal levels of GFR. As the GFR falls progressively, however, creatinine clearance deviates further and further from the true GFR.

Creatinine clearance is usually about 110 mL/min in the 20–40-year-old age-group. Thereafter, it falls slowly but progressively to about 70 mL/min in people over 80. In children, the GFR should be related to surface area; when this is done, results are similar to those found in young adults.

Measurement of plasma [creatinine] is more precise than creatinine clearance as there are two extra sources of imprecision in clearance measurements, i.e. the data for urine volume per minute and for the measurement of urine [creatinine]. Accuracy of urine collections is very dependent on patients' cooperation and the care with which the procedure has been explained or supervised; inaccuracies of 20–30% are not uncommon in the timed collection of urine specimens. The combination of these errors causes an imprecision (1 SD) of about 10% under ideal conditions with 'good' collectors; this increases to 20–30% under less ideal conditions. When assessing the progress of renal disease, it will be apparent that creatinine clearance measurements leave much to be desired.

If endogenous production of creatinine remains constant, the amount of it excreted in the urine each day becomes constant and the plasma [creatinine] will then be inversely proportional to creatinine clearance. In most circumstances, therefore, we recommend that assessment of glomerular function be made and changes in GFR over time be monitored, biochemically, by measurement of plasma [creatinine] rather than by measurement of creatinine clearance, because:

1 Plasma [creatinine] normally remains fairly constant throughout adult life, whereas creatinine clearance declines with advancing age.

2 Plasma [creatinine] correlates as well with GFR as does creatinine clearance in patients with renal disease.

3 Measurements of plasma [creatinine] are as effective in detecting early renal disease as creatinine clearance.

4 Plasma [creatinine] measurements enable the progress of renal disease to be followed with better precision than creatinine clearance.

Plasma urea (reference range, 2.5–6.6 mmol/L, in males under 50)

Urea is formed in the liver from ammonia released by deamination of amino acids. Over 75% of non-protein nitrogen is excreted as urea, mainly by the kidneys; small amounts are lost through the skin and the GI tract.

Urea measurements are widely available. They are quick, accurate, precise and inexpensive to perform. Plasma [urea] is often included in the group called plasma 'electrolytes', and has come to be accepted as giving a measure of renal function. However, as a test of renal function, it is inferior to plasma [creatinine] since 50% or more of urea filtered at the glomerulus is passively reabsorbed through the tubules, and this fraction increases if urine flow rate decreases.

High plasma urea (Table 9.2)

It is convenient to subdivide the causes of a high plasma [urea] into pre-renal, renal and post-renal.

Pre-renal uraemia may develop whenever there is impaired renal perfusion as there is then reduced urine flow and increased passive tubular reabsorption of urea. Thus shock, e.g. due to burns, haemorrhage or loss of water and electrolytes (e.g. severe diarrhoea), may lead to increased plasma [urea]. Renal blood flow also falls in congestive cardiac failure and when intravascular volume is reduced, with interstitial oedema accompanying hypoproteinaemia; this is very liable to occur if such patients are treated with potent diuretics.

Increased production of urea in the liver occurs on high protein diets, or as a result of increased protein catabolism (e.g. due to trauma, major surgery, extreme starvation). It may also occur after haemorrhage into the upper GI tract, which gives rise to a 'protein meal' of blood.

Urea infusion, used (like mannitol) as a diuretic in the treatment of cerebral oedema, is an iatrogenic cause of pre-renal uraemia.

Plasma [urea] increases relatively more than plasma [creatinine] in pre-renal uraemia due to impaired renal perfusion. This is because tubular reabsorption of urea is increased significantly in these patients, whereas relatively little reabsorption of creatinine occurs.

Renal uraemia may be due to acute or chronic renal failure, with reduction in glomerular filtration. Plasma [urea] increases until a new steady-state is reached at which urea production equals the amount excreted in the urine, or continues to rise in the face of near-total renal failure. Although frequently measured as a test

Table 9.2 Causes of an abnormal plasma [urea]

Reduced plasma [urea]	Low protein diet, severe liver disease, water retention
Increased plasma [urea]	
Pre-renal causes	High protein diet, GI haemorrhage ('meal' of blood)
	Any cause of increased protein catabolism (e.g. trauma, surgery, extreme starvation)
	Any cause of impaired renal perfusion (e.g. ECF losses, cardiac failure, hypoproteinaemia)
	Iatrogenic (urea infusion)
Renal causes	Any cause (acute or chronic) of a reduced GFR
Post-renal causes	Any cause of obstruction to urine outflow (e.g. benign prostatic hypertrophy, malignant stricture or obstruction, stone)

of renal function, it is always important to remember that plasma [urea] may be increased for reasons other than renal disease (pre-renal and post-renal uraemia).

Post-renal uraemia, due to outflow obstruction, may occur at different levels (i.e. in the ureter, bladder or urethra) and be due to various causes (e.g. renal stones, prostatism, genitourinary cancer). Back-pressure on the renal tubules enhances back-diffusion of urea so plasma [urea] rises disproportionately more than plasma [creatinine].

Post-renal uraemia and pre-renal uraemia due to impaired renal perfusion may themselves cause damage to the kidney and thus renal uraemia. It can, therefore, be difficult sometimes to determine the underlying cause of an increased plasma [urea], even after taking into consideration the history of the patient's illness, the findings on physical examination and other data (e.g. plasma [creatinine], urine volume and composition).

Low plasma urea (Table 9.2)

Less urea is synthesized in the liver if there is reduced availability of amino acids for deamination, as may occur in starvation or malabsorption. However, in extreme starvation plasma [urea] may rise, as increased muscle protein breakdown then provides the major source of fuel. In patients with severe liver disease (usually chronic), urea synthesis may be impaired, leading to a fall in plasma [urea].

Plasma [urea] may fall as a result of water retention associated with inappropriate AVP secretion or dilution of plasma with intravenous fluids. If a blood specimen is taken from a site close to an intravenous infusion, the low plasma [urea] that results is liable to be grossly misleading.

Urine urea

Urine urea excretion reflects both dietary protein content and endogenous protein catabolism. By determining the 24-hour excretion, a measure of urinary nitrogen loss can be obtained (p. 241).

Tubular function

The healthy kidney has a considerable reserve capacity for reabsorbing water, and for excreting H^+ and other ions, only exceeded under exceptional physiological loads. Moderate impairment of renal function may reduce this reserve, revealed when loading tests are employed to stress the kidney. Tubular function tests, therefore, are not often used unless there is reason to suspect that a specific abnormality is present. The functions tested most often are renal concentrating power and the ability to produce an acid urine.

Urine osmolality and renal concentration tests

Urine osmolality varies widely in health, between about 60 and 1250 mmol/kg, depending upon the body's requirement to produce a maximally dilute or a maximally concentrated urine. The failing kidney loses its capacity to concentrate urine at a relatively late stage, compared with when a rise in plasma [creatinine] or [urea] can first be detected.

A patient with polyuria due to chronic renal failure is unable to produce either a dilute or a concentrated urine. Instead, urine osmolality is generally within 50 mmol/kg of the plasma osmolality (i.e. between about 240 and 350 mmol/kg). This has important implications. To excrete the obligatory daily solute load of about 600 mmol requires approximately two litres of water at a maximum urine osmolality of 350 mmol/kg, compared to 500 mL of the most concentrated urine achieved by the normal kidney. Hence, patients with chronic renal disease require a daily water intake of at least 2 L to maintain their water balance. On the other hand, a large intake of water can lead to dangerous hyponatraemia since water excretion is limited by the fact that the diseased kidney is unable to produce a sufficiently dilute urine.

Urine osmolality is directly proportional to the osmotic work done by the kidney, and is the correct measure of concentrating power. Urine sp. gr. is usually directly proportional to osmolality, but gives misleadingly high results if there is significant glycosuria or proteinuria.

Renal concentration tests are not normally required in patients with established chronic renal failure; indeed, concentration tests may be positively dangerous. However, the tests may be indicated in patients with polyuria and polydipsia in whom common causes of these symptoms (e.g. diabetes mellitus) have first been excluded. Causes of failure to concentrate urine are shown in Table 9.3.

In cases of polyuria, measurement of the osmolality of two early morning urine specimens, or several specimens passed during the day, should be made before proceeding to formal concentration tests. If urinary osmolality greater than 800 mmol/kg (or sp. gr. more than 1.020) is observed in any specimen, as should be the case in most patients who can concentrate urine normally, there is no point in performing further tests of concentrating ability.

Formal tests of renal concentrating power measure the maximal concentration of urine produced in response either to fluid deprivation or to intramuscular injection of desaminocys-1-8-D-arginine vasopressin (DDAVP), a synthetic analogue of the antidiuretic hormone (AVP); the tests have the same antidiuretic

Table 9.3 Causes of failure to concentrate urine

Causal mechanism	Examples of causes
Insufficient secretion of AVP	Lesions of the supra-optic–hypothalamic–hypophyseal tract (e.g. trauma, neoplasm)
Inhibition of AVP release	Psychogenic diabetes insipidus, lesions of the thirst centre causing polydipsia
Inability to respond to AVP	Renal tubular defects (e.g. nephrogenic diabetes insipidus, Fanconi syndrome)
Inability to maintain renal medullary hyperosmolality	Chronic renal failure, hydronephrosis, lithium toxicity, hypokalaemia, hypercalcaemia, renal papillary necrosis (e.g. analgesic nephropathy)
Increased solute load per nephron	Chronic renal failure, diabetes mellitus

effect. If the patient is receiving drugs (e.g. carbamazepine, chlorpropamide, DDAVP), these should be stopped at least 48 hours before testing renal concentrating power.

It is usual to follow a set pattern of testing patients in hospital, when they are being investigated for polyuria that is thought to be due to hypothalamic or posterior pituitary disease, or to renal tubular dysfunction. A fluid deprivation test is performed first. Then, *if the patient is unable to concentrate the urine adequately* following fluid deprivation, a DDAVP test follows on immediately. The sequence of events might be as described below.

Fluid deprivation test

There are many ways of performing this test, differing in detail but all involving fluid deprivation over several hours, with the patient under observation in hospital to ensure that no fluid is taken; local directions for test performance should be followed. For instance, beginning at 2200 h, the patient is told not to drink overnight and urine specimens are collected whilst the patient continues not to drink between 0800 h and 1500 h the next day. During the test, the patient should be weighed every 2 hours and the test stopped if weight loss of 3–5% occurs.

Blood and urine specimens are collected for measurement of osmolality. Normally, there is no increase in plasma osmolality (reference range, 280–290 mmol/kg) over the period of water deprivation whereas urine osmolality rises to 800 mmol/kg or more. A rising plasma osmolality and a failure to concentrate urine are consistent with either a failure to secrete AVP or a failure to respond to AVP at the level of the distal nephron. When this pattern of results is obtained, it is usual to proceed immediately to perform the DDAVP test.

DDAVP test

The patient is allowed a moderate amount of water to drink at the end of the fluid deprivation test, to alleviate thirst. An intramuscular injection (4 µg) of DDAVP is then given and urine specimens are collected at hourly intervals for a further three hours and their osmolality measured.

Interpretation of tests of renal concentrating ability

These tests are of most value in distinguishing between hypothalamic–pituitary, psychogenic and renal causes of polyuria (Table 9.3). These will be discussed seriatim.

Patients with *diabetes insipidus of hypothalamic–pituitary origin* produce insufficient AVP; they should, therefore, respond to the DDAVP test but not to fluid deprivation. As a rule, these patients show an increase in plasma osmolality during the fluid deprivation test, to more than 300 mmol/kg, and a low urine osmolality (200–400 mmol/kg). There is a marked increase in urine osmolality, to 600 mmol/kg or more, in the DDAVP test.

Patients with *psychogenic diabetes insipidus* should respond to both fluid deprivation and to DDAVP. In practice, however, medullary hypo-osmolality often prevents the urine osmolality from reaching 800 mmol/kg after fluid deprivation or DDAVP injection in these tests, as normally performed. Also, the chronic suppression of the physiological mechanism that controls AVP release may impair the normal hypothalamic response to dehydration. These patients have a plasma osmolality that is initially low but which rises to normal during the tests. However, fluid deprivation may have to be continued for much more than 24 hours in these patients before renal medullary hyperosmolality is restored; only then do they show normal responses to fluid deprivation or to DDAVP injection.

Polyuria of renal origin may be due to inability of the renal tubule to respond to AVP, as in nephrogenic diabetes insipidus. In a number of other conditions, the kidney loses its ability to maintain medullary hyperosmolality but these should have been excluded before renal concentration tests are performed. In nephrogenic diabetes insipidus, there is failure to produce a concentrated urine in response both to fluid deprivation and to DDAVP injection, the urinary osmolality usually remaining below 400 mmol/kg; in these patients, plasma osmolality increases as a result of fluid deprivation.

Urinary acidification tests

Urine is normally acidic (as compared with plasma) in healthy subjects on a meat-containing diet. An alkaline urine may be found in vegans, in patients ingesting alkali, or in patients with urinary tract infections. 'Side-room' tests can be used to give a rough estimate of urine pH over the range 5–9 pH units. It is important to measure urine pH on freshly voided urine specimens.

Urine acidification is a function of the distal nephron which can secrete H^+ until the limiting intraluminal pH of approximately 5.0 or less is reached. Acidification occurs as a result of the kidney reabsorbing large amounts of the HCO_3^- that has been filtered at the glomerulus, and excreting H^+ produced as nonvolatile acids during tissue metabolism. The amount of H^+ which can be secreted into the tubules before the limiting intraluminal pH is reached depends upon the presence of urine buffers. The H^+ in urine is only partly eliminated as such, it being mostly excreted as NH_4^+ or H^+ combined with buffer ions, principally inorganic phosphate (Fig. 9.1).

It is possible to assess the capacity of the kidney to produce an acid urine after a metabolic acidosis has been induced by administering ammonium chloride (NH_4Cl). In response to the NH_4Cl load, urine pH normally falls to below 5.3 in at least one specimen. It is essential to check that a satisfactory acidosis was induced and this is assumed to have occurred if plasma [total CO_2] falls by about 4 mmol/L after NH_4Cl ingestion. More elaborate tests of urinary acidification (e.g. determining the renal threshold for HCO_3^-) are needed to differentiate between proximal and distal renal tubular acidosis.

Renal tubular acidosis

At least two distinct tubular abnormalities may give rise to conditions in which there is acidosis of renal origin but little or no change in plasma [creatinine], or other measures of the GFR.

Distal renal tubular acidosis is the commoner type. It is due to an inability to maintain a gradient of $[H^+]$ across the distal tubule and collecting ducts. It is

---

Case 9.1

A 58-year-old man, a known manic depressive who was being treated with lithium carbonate, was admitted to a hospital psychiatric ward with a recent history of lethargy and confusion. On examination, he was found to be very dehydrated, and the results of chemical investigations were:

Plasma analysis	Result	Reference range	Units
[Urea]	16.1	2.5–6.6	mmol/L
[Na$^+$]	197	132–144	mmol/L
[K$^+$]	3.6	3.3–4.7	mmol/L
[Total CO$_2$]	28	24–30	mmol/L
[Glucose]	6.2		mmol/L

Urine: osmolality, 209 mmol/kg

No reference range is given for plasma [glucose] as it was not a fasting specimen (for which the range is 3.6–5.8 mmol/L). No reference range is given for urine osmolality as this should reflect the need to conserve or to lose water, depending on a patient's plasma osmolality (reference range for plasma osmolality is 280–290 mmol/kg).

Is this patient's urine osmolality appropriate, given his history and the results of plasma measurements? What do you think might be the diagnosis, and can you identify any relevant factors? This patient is discussed on p. 143.

---

usually caused by an inherited abnormality, but may occur in certain forms of acquired renal disease. Bone disease, commonly osteomalacia, results from the buffering of H$^+$ by bone, and there is often hypercalciuria and nephrocalcinosis. Loss of Na$^+$ and K$^+$ in the urine and hypokalaemia are common. Urinary pH rarely falls below 6.0 and never below 5.3 in the ammonium chloride test of urinary acidification.

Proximal renal tubular acidosis is much less common. It is due to proximal tubular loss of HCO$_3^-$ caused by a low renal threshold for HCO$_3^-$. Occasionally this is an isolated abnormality. More often it occurs as one of the features in some patients with Fanconi syndrome (see below). If these patients are given enough NH$_4$Cl to reduce plasma [total CO$_2$] below the renal threshold for HCO$_3^-$, urinary pH may fall below 5.3.

The amino acidurias

Specific disorders affecting the proximal tubules may cause impaired reabsorption of amino acids, or glucose, or phosphate, etc. In some conditions these defects occur singly; in others, multiple defects are present. Chemical investigations are needed for specific identification of these abnormalities and may include amino acid chromatography, or investigation of calcium and phosphate metabolism (Chapter 13), or an oral glucose tolerance test (p. 166).

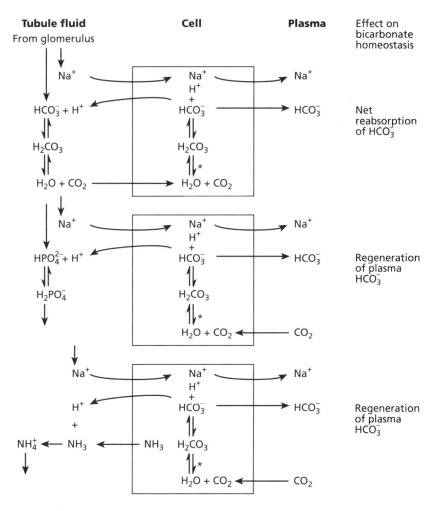

| Tubule fluid | Cell | Plasma | Effect on bicarbonate homeostasis |

Fig. 9.1 Three different mechanisms that are involved in the reclamation or regeneration of bicarbonate, filtered at the glomerulus. The proximal renal tubule, the site where carbonic anhydrase is located on the brush border and the only site where *reclamation* takes place, is quantitatively the most important of the three contributors to bicarbonate homeostasis. The other points of action of carbonic anhydrase, within the tubule cells, are indicated by asterisks.

Regeneration of bicarbonate (shown in the middle and lower diagrams) is effected by two different mechanisms, both of which result in an exchange of H^+ in the cell for Na^+ in the tubule fluid; it is these mechanisms that are impaired in chronic renal failure.

There are four groups of acids — the neutral, acidic and basic amino acids, and the imino acids proline and hydroxyproline. Each has its own specific mechanism for transport across the proximal tubular cell. Normally, the renal tubules reabsorb all the filtered amino acids except for small amounts of glycine, serine, alanine and glutamine. Amino aciduria may be due to:

1 Disease of the renal tubule (*renal or low threshold type*).

2 Raised plasma [amino acids] (*generalized or overflow type*).

Renal amino aciduria may be due to impairment of one of the specific transport mechanisms. For example, *Hartnup disease* is a rare hereditary disorder in which epithelial (GI tract *and* renal) transport of the monoamino-monocarboxylic (neutral) amino acids is affected; it may give rise to tryptophan deficiency and niacin deficiency (p. 237). In *cystinuria* there is a hereditary defect in the epithelial transport of cystine and the basic amino acids lysine, ornithine and arginine; it is a rare cause of renal (cystine) stones. Renal amino aciduria may also occur as a non-specific abnormality due to generalized tubular damage, and together with reabsorption defects affecting glucose or phosphate, or both.

The overflow types of amino aciduria result when the renal threshold for amino acids is exceeded, due to overproduction or to accumulation of amino acids in the body (e.g. heavy metal poisoning, p. 375; acute hepatic necrosis).

Fanconi syndrome is a syndrome that may be inherited or secondary to a number of uncommon disorders (e.g. heavy metal poisoning, multiple myeloma). The syndrome comprises multiple defects of proximal tubular function. There are excessive urinary losses of amino acids (generalized amino aciduria), phosphate, glucose and sometimes HCO_3^-, which gives rise to a proximal renal tubular acidosis. Distal tubular functions may also be affected. Sometimes globulins of low mol mass may be detectable in urine, in addition to the amino aciduria. One of the inherited causes of the Fanconi syndrome is cystinosis.

Cystinosis (Lignac–Fanconi disease) is a rare disease in which cystine is deposited in the cells of the lymphoreticular system. Renal tubular damage also occurs and there is a generalized amino aciduria, glucosuria and phosphaturia. Affected infants fail to thrive and develop vitamin D-resistant rickets. Cystinosis should not be confused with cystinuria.

Renal handling of sodium and potassium

Sodium excretion

The kidneys are essential for maintaining sodium balance, normally filtering about 21 000 mmol Na^+/day. Thus, on a diet of 100 mmol Na^+, and in the absence of any pathological loss of Na^+, the kidney would match this intake with an excretion of 100 mmol Na^+, which represents about 0.5% of the filtered Na^+ load (fractional excretion or Fe_{Na} of 0.5%). A reduction in the GFR to one-tenth of normal means that, on the same diet, the Fe_{Na} would need to be 10-fold higher (i.e. 5%) to maintain Na^+ balance.

As the GFR declines in chronic renal failure, the Fe_{Na} needs to increase progressively to maintain Na^+ balance. The limit of adaptation is determined by the maximum possible Fe_{Na}, which cannot generally exceed 20–30% of the filtered Na^+ load. Once this limit is reached, any further reduction in GFR, or an increase in dietary Na^+, leads to Na^+ retention. Most patients with chronic renal failure tolerate normal levels of dietary Na^+ if the GFR is more than 10 mL/min. However, if the GFR is below this level, Na^+ retention occurs leading to expansion of the ECF, weight gain and worsening hypertension. In the presence of other Na^+-retaining states (e.g. congestive cardiac failure or cirrhosis), Na^+ retention will be even more pronounced. Treatment depends upon Na^+ restriction and careful use of diuretic therapy.

Excessive Na^+ loss may occur in chronic renal failure. The kidneys' capacity to adapt to changes in Na^+ intake is limited and a requirement to conserve Na^+ (e.g. in response to excessive use of diuretics or if the patient has severe diarrhoea) may not be met by the damaged kidneys. This leads on to a further fall in GFR. In chronic pyelonephritis and other disorders primarily affecting the renal tubules, large amounts of Na^+ may be lost in the urine and severe Na^+ and water depletion can occur.

The ability to conserve Na^+ can be tested by giving a diet containing 20 mmol Na^+/day. Normally, urinary Na^+ excretion falls within a week to the amount present in the diet. This test should always be carefully monitored, by daily measurement of plasma $[Na^+]$ and [creatinine] or [urea], since severe Na^+ depletion can be induced.

Potassium excretion

About 90% of K^+ in the glomerular filtrate is normally reabsorbed in the proximal tubules, the distal tubules regulating the amount of K^+ excreted in the urine. The rate of secretion of K^+ by the distal tubules is influenced by the trans-tubular potential and by the tubular cell $[K^+]$, and is usually maintained adequately provided the daily urine flow rate is greater than 1 L.

In the presence of a normal GFR, about 550 mmol K^+ are filtered daily at the glomerulus. An average dietary intake of K^+ is about 80 mmol/day and external K^+ balance is normally achieved by excreting about 15% of the filtered K^+ (Fe_K). A reduction in GFR to about 10 mL/min requires an increase in Fe_K to 150%; the net addition of K^+ to the tubular filtrate through distal tubular secretion is needed to achieve this, and generally the normal daily intake of K^+ can be tolerated if the GFR is 10 mL/min. At a GFR of about 5 mL/min, however, the limit of adaptation is reached, leading to K^+ retention and hyperkalaemia. The ability of the GI tract to increase excretion of K^+ helps to delay the onset of hyperkalaemia.

In some patients hyperkalaemia may develop with a GFR above 10 mL/min. For instance, this occurs in diabetic patients with defective renin production and, therefore, deficient aldosterone production. It also occurs when the renal tubule becomes unresponsive to aldosterone action.

Excessive renal losses of K^+ rarely occur in chronic renal disease, but the Na^+ depletion which sometimes develops in renal disease may be associated with secondary aldosteronism, which in turn causes excessive loss of K^+.

Measurement of urinary K^+ output can prove very helpful in patients suspected of losing abnormal amounts of K^+. If dietary K^+ is reduced to 20 mmol/day, urinary output normally falls to this level within 1 week but occasionally it takes 2 weeks. Persistence of a relatively high urinary K^+ output in the presence of hypokalaemia strongly suggests that the kidney is unable to conserve K^+ adequately.

Acute renal failure

By definition, there is renal disease of acute onset, severe enough to cause failure of renal homeostasis. A few patients maintain a normal urine volume throughout the course of the illness, but usually oliguric, diuretic and recovery phases can be recognized. Chemical investigations help to determine the severity of the disease and to follow its course, but do not help much in determining the cause.

Oliguric phase

Less than 400 mL urine is produced each day; there may be anuria in renal failure due to outflow obstruction. The oliguria is mainly due to a fall in GFR. The urine that is formed usually has an osmolality similar to plasma and a relatively high $[Na^+]$, since the composition of the small amount of glomerular filtrate produced is little altered by the damaged tubules.

Plasma $[Na^+]$ is usually low due to a combination of factors, including intake of water in excess of the amount able to be excreted, increase in metabolic water from increased tissue catabolism, and a shift of Na^+ from ECF to ICF. Plasma $[K^+]$, on the other hand, is usually increased due to the impaired renal output and increased tissue catabolism, aggravated by the shift of K^+ out of cells that accompanies the metabolic acidosis which develops due to failure to excrete H^+ and to the increased formation of H^+ from tissue catabolism.

Retention of urea, creatinine, sulphate and other waste products occurs. The rate at which plasma [urea] rises is affected by the rate of tissue catabolism; this, in turn, depends on the cause of the acute renal failure. In renal failure due to trauma (including renal failure developing after surgical operations), plasma [urea] tends to rise more rapidly than in patients with renal failure due to medical causes such as acute glomerulonephritis.

To differentiate the low urinary output of suspected acute renal failure from that due to severe circulatory impairment with reduced blood volume, the tests summarized in Table 9.4 may be helpful. However, none of these tests can be completely relied upon to make the important and urgent distinction between renal failure and hypovolaemia.

For monitoring patients in the oliguric phase of acute renal failure, plasma [creatinine] or [urea] and plasma $[K^+]$ are particularly important and need to be determined at least once daily. Decisions to use haemodialysis are reached at least partly on the basis of the results of these tests. The volume of urine and its electrolyte composition (and the volume and composition of any other measurable sources of fluid loss) should also be assessed in order to determine fluid replacement requirements.

Diuretic phase

With the onset of this phase, urine volume increases but the clearance of urea,

Table 9.4 Investigation of low urinary output

Investigation	Simple hypovolaemia	Acute renal failure
Urine osmolality	Usually > 600 mmol/kg	Usually < 350 mmol/kg
Urine [urea] : plasma [urea]	Usually > 10	Usually < 5
Urine $[Na^+]$	Usually < 10 mmol/L	Usually > 20 mmol/L

creatinine and other waste products may not improve to the same extent. Plasma [urea] and [creatinine] may therefore continue to rise, at least at the start of the diuretic phase. Large losses of electrolytes may occur in the urine and require to be replaced orally or parenterally. Measurement of these losses is needed so that correct replacement therapy can be given; this requires *complete* urine collections, for urine [Na^+] and [K^+] measurement, and calculation of daily outputs.

Plasma [K^+] tends to fall as the diuretic phase continues, due to the shift of K^+ back into the cells and to marked losses in urine resulting from impaired conservation of K^+ by the still-damaged tubules. Usually, Na^+ deficiency occurs also, due to failure of renal conservation. Throughout the diuretic phase, therefore, it is important to measure plasma [creatinine] or [urea] and both plasma [Na^+] and [K^+] at least once daily, and to monitor the output of Na^+ and K^+ in the urine.

Chronic renal failure

Most of the functional changes seen in chronic renal failure can be explained in terms of a full solute load falling on a reduced number of normal nephrons. The GFR is invariably reduced, associated with retention of urea, creatinine, urate, phosphates, various phenolic and indolic acids and other organic substances. The progress and severity of the disease are usually monitored by measuring plasma [creatinine] or [urea], or both, periodically.

Sodium, potassium and water

The renal handling of Na^+, K^+ and water by normal kidneys and in chronic renal failure have already been considered.

Acid–base disturbances

The total excretion of H^+ is impaired, mainly due to a fall in the renal capacity to form NH_4^+. Metabolic acidosis is present in most patients but its severity remains fairly stable in spite of the reduced urinary H^+ excretion. There may be an extra-renal mechanism for H^+ elimination, possibly involving buffering of H^+ by calcium salts in bone; this would help to account for the demineralization of bone that often occurs in chronic renal failure.

Calcium and phosphate

Plasma [calcium] tends to be low, often due at least partly to reduced plasma [albumin]. Plasma [phosphate] is high, mainly due to a reduction of GFR.

Virtually all patients with chronic renal failure have secondary or, much less often, tertiary hyperparathyroidism, and they may develop osteitis fibrosa. Plasma [calcium], which is decreased or close to the lower reference value in patients with secondary hyperparathyroidism, increases later if tertiary hyperparathyroidism develops. Many patients with a low plasma [calcium] have reduced activity of renal 1α-hydroxylase and develop osteomalacia or rickets. A few patients show a third type of bone abnormality, with increased bone density (osteosclerosis). It is not clear why any particular one of these various types of renal osteodystrophy should develop in an individual patient (p. 212).

Case 9.2

A previously healthy 32-year-old bricklayer was admitted to hospital in shock, with severe crush injuries to his legs, caused by the collapse of a building on to him. As part of the monitoring of his progress, 3 days later the following results were obtained:

Plasma analysis	Result	Reference range	Units
[Urea]	42	2.5–6.6	mmol/L
[Na^+]	141	132–144	mmol/L
[K^+]	6.8	3.3–4.7	mmol/L
[Total CO_2]	12	24–30	mmol/L
Osmolality	330	280–290	mmol/kg

Urine: Volume in the previous 24 hours, 200 mL
Analyses on this specimen gave [urea], 280 mmol/L;
[Na^+], 62 mmol/L;
osmolality, 330 mmol/kg

How would you explain these findings? This patient is discussed on p. 143.

Other metabolic abnormalities

Other findings in chronic renal failure may include impaired glucose tolerance and raised plasma [magnesium]. These are of no particular diagnostic significance.

Uraemic toxins

Many substances accumulate in patients with uraemia, and many explanations have been offered for the symptoms and complications that develop. The subject remains confused, despite much study of the effects of haemodialysis and peritoneal dialysis, modifications to the diet, and renal transplantation. The main point of agreement is that urea is one of the least toxic of the substances so far investigated.

Renal transplantation

Following a transplant operation, renal function should be monitored by daily measurements of the plasma and urinary concentrations of creatinine, Na^+ and K^+, and recording of the urine volume. Clinical signs of rejection are accompanied by an increase in plasma [creatinine] and fall in urinary [Na^+].

Many other chemical measurements have been assessed in the search for more sensitive and specific early indicators of transplant rejection. These include daily measurement in urine of various low mol mass plasma proteins (e.g. β_2-microglobulin, lysozyme, retinol-binding protein), and renal tract enzyme activities including N-acetyl-β-D-glucosaminidase (NAG). With all these substances, increased urinary excretion may provide a much earlier indication of transplant rejection than plasma [creatinine]. However, so far these relatively complex tests have mostly been lacking in specificity; other causes of their increase include treatment with certain antibiotics and urinary tract infection.

In the UK, most experience has been obtained with measurements of NAG, an enzyme located in the lysosomes of the proximal renal tubules. Total urinary NAG activity rises, and the isoenzyme pattern changes, prior to transplant rejection.

Proteinuria

Glomerular filtrate normally contains about 30 mg/L protein; this corresponds to a total filtered load of about 5 g/24 h. Since less than 200 mg protein is normally excreted in the urine each day, tubular reabsorption must be very efficient in health.

Proteinuria is described as *glomerular* proteinuria if the glomerulus becomes abnormally leaky, or as *tubular* proteinuria when tubular reabsorption of protein becomes defective. Abnormal amounts of some plasma proteins may lead to an *overflow* proteinuria. Protein may also enter the urinary tract distal to the kidneys (e.g. due to inflammation) leading to *post-renal* proteinuria; if post-renal proteinuria is suspected, urine microscopy (including cytology) and culture should be carried out.

'Side-room' testing of urine for protein should be part of the full clinical examination of every patient. It must be stressed, however, that 'side-room' tests are not sufficiently sensitive to detect pathologically significant 'microalbuminuria' (p. 172).

Overflow proteinuria

Several conditions may give rise to abnormal amounts of low mol mass proteins (i.e. less than about 70 kDa) in plasma and in urine. These proteins are filtered at the glomerulus and may then be neither reabsorbed completely nor catabolized completely by the renal tubular cells. The principal examples are listed in Table 9.5.

Glomerular proteinuria

Table 9.6 classifies glomerular proteinuria separately from tubular proteinuria, but many patients show features of both glomerular and tubular protein loss. Where quantitative measurements of urine protein loss are required (e.g. when monitoring treatment for the nephrotic syndrome), 'side-room' tests are insufficiently precise; 24-hour collections of urine should be examined in the laboratory.

Some patients, typically with protein excretion rates of less than 1 g/24 h, have *benign or functional proteinuria*. This probably results from blood flow changes through the glomeruli and is found in association with exercise, fever and

Table 9.5 Overflow proteinuria

Protein	Molecular mass (Da)	Cause
Amylase	45 000	Acute pancreatitis
Bence Jones protein	44 000	Multiple myeloma
Haemoglobin	68 000	Intravascular haemolysis
Lysozyme	15 000	Myelomonocytic leukaemia
Myoglobin	17 000	Crush injuries

Table 9.6 Glomerular and tubular proteinuria

Classification	Examples of causes
Glomerular proteinuria May or may not be of pathological significance	Orthostatic proteinuria, effort proteinuria, febrile proteinuria
Pathological significance	Glomerulonephritis, all forms; pathological causes of altered haemodynamics (e.g. renal artery stenosis)
Tubular proteinuria	Chronic nephritis and pyelonephritis, acute tubular necrosis, renal tubule defects (e.g. renal tubular acidosis), heavy metal poisoning, renal transplantation

congestive cardiac failure. Amongst these conditions, it is particularly important to recognize orthostatic proteinuria.

Orthostatic proteinuria

This is a benign condition that affects children and young adults; they exhibit proteinuria only after they have been standing up. For orthostatic (or postural) proteinuria to be diagnosed, protein will not be detectable in an early morning urine specimen when tested by normal 'side-room' methods (i.e. urine contains less than 100 mg/L). The subject is instructed to empty the bladder just before going to bed, and the test for protein is performed on a specimen of urine passed the following morning, *collected immediately after getting up*.

Orthostatic proteinuria is usually observed in only some of the urine specimens passed when up and about. For these individuals the prognosis is good, but it is less good for subjects in whom proteinuria is always detected when they are up and about.

Glomerulonephritis

This is the commonest group of causes of persistent proteinuria. Plasma proteins escape in varying amounts, depending on their mol mass, on the amount of glomerular damage, and on the capacity of the renal tubule cells to reabsorb or metabolize the proteins that have passed the glomerulus.

The degree of proteinuria does not provide an index of the severity of renal disease. However, it is convenient to distinguish *mild or moderate proteinuria*, in which the loss is not sufficient to cause protein depletion, from *severe proteinuria*, in which the protein loss exceeds the body's capacity to replace losses by synthesis (usually 5–10 g/24 h). Severe, persistent proteinuria is one feature of the nephrotic syndrome, in which urinary protein loss is sometimes more than 30 g/24 h.

Differential protein clearance (selectivity) measurements are sometimes performed in patients with the nephrotic syndrome, since those with selective proteinuria (e.g. due to minimal change disease) are more likely to respond to steroid therapy than those with unselective proteinuria. Selectivity measurements are based on the fact that glomerular permeability to a plasma protein depends largely on its mol mass, small molecules being cleared more rapidly than large.

Differences in clearance can be investigated by measuring the ratio of the clearances of two proteins of widely different mol mass, e.g. transferrin (M_r, 80 kDa) and α_2-macroglobulin (M_r, 820 kDa). If the ratio is high, this means that large molecules are failing to pass into the glomerular filtrate and that the proteinuria is selective; if the ratio is low, the proteinuria is unselective.

Tubular proteinuria

This may be due to tubular or interstitial damage resulting from a variety of causes. The proteinuria is due to failure of the tubules to reabsorb some of the plasma proteins filtered by the normal glomerulus, or possibly due to abnormal secretion of protein into the urinary tract. The proteins excreted in tubular proteinuria mostly have a low mol mass, e.g. β_2-microglobulin (M_r, 11.8 kDa) and lysozyme (M_r, 15 kDa). The loss of protein is usually mild, rarely more than 2 g/24 h.

Urinary β_2-microglobulin excretion is normally very small (under 0.4 mg/ 24 h). Its measurement has been used as a sensitive test of renal tubular damage. The test is of limited value for this purpose, however, if there is evidence of renal insufficiency, e.g. increased plasma [creatinine].

Renal stones

Physicochemical principles govern the formation of renal stones, and are relevant to the choice of treatment aimed at preventing progression or recurrence. Stones may cause renal damage, often progressive; renal function tests then show deterioration.

The solubility of a salt depends on the product of the activities of its constituent ions. Frequently, the solubility product in urine is exceeded without the formation of a stone, provided there is no 'seeding'. 'Seeding' promotes crystal formation in relation to particles present in urine, such as debris or bacteria. Formation of stones may be prevented by inhibiting substances that are normally present in the urine.

People living or working in hot conditions are liable to become dehydrated, and show a greater tendency to form renal stones. Urinary tract infection may be the precipitating factor. There are also several metabolic factors that can cause stones to form in the renal tract. However, in many patients, no cause can be found to explain why stones have formed. The main types of renal stone are listed in Table 9.7.

Hypercalciuria

Stones in the upper renal tract occur in 5–10% of adults in Western Europe and the USA. These are mostly either pure calcium oxalate or a mixture of calcium oxalate and phosphate. Not every patient with renal stones, however, has hypercalciuria since there is considerable overlap between the 24-hour urinary calcium excretion of healthy individuals on their normal diet (up to 12 mmol/24 h) and the urinary calcium excretion of stone-formers.

The causes of urinary calcium excretion in excess of 12 mmol/24 h, in patients taking their normal diet, include idiopathic hypercalciuria, primary hyperparathyroidism (p. 203), vitamin D overdosage and increased formation of

Table 9.7 Renal stones

Type of stone	Frequency in UK (%)	Metabolic cause or relevant factors*
Calcium oxalate stones and mixed (calcium oxalate and phosphate) stones	80–85	Hypercalciuria (see text), excessive absorption of dietary oxalate, primary hyperoxaluria
Triple phosphate stones†	5–10	Urinary tract infection (fall in $[H^+]$)
Urate stones	5–10	Gout, myeloproliferative disorders, high protein diet, uricosuric drugs
Cystine stones	Approx. 1	Cystinuria
Xanthine stones	< 1	Xanthinuria

*Although not specifically listed in the table, dehydration is an important factor that is common to all cases of stone formation.
†'Triple phosphate' stones contain magnesium ammonium phosphate and calcium phosphate; they tend to form in alkaline urine.

1 : 25-DHCC (p. 206), prolonged immobilization, and renal tubular acidosis. Up to 10% of renal calculi, depending on the series, have been attributed to primary hyperparathyroidism. It is important to investigate patients with renal calculi for primary hyperparathyroidism since it is amenable to curative treatment. Idiopathic hypercalciuria is the commonest single cause of renal stones, but little is known about the basic abnormality in this disorder.

Oxalate, cystine and xanthine excretion

The majority of urinary calculi contain oxalate, but excessive excretion of oxalate is primarily responsible for the formation of stones in only a small percentage of cases. Other occasional causes of stone formation include cystinuria (p. 134) and xanthinuria (p. 246).

Primary hyperoxaluria is a rare condition in which there is increased excretion of oxalate and of glyoxylate, the latter due to deficiency of the enzyme responsible for converting glyoxylate to glycine. Patients with disease of the terminal ileum may have an increased tendency to form oxalate stones, due to the hyperoxaluria caused by increased absorption of dietary oxalate.

Chemical investigations on patients with renal stones

Stones should be analysed for some or all of the constituents listed in Table 9.7 as this can be helpful. Care must be taken, however, to ensure that the specimen sent to the laboratory for analysis really is a stone that came from the patient — patients have been known to fool doctors by producing small bits of gravel and saying that they have passed them as stones. The following tests may also be helpful in reaching a diagnosis:

1 *Plasma* calcium, albumin, phosphate, total CO_2 and urate concentrations, and alkaline phosphatase activity. Full acid–base assessment is rarely needed.

2 *Urine* 'side-room' tests (pH and protein), and 24-hour excretion of calcium,

phosphate and urate. Occasionally, urinary excretion of oxalate, cystine or xanthine may be required, or urinary acidification tests.

3 *Renal function tests* — plasma [creatinine], or creatinine clearance, and
plasma [urea].

In addition to chemical tests, microbiological examination of urine is usually
performed and radiological investigations of the urinary tract.

Comments on Case 9.1 (p. 131)

The values for the calculated plasma osmolality, using the formulae given on
p. 36, are 423 and 408 mmol/kg, respectively. These high values accord with the
findings on clinical examination. The kidneys would have been expected to be
producing a very concentrated urine, and the low urinary osmolality (lower than
the plasma value) indicates either that AVP is not being secreted (leading to
diabetes insipidus) or that the kidneys are not responding to AVP (nephrogenic
diabetes insipidus).

It was not known whether or not the patient felt thirsty, but patients with any
kind of diabetes insipidus, if unable or unwilling to respond to the thirst stimulus,
rapidly become dehydrated. This patient was confused. In addition he was on
lithium treatment; lithium has a narrow therapeutic : toxic ratio and its dosage
should be reviewed periodically (p. 368). Lithium is also a known cause of
nephrogenic diabetes insipidus.

Comments on Case 9.2 (p. 138)

This man had developed acute renal failure as a result of his crush injury. The
combination of hypovolaemia, plus the release of myoglobin from the crushed
muscles, led to acute renal shutdown with a high plasma [urea]. The plasma $[K^+]$
increased as a result of the acute renal failure; there might also have been
significant K^+ leakage from damaged cells contributing to this increase. The low
plasma [total CO_2] reflected the metabolic acidosis which is a feature of acute
renal failure.

The urine volume was very low as glomerular filtration had almost completely
ceased. This low volume was accompanied by a urine with a composition inappropriate for someone who was severely volume-depleted, i.e. it was dilute and
contained a relatively high $[Na^+]$. AVP and aldosterone levels would both be
expected to have been high in this patient, leading to urine which was both
concentrated and low in $[Na^+]$.

In general terms, the formation of a urine which is both dilute and contains
relatively high $[Na^+]$, in a patient with an acute increase in plasma [urea], favours
an acute failure of renal function rather than pre-renal uraemia (in which renal
function may be intrinsically normal). A urine osmolality > 500 mmol/kg and a
urine $[Na^+]$ < 20 mmol/L would tend to favour a pre-renal (reversible) cause for
the uraemia, whereas a urine osmolality < 400 mmol/kg and a urine $[Na^+]$
> 40 mmol/L would tend to favour a renal cause for the uraemia.

Chapter 10
Gastrointestinal Tract Disease

Chemical tests play a relatively minor part in the investigation of patients with gastrointestinal (GI) tract disease. Microbiological investigations, radiological investigations, endoscopy, and biopsy procedures have much more to offer. The chemical tests that have proved most valuable and reliable, for the investigation of particular conditions, and which are widely available or able to be arranged without undue difficulty, are given in Table 10.1.

Several GI polypeptides have been identified (Table 10.2); they have various hormonal and local effects. Some have been found not only in cells and nerve fibres widely distributed in the GI tract but also in the CNS. Some GI peptides have endocrine effects acting on organs at a distance. Others appear to act locally, by diffusion to their target organs through the extracellular space; these are called paracrine effects.

Table 10.1 The principal examples of chemical tests described in this chapter for the investigation of GI tract disease

Condition to be investigated	Chemical investigations
Peptic ulcer	
Zollinger–Ellison syndrome	Pentagastrin test, plasma [gastrin]
Completeness of vagotomy	Insulin-hypoglycaemia test
Acute pancreatitis	Plasma amylase activity
Chronic pancreatitis	
Direct (invasive) tests	Secretin/CCK-PZ test, Lundh test
Indirect tests	BT-PABA/[^{14}C]-PABA test, fluorescein dilaurate test
Intestinal malabsorption	
Carbohydrate absorption	Xylose absorption test
Disaccharide absorption	Disaccharide tolerance tests
Amino acid transport	Urine chromatography
Fat absorption	Faecal fat excretion, triglyceride breath test
Bacterial colonization	Urinary indican excretion, [^{14}C]-xylose breath test
Intestinal permeability	Cellobiose : mannitol ratio
Loose, watery stools, after excluding infectious causes	Faecal pH, osmotic gap, sodium : potassium ratio
Verner–Morrison syndrome	Plasma [VIP]
Carcinoid syndrome	Urinary 5-hydroxyindoleacetic acid

Table 10.2 Examples of gastrointestinal peptides

Peptide and GI location	Probable functions
Gastric antrum and duodenum	
Gastrin (in cells called G cells)	Stimulates gastric H^+ production. Also trophic to the gastric mucosa
Duodenum and jejunum	
Secretin	Stimulates water and HCO_3^- secretion from the pancreas
Cholecystokinin (CCK)*	Stimulates secretion of enzymes by the pancreas, and contraction of the gallbladder
Glucose-dependent insulinotrophic peptide (GIP)	Stimulates post-prandial release of insulin
Motilin	Stimulates intestinal motor activity
Pancreas	
Pancreatic polypeptide	Inhibits enzyme release from the pancreas, and relaxes gallbladder
Ileum and colon	
Enteroglucagon	Increases small intestinal mucosal growth and slows the rate of intestinal transit
All areas of the GI tract	
Vasoactive intestinal peptide (VIP)*	Secretomotor actions, also vasodilation, and relaxation of intestinal smooth muscle

* CCK and VIP are examples of peptides found both in the GI tract and in the CNS.

The functional relationships of the GI peptides are not fully understood, and the diagnostic value of measuring their concentrations in plasma is in most cases still unknown. However, the Zollinger–Ellison syndrome (p. 147), the Verner–Morrison syndrome (p. 158) and coeliac disease (p. 337) are three conditions in which abnormal secretion of GI peptides will be discussed.

Peptic ulcer

Gastric acid secretion may be measured in the basal (unstimulated) state and following stimulation by pentagastrin or by insulin-induced hypoglycaemia.

Pentagastrin test

Gastrin is a polypeptide released by specialized cells in the antral and duodenal mucosa. It is a potent stimulator of gastric acid production. Pentagastrin is a pentapeptide with the four C-terminal amino acids identical to those of gastrin. Like gastrin, it stimulates acid production strongly. The pentagastrin test assesses acid production under basal and under maximally stimulated conditions.

To perform the test, the patient should be fasting and should not have received any anti-secretory drugs (e.g. H_2 antagonists) for at least 48 hours. A radio-opaque nasogastric tube is passed into the stomach, the position of the tube checked radiographically, and the resting juice (the juice present in the stomach of the fasting patient) aspirated. The basal output of gastric juice ('basal juice') is then assessed by collecting the fluid output for the next 60 minutes with the patient resting, after which pentagastrin (6 µg/kg body weight) is injected subcutaneously and the 'post-pentagastrin secretion' collected for 60 minutes as four separate 15-minute specimens.

The volume and pH of each sample are measured and the acid content determined. The 'peak acid output' is usually reported as the rate of acid secretion (expressed as mmol/h) derived from the two adjacent 15-minute specimens that together show maximal output. The presence of bile or blood in any of the samples should be noted.

Resting juice is normally less than 50 mL in volume, with a low acid content, and the basal acid secretion is usually less than 5 mmol/h. The response in healthy subjects to the administration of pentagastrin is variable. Following pentagastrin, the 'peak acid output' is usually less than 45 mmol/h in males and less than 35 mmol/h in females. It is difficult to define the lower reference value for 'peak acid output', but acid is usually detectable. The pentagastrin test is not often used nowadays but it may be of value in:

1 The investigation of patients with suspected gastrinoma (see below).
2 Differentiating superficial gastritis, in which acid output is mildly reduced, from atrophic gastritis in which there is achlorhydria even after pentagastrin stimulation, as occurs in pernicious anaemia (except in the rare juvenile form).
3 The investigation of gastric hypertrophy detected by endoscopy. Reduced acid secretion is found in giant hypertrophic gastritis (Ménétrier's disease), but secretion is increased if hypotrophic, hypersecretory gastropathy is the cause.

Acid secretion studies are rarely of value in patients with peptic ulcer, and of no value in differentiating a non-malignant gastric ulcer from gastric carcinoma.

Insulin-hypoglycaemia test

This test is used for investigating patients with peptic ulcer before and shortly after treatment by vagotomy, to determine whether vagal section has been adequate. Hypoglycaemia normally stimulates a vagus-mediated output of gastric acid that is abolished if the vagi are completely severed. However, since hypoglycaemia also promotes gastrin release (and hence acid production) via the release of adrenaline, if a small amount of acid secretion occurs in response to hypoglycaemia this does not necessarily indicate that vagotomy has been incomplete.

Intubation is performed as in the pentagastrin test. Resting juice is aspirated and 'basal juice' collected for 60 minutes. Insulin (0.2 units/kg body weight) is then injected subcutaneously, and gastric juice collected for 2 hours. Plasma [glucose] is measured before the injection of insulin and 15, 30, 45 and 60 minutes afterwards. The patient must be kept under observation throughout the test and glucose solutions must be immediately available, for oral or intravenous administration, as appropriate, if severe hypoglycaemic symptoms develop.

No significance can be attached to the results of this test unless hypoglycaemia occurs, usually defined as a plasma [glucose] less than 2.2 mmol/L in at least one of the blood specimens. If the $[H^+]$ in any of the specimens increases by more than 20 mmol/L over the basal level, it can be assumed that vagal section has been incomplete. Also, if the acid output in any four consecutive 15-minute specimens totals 10 mmol or more, this indicates that vagotomy is incomplete and that there is a strong chance that ulceration will recur.

Plasma gastrin

Gastrin occurs in many molecular forms. The first to be described comprised 17 amino acids and is known as G17 or 'little gastrin'; both larger and smaller forms occur. Plasma [gastrin] normally reflects the rate of gastrin secretion by the G cells of the antral and duodenal mucosa.

The most potent physiological stimulus for gastrin release is the combined effect of distension of the stomach and the presence in it of certain small peptides and amino acids released by digestion of protein. A fall in gastric $[H^+]$ caused by the presence of food or HCO_3^- in the stomach, or vagal stimulation, or bombesin release are other factors which increase gastrin secretion. Fasting causes a reduction in plasma [gastrin].

Plasma [gastrin], after an overnight fast, should be measured in patients with persistent, recurrent or multiple peptic ulceration, in whom the provisional diagnosis is gastrinoma and in whom a high acid secretion has already been demonstrated. Gastrin is very labile. The fasting blood sample should be taken into a plastic heparinized tube containing aprotinin (an inhibitor of proteases), the plasma separated within 15 minutes of venepuncture and frozen immediately. If there is any visible sign of haemolysis, another specimen must be obtained.

In diseases causing hyperacidity (e.g. duodenal ulcer), plasma [gastrin] is reduced except in the case of gastrinoma; most of these patients have increased levels. However, increased fasting plasma [gastrin] is not by itself diagnostic of gastrinoma as it occurs also where there is achlorhydria or hypochlorhydria, which may be due to gastritis, treatment with H_2 antagonists or omeprazole, pernicious anaemia or previous vagotomy. Increased plasma [gastrin] may also be found in patients with hypercalcaemia or G-cell hyperplasia, or following gastric surgery as a result of which antral mucosa may have become isolated from gastric contents.

Zollinger–Ellison syndrome

This syndrome is due to a gastrinoma, i.e. neoplasia of either pancreatic gastrin-producing cells or gastric gastrin-producing cells, the former being the more common site. Increased gastrin production leads to chronic hypersecretion of gastric acid which, in turn, causes peptic ulceration and sometimes diarrhoea and fat malabsorption. The steatorrhoea is thought to be due to high $[H^+]$ in the intestinal lumen; this inhibits the action of pancreatic lipase. Patients with a gastrinoma often present with multiple and recurrent peptic ulcers and diarrhoea. However, in some patients an isolated simple duodenal ulcer or diarrhoea may be the presenting feature.

The diagnosis is often made by finding a grossly elevated fasting plasma [gastrin], usually greater than 200 ng/L, and by excluding other causes of a raised level such as hypercalcaemia, achlorhydria or treatment with H_2 antagonists. However, up to 30% of patients with a gastrinoma may have normal or only slightly increased plasma [gastrin], and studies of acid secretion probably represent the most important diagnostic test in these patients.

In patients with a gastrinoma, more than 1 L of fluid is usually collected if gastric juice is aspirated overnight, containing at least 100 mmol/L HCl. In the pentagastrin test there is usually a high basal output of gastric H^+ (greater than 15 mmol/h or an acid concentration greater than 100 mmol/L) and pentagastrin causes little further stimulation; the basal secretion rate is often over 60% of the 'peak acid output'.

Secretin test for gastrinoma

About 15% of patients with a gastrinoma have only slightly increased plasma [gastrin] and gastric acid secretion; similar findings may be obtained in patients with antral G-cell hyperplasia. The secretin test may help to distinguish between antral G-cell hyperplasia and gastrinoma (Fig. 10.1).

In this test the patient is fasted overnight and blood specimens are collected via an indwelling cannula 5 minutes before and at the time of injecting secretin (1 unit/kg). Further blood specimens are collected at 2, 5, 10, 20 and 30 minutes after the injection and plasma [gastrin] is measured in all samples. In patients with gastrinoma, there is usually at least a twofold increase in plasma [gastrin], whereas

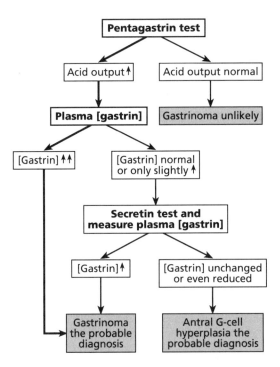

Fig. 10.1 The investigation of patients in whom a provisional diagnosis of gastrinoma (Zollinger–Ellison syndrome) has been made. Note that patients must not be taking drugs that interfere with the secretion of gastrin or of acid before these tests (e.g. H_2 antagonists).

in patients with G-cell hyperplasia there is usually a decrease or no change in plasma [gastrin].

Urease activity in the stomach

In nearly all patients with duodenal ulcer, and in the majority with non-malignant gastric ulcer, *Helicobacter pylori* is present in the gastric mucosa. This organism has considerable urease activity and can stimulate acid production by converting urea into ammonia and CO_2 in the stomach. Urease activity can be determined in a gastric biopsy specimen, or indirectly by means of a breath test which is non-invasive.

In the breath test, the patient fasts overnight and is then given [^{14}C]-urea (370 kBq) by mouth. Breath samples are taken at frequent intervals into hyamine hydroxide to trap CO_2 and the ^{14}C content of the samples is determined. Patients infected with *Helicobacter pylori* have increased excretion of $^{14}CO_2$. This test is not diagnostic, but it can be used to monitor the effects of antibacterial treatment in these patients.

Acute pancreatitis

There are two forms of the disease, a predominantly oedematous form and a relatively serious, haemorrhagic form in which tissue necrosis is more severe. Acute pancreatitis is commonly associated with gallstones or alcoholism; vascular and infective causes have also been recognized. Confirmation of the clinical diagnosis mainly depends on plasma amylase activity measurements.

Plasma amylase

Amylase in plasma arises mainly from the pancreas (P-isoamylase) and the salivary glands (S-isoamylase). Total plasma amylase activity is most often measured to investigate disease of the pancreas and is usually greatly increased in acute pancreatitis, but not always. Maximum values of more than five times the upper reference value are found in about 50% of cases, and usually occur on the first or second day of the illness. Such high values are considered by some to be pathognomonic of acute pancreatitis, but this is not correct. Similarly high values sometimes occur in the afferent loop syndrome, mesenteric infarction and acute biliary tract disease, as well as in acute parotitis. Smaller and more transient increases may occur in almost any acute abdominal condition (e.g. perforated peptic ulcer), or after injection of morphine and other drugs that cause spasm of the sphincter of Oddi; also, moderate increases have been reported in patients with diabetic ketoacidosis. In patients with acute pancreatitis, plasma amylase activity usually returns to normal within 3–5 days.

Plasma P-isoamylase activity is a more sensitive and specific test than total amylase for the detection of acute pancreatitis but it is less widely measured. Plasma lipase and trypsin activities are also increased, but these enzymes are rarely measured routinely for the investigation of patients with acute abdominal pain.

Urine amylase

Amylase (M_r, 45 kDa) activity is normally detectable in urine in small amounts.

Also, in most conditions where plasma amylase activity is increased, urinary amylase activity rises. However, this test offers no advantages over plasma amylase measurements for the investigation of acute pancreatitis and the diagnostic value of measuring urinary amylase activity has not been improved by measuring the amylase : creatinine clearance ratio. Measurements of urinary amylase activity have not gained widespread acceptance, except as part of the investigation of macro-amylasaemia.

Macro-amylasaemia

This is a rare disorder in which part of the plasma amylase activity is attributable to an enzyme molecule with a much larger mol mass than 45 kDa, the mol mass of both P- and S-isoamylase. The increased plasma amylase activity is due to reduced renal clearance of this large molecule. In some cases, macro-amylase is probably a polymer but in others it is due to complex formation between amylase and an immunoglobulin.

Macro-amylasaemia may cause diagnostic difficulty due to the presence of an unexplained and persistently moderately increased plasma amylase activity. The diagnosis may be made when the increased plasma amylase activity is found to be persistent and accompanied by a normal urinary amylase activity. Further confirmation of the diagnosis requires more complex tests.

Other chemical tests

Plasma [calcium] may be considerably reduced in severe cases of acute pancreatitis, but sometimes not for a few days. It probably falls as a result of the formation of insoluble salts of fatty acids in areas of fat necrosis.

Plasma [methaemalbumin] is sometimes increased in severe cases of acute pancreatitis, giving rise to methaemalbuminaemia. Normally, at most only a trace of methaemalbumin is detectable in plasma.

Chronic pancreatitis

Failure to secrete adequate amounts of pancreatic enzymes may not occur until the disease is advanced, but may then give rise to malabsorption, especially steatorrhoea. Various chemical methods, many of them time-consuming and lacking in sensitivity, have been used for the investigation of these patients. Direct assessment of pancreatic secretion, following duodenal intubation, continues to be performed but alternative, non-invasive or indirect, procedures are increasingly preferred. However, none of the function tests to be described in this section has proved entirely satisfactory in practice for the diagnosis of chronic pancreatitis. Instead, some advocate the measurement of faecal fat excretion, a test of intestinal absorption (see below), before and during treatment of the patient with oral pancreatic enzyme supplements as a means of helping to diagnose chronic pancreatitis.

Secretin/CCK-PZ test

Direct stimulation of pancreatic secretion can be achieved by injecting secretin together with or followed by cholecystokinin-pancreozymin (CCK-PZ). Some patients are sensitive to CCK-PZ and caerulein may be used instead. Caerulein is a decapeptide with CCK-PZ-like activity. The test can be performed in various ways. The following account indicates principles that are generally applicable.

The patient fasts overnight and a double-lumen radio-opaque tube is passed in the morning under radiological control. One opening is positioned for aspiration of gastric secretions, and the other close to the opening of the pancreatic duct so that it can collect duodenal contents from the second part of the duodenum. Continuous suction is applied to both tubes, the gastric juice being aspirated to prevent it contaminating the pancreatic juice. Specimens of duodenal contents are collected and preserved on ice, as follows:

1 Basal specimens are collected for two periods of 10 minutes.

2 After intravenous secretin, six more 10-minute collections are made.

3 After intravenous CCK-PZ, two more 10-minute collections are made.

The 10 specimens are kept cool and taken to the laboratory immediately the test ends. The volume, [HCO_3^-], and trypsin or amylase activity are measured on each specimen. Trypsin and amylase are technically easier to measure than lipase.

Healthy subjects show a wide variation in the pattern of results, partly due to difficulties in securing complete collections of specimens. The post-secretin specimens usually show a maximal hourly secretory rate of at least 2.0 mL/kg body weight and the [HCO_3^-] normally rises above 75 mmol/L. The results for pancreatic juice enzyme activity measurements depend so much on the method used by the laboratory that it is necessary to consult locally to find out what represents a normal response (i.e. how great an increase in enzyme activity should follow CCK-PZ injection).

Abnormal results are obtained in most cases of chronic pancreatitis, enzymic activity and [HCO_3^-] tending to fall before there is any obvious reduction in the volume of juice. Results are also abnormal in some cases of pancreatic carcinoma; although all three variables (enzymic activity, [HCO_3^-] and volume) may be affected, a low volume of juice is a particularly marked feature of pancreatic carcinoma when the tumour is at the head of the pancreas and producing obstruction. Tumours in the tail of the pancreas do not give rise to abnormal results in this or similar tests (e.g. Lundh test).

Other direct tests of pancreatic function

The Lundh test involves stimulation of pancreatic secretion by a meal containing carbohydrate, protein and fat. The duodenal contents are then collected for 2 hours and the activity of trypsin or amylase (or lipase) measured. Low enzymic activity indicates pancreatic exocrine insufficiency. This test is less sensitive than the secretin–CCK-PZ test.

Both the secretin–CCK-PZ test and the Lundh test can be used as stimuli to produce increases in pancreatic enzymes in the blood. Tests based on plasma amylase, lipase and trypsin activity or concentration measurements have been described. Of these, *serum immunoreactive trypsin (IRT)* concentration has so far proved the most promising. Patients with chronic pancreatitis frequently have a low fasting serum [IRT], and the test has been suggested as a screening investigation for chronic pancreatitis. If the fasting value is normal and duct obstruction is suspected, serial measurements at 30-minute intervals for 2 hours after a Lundh test meal may show a marked increase in serum [IRT] if obstruction is present.

Lactoferrin is an iron-containing glycoprotein secreted by the pancreas. Its concentration has been reported to be higher than normal in pancreatic juice collected from patients with chronic pancreatitis, and normal in pancreatic carcinoma. Similar results have been obtained for [lactoferrin] in duodenal juice.

BT-PABA–[^{14}C]-PABA test (Fig. 10.2)

This is an *indirect* test of pancreatic function. Such tests are less specific and less sensitive than the direct stimulation tests but are relatively easy to perform. They assess the pancreatic response to a meal (e.g. the Lundh test meal). The BT-PABA–[^{14}C]-PABA test depends on the fact that pancreatic chymotrypsin specifically hydrolyses the synthetic peptide N-benzoyl-L-tyrosyl-p-aminobenzoic acid (BT-PABA), to release PABA, which is then absorbed from the intestine, partly metabolized by the liver, and excreted in the urine as PABA and its metabolites.

The patient is given BT-PABA (0.5 g) together with [^{14}C]-PABA (5 µCi) at the same time as a test meal to achieve pancreatic stimulation. The [^{14}C]-PABA is added to correct for individual absorption, metabolism and excretion characteristics of PABA following its release from BT-PABA in the intestine. Urine is collected for 6 hours and urinary PABA and ^{14}C content measured; both results are expressed as a percentage of their oral dose. These percentages are then used to calculate a ratio, the PABA : ^{14}C excretion index (reference range 0.84–1.16). In chronic pancreatitis, hydrolysis of BT-PABA is impaired and the excretion index low.

The results of the BT-PABA/[^{14}C]-PABA test correlate well with the CCK-PZ and Lundh tests. It has the advantage of being non-invasive, and suitable for the

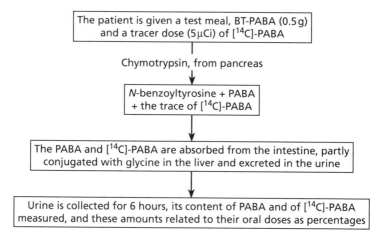

Fig. 10.2 The principles of the BT-PABA–[^{14}C]-PABA test. The results are expressed as a ratio of the percentages of the doses of PABA and of [^{14}C] excreted, the PABA : [^{14}C] excretion index (reference range 0.84–1.16).

investigation of out-patients, but is contraindicated in children, in pregnancy and in patients with renal failure. In those versions of the test that omit [^{14}C]-PABA and only measure the urinary PABA excretion in 6 hours, falsely abnormal results may be found in liver and small bowel disease.

Fluorescein dilaurate test (Fig. 10.3)

This is another indirect test of pancreatic function. Also called the pancreolauryl test, it depends on the hydrolysis of fluorescein dilaurate (which has low solubility in water) by cholesterol ester hydrolase, an enzyme normally present in pancreatic juice. The product, fluorescein, is water-soluble and is readily absorbed from the intestine; it is then conjugated in the liver and excreted as its glucuronide in the urine, where its fluorescence is measured.

The patient is given 0.5 mmol fluorescein dilaurate together with a test meal to stimulate secretion of pancreatic enzymes and urine is collected for the next 10 hours. The test is repeated the next day, but on this occasion the patient is given the equivalent dose of free fluorescein; this second test seeks to correct for individual variations in absorption from the intestine, hepatic conjugation and renal excretion. The ratio of the amounts of fluorescein excreted after administration (i) of fluorescein dilaurate and (ii) of free fluorescein is expressed as a percentage. Normally, the ratio is over 30%. Ratios of less then 20% are considered abnormal, while results between 20 and 30% are equivocal.

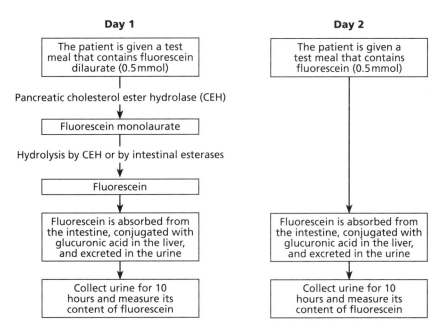

Fig. 10.3 The principles of the fluorescein dilaurate test. The ratio of the amounts of fluorescein excreted on days 1 and 2 is determined (normally this is over 30%).

Tests of intestinal absorption

Carbohydrate absorption

Xylose absorption test. In this test D-xylose, a pentose, is normally absorbed rapidly from the small intestine by a different mechanism from most dietary carbohydrates. It is partly metabolized in the liver, the rest being excreted in the urine. It can be used to test the intestine's ability to absorb monosaccharides. There is no standard protocol for performing the xylose absorption test, as the following description shows. It is therefore necessary to consult the laboratory for details of the local procedure, and for information on how to interpret the results.

Various doses of xylose have been used, but a 5 g dose has been widely adopted (e.g. in preference to 25 g) as being less likely to provoke nausea. The dose is given to the patient after an overnight fast and the patient must not eat during the test. The response can be assessed on the basis of serum or blood [xylose] 1 or 2 hours after ingestion, or by measuring urinary xylose excretion. Urine specimens may be collected over a 5-hour period or the collection period divided into two, the first being completed after 2 hours and the second over the 2–5-hour period. Blood measurements are to be preferred as they are independent of renal function; they also avoid the difficulties of ensuring complete, accurately timed urine collections.

Impaired absorption and excretion of xylose have often been reported in patients with disease of the small intestine. Low values may also be observed in patients who have bacterial colonization of the small intestine, since the bacteria may metabolize xylose. Low urinary values occur in patients with renal disease, due to impaired excretion of xylose; blood or serum [xylose] should be measured if the patient's plasma [urea] exceeds 8 mmol/L.

The availability of jejunal biopsy has greatly reduced the need to perform xylose absorption tests. However, the test can be used to monitor the response to therapy (e.g. the response of patients with coeliac disease to starting treatment by means of a gluten-free diet).

Disaccharide tolerance tests

Disaccharidase deficiency may be exhibited as intolerance to one or more of the disaccharides, lactose, maltose or sucrose. The defect may be congenital or acquired. Several tests of carbohydrate absorption are based on the ability to hydrolyse and absorb disaccharides. These are performed to determine whether there is impairment of absorption of ingested disaccharides, and to help define whether any impairment is due to intestinal disaccharidase deficiency.

Disaccharidase activity can be measured in small intestinal mucosa biopsy specimens. This is the most reliable way of specifically diagnosing small intestinal disaccharidase deficiency.

Tests based on plasma glucose measurements

After an overnight fast, blood is collected for measurement of plasma [glucose] before the test is started. An oral dose of 50 g disaccharide (usually lactose or sucrose) is then given, and plasma [glucose] measured at 30-minute intervals for the next 2 hours. In healthy individuals, plasma [glucose] should increase by at least 1.1 mmol/L; in disaccharidase deficiency, the rise is usually less. To eliminate the possibility that generalized mucosal disease is present, the test should be repeated using a mixture containing 25 g of each of the monosaccharides that made up the disaccharide used in the first part of the test.

Breath hydrogen test

This is based on the fact that any carbohydrate not absorbed in the small intestine is liable to be metabolized in the large intestine by bacteria with the production of hydrogen; this diffuses rapidly across the colonic mucosa into the blood and can be measured in the breath by gas chromatography.

To perform the test, 50 g disaccharide (e.g. lactose, sucrose) is given orally and the breath H_2 determined at half-hourly intervals from the start of the test for the next 2–5 hours. An increase in breath H_2 of more than 20 μL/L expired air over the basal level indicates malabsorption of the disaccharide. False-negative results may be produced in the absence of colonic organisms responsible for H_2 production, due to antibiotic treatment. False-positive results may be caused by bacterial colonization of the small intestine.

Faecal acidity

Measurement of faecal [H^+] may assist in diagnosis since the pH of faeces may fall to below 5.5 due to bacterial metabolism of unabsorbed carbohydrate.

Amino acid absorption

Certain specific disorders affect both intestinal and renal epithelial transport. In Hartnup disease (p. 134) there is impaired transport of neutral amino acids, and deficiency of some essential amino acids (especially tryptophan) may occur. In cystinuria (p. 134) the basic amino acids and cystine are affected; however, there is no associated nutritional defect despite the fact that lysine is an essential amino acid. These disorders are investigated by examining the pattern of amino acids excreted in the urine by chromatography.

Fat absorption

Efficient absorption of fat requires both effective solubilization of fats and lipolysis, followed by the absorption of hydrolysed products across the jejunum. Bile salts play an important role in lipid absorption. Primary bile acids are formed in the liver, conjugated with glycine and taurine, and secreted into bile. Together with phospholipids, bile salts form micelles which render dietary fats soluble; bile salts also promote the action of pancreatic lipase and co-lipase. The micelles also solubilize the products of lipolysis and enable their absorption.

During absorption of a fat-containing meal, bile acids must be present in the upper small intestine in concentrations sufficient to allow the formation of micelles. The bile salts are mostly reabsorbed in the terminal ileum by an active process and are transported back to the liver where they are re-excreted in bile, thus completing an enterohepatic circulation. Insufficient bile acids may give rise to malabsorption of fat (Table 10.3).

Table 10.3 Malabsorption due to insufficient bile salts

Reason for bile salt insufficiency	Examples of causes of the insufficiency
Impaired synthesis of bile acids	Cirrhosis of the liver
Impaired delivery of bile acids to the intestine (due to obstruction to the outflow of bile)	Choledocholithiasis, carcinoma of the head of the pancreas
Interruptions to the enterohepatic circulation	
(a) Impaired absorption of bile acid conjugates from the terminal ileum	Ileal disease (e.g. Crohn's disease), resection of the terminal ileum
(b) Impaired ability of the liver to clear bile acid conjugates from the portal blood and to secrete them again into the bile	Cholestasis associated with hepatic cirrhosis
Splitting of bile acid conjugates in the upper small intestine (reducing their effective concentration at the site of fat absorption)	Bacterial colonization of the upper small intestine (the 'stagnant gut syndrome')

Fat-soluble vitamins (A, D, E and K) share absorptive mechanisms with other dietary lipids. Malabsorption of fat-soluble vitamins, which is most commonly manifest as vitamin D deficiency (p. 208), occurs in conditions causing fat malabsorption.

Faecal fat

In the simplest form of the test, all faecal specimens passed over a 5-day period are collected and sent to the laboratory. The specimens are combined and total fat content estimated. No attempt is made to subdivide the measurement into unhydrolysed and hydrolysed fat. Important drawbacks of the test are the difficulty (even under the best conditions) of ensuring complete 5-day collections of faeces, and the inherently unpleasant nature of the test. Tests based on the separate estimation of unhydrolysed triglyceride ('unsplit fat') and hydrolysed triglyceride ('split fat') in the faeces have proved unreliable as a means of differentiating between pancreatic and non-pancreatic causes of fat malabsorption; this is because intestinal bacteria can also hydrolyse triglycerides.

Before starting a faecal fat test, the patient should have been on a normal mixed diet containing between 50 and 100 g fat/day for at least 3 days. Patients should ideally be admitted to a metabolic ward and a non-absorbable dye marker (e.g. carmine) or inert indicator (e.g. chromium sesquioxide) given to improve the accuracy of faecal collections or fat concentration measurements, respectively. Preservation of faecal specimens prior to chemical analysis is by refrigeration.

Provided fat intake does not exceed 100 g/day, the normal faecal fat excretion by healthy individuals is up to 5 g/ 24 h. It may be increased in patients with pancreatic disease and in patients with intestinal malabsorption. Sometimes the output is very high, as much as 25–40 g/24 h. In pancreatic disease, faecal fat excretion is only increased when pancreatic function has fallen to less than 10% of normal.

Triglyceride 'breath test'

This test avoids the difficulties and unpleasantness of collecting faeces over several days. Following digestion and absorption of an oral dose of $[^{14}C]$-triolein (the marker is in the fatty acid component), part of the fatty acid is metabolized to $^{14}CO_2$ which is then excreted in expired air. A high $^{14}CO_2$ excretion is associated with normal fat absorption, whereas $^{14}CO_2$ excretion is low in patients with fat malabsorption. This test is convenient and rapid, but technically difficult.

Miscellaneous tests of intestinal function

Bacterial colonization of the small intestine

The small intestine is usually virtually sterile. However, when there is stasis (e.g. blind loop, stricture) or a colonic fistula or, occasionally, when immune mechanisms are impaired, anaerobic bacteria colonize the small intestine. This often causes fat malabsorption, due at least partly to deconjugation of bile acid conjugates by the bacteria. Vitamin B_{12} deficiency may also develop, due to its consumption by the bacteria.

Diagnosis of bacterial colonization of the small intestine requires intubation for the collection of specimens on which microbiological procedures are then performed. However, some non-invasive tests have been devised for detecting the possible presence of bacterial colonization.

Urinary indican

Most of the tryptophan released by the digestion of protein is normally absorbed. Unabsorbed tryptophan is metabolized by the intestinal flora to indoles; these are absorbed, metabolized in the liver to indicans, and excreted in the urine. Urinary indican excretion may be increased when there are abnormal amounts of tryptophan in the colon due to disease of the small intestine, or when there is bacterial colonization of the small intestine, or when there is a tryptophan transport defect (e.g. Hartnup disease). In the absence of severe steatorrhoea, a urinary indican excretion of more than 200 mg/24 h is indicative of bacterial colonization of the small intestine.

Breath tests

The *$[^{14}C]$-xylose breath test* depends on the ability of anaerobic bacteria to metabolize $[^{14}C]$-xylose with the production of $^{14}CO_2$ which is then absorbed from the intestine, transported to the lungs and excreted in the expired air. Some $^{14}CO_2$ is normally produced by the liver as a result of metabolism of $[^{14}C]$-xylose, following absorption, but increased $^{14}CO_2$ production is associated with bacterial colonization. To perform the test, $[^{14}C]$-xylose (1 g, 10 µCi) is given by mouth and breath samples are collected hourly for the next 6 hours. Abnormally increased breath $^{14}CO_2$ occurs within the first 60 minutes in 85% of patients with bacterial colonization. However, if gastric emptying is delayed, the increase in $^{14}CO_2$ excretion may not become abnormal for three hours.

The *$[^{14}C]$-glycocholate breath test* depends on the fact that some bacteria metabolize $[^{14}C]$-glycocholate with the production of $^{14}CO_2$. The test is performed in a manner similar to the [^{14}C]-xylose breath test. The comparisons between these two tests indicate that the [^{14}C]-xylose breath test is the more reliable.

Intestinal permeability

In small intestinal disease, absorptive function may be diminished but permeability (via intercellular junctions) is often increased. In coeliac disease, intestinal permeability may be further increased by applying a high osmotic load. Permeability can be assessed by determining the *cellobiose : mannitol ratio*. Cellobiose is a disaccharide that is not normally hydrolysed in or absorbed from the small intestine. Mannitol is a sugar alcohol that is normally absorbed across the enterocyte. In coeliac disease, mannitol absorption is diminished and its urinary excretion is diminished, whereas permeability to cellobiose is increased; it is absorbed through intercellular junctions, especially if intestinal osmolality is high, and is then excreted in the urine.

To determine the cellobiose : mannitol ratio, cellobiose (5 g), mannitol (2 g), sucrose (20 g) and lactose (20 g) are dissolved in 100 mL water and given to the patient. Sucrose and lactose are included to produce a high osmolality in the intestine. Urine is collected over the next 5 hours and the cellobiose : mannitol ratio measured. The ratio is increased in intestinal disease. The test has not been widely used because it causes nausea, and because the measurements of cellobiose and mannitol present difficulties. However, it can be used to monitor treatment of coeliac disease.

Intestinal permeability can also be assessed by giving [^{51}Cr]-EDTA (100 μCi) by mouth and then collecting urine for 24 hours. Increased urinary excretion of [^{51}Cr]-EDTA occurs in intestinal disease. Glomerular function should be assessed before performing this test, as its interpretation depends on there being normal glomerular function.

Reabsorption of water and inorganic constituents

About 8 L of intestinal secretions are produced each day and must be largely reabsorbed or deficiency states rapidly develop. Reabsorption takes place mainly in the jejunum and ileum, but also in the colon. Acute and severe disturbances may occur in patients following operations, especially operations on the GI tract, and losses of K^+ often become very large.

Non-surgical intestinal causes of electrolyte imbalance include severe diarrhoea and cholera, in which there is a defect of Na^+ reabsorption in the jejunum. In the *Verner–Morrison syndrome*, there is severe watery diarrhoea and hypokalaemia, associated with hypersecretion of vasoactive intestinal peptide (VIP). In these patients, fasting plasma [VIP] is high, whereas it is normal or low in patients with diarrhoea due to other causes.

The systematic investigation of malabsorption by chemical tests

Efficient digestion and absorption require the stomach, pancreas, hepatobiliary system and the small intestine all to be functioning normally. Severe defects in the function of any one of these organs may cause intestinal malabsorptive disease; the

Table 10.4 Examples of the ways in which GI diseases cause malabsorption

Dietary constituent	Disease of the GI tract	Why malabsorption may occur
Polysaccharides	Chronic pancreatitis	Amylase deficiency
Disaccharides	Intestinal mucosal defect	Disaccharidase deficiency
Proteins	Chronic pancreatitis	Pancreatic peptidase deficiency
Amino acids	Intestinal mucosal defect	Specific amino acid transport abnormalities
Lipids	Chronic pancreatitis	Lipase and/or co-lipase deficiency
	Insufficient bile salts	Micelle formation impaired
	Gastrinoma	High intestinal [H^+] inhibits pancreatic lipase
	Abetalipoproteinaemia	Transfer of lipids to plasma impaired

Note, in addition, that any generalized intestinal disease is liable to cause malabsorption of all dietary constituents.

patient may complain of diarrhoea or weight loss. The causes of carbohydrate, protein and amino acid, and lipid malabsorption are summarized in Table 10.4; most of these have been referred to in this chapter, but a few are considered elsewhere in this book.

Clinical diagnosis

Prior to performing chemical tests of GI function, it is important to consider the history of the patient's illness and the findings on physical examination, and to formulate a provisional diagnosis and list the differential diagnoses. Then, by grouping intestinal malabsorptive disease into the following categories, the selection of investigations and interpretation of their results are simplified:

1 *Pancreatic disease* may cause malabsorption of protein, fat or carbohydrate, due to deficiency of digestive enzymes.

2 *Biliary disease* may cause malabsorption of fat and fat-soluble vitamins, due to lack of bile acids.

3 *Intestinal mucosal disease* may affect digestion or transport, or both, of many dietary constituents, and reabsorption of bile acids. The effects may be general, or relatively specific.

4 *Bacterial colonization of the small intestine* may cause a functional deficiency of bile acids, and so interfere with absorption of fats. It may also interfere with the digestion of protein or absorption of amino acids, and decrease the availability of water-soluble vitamins.

Initial investigations

Microbiological examination, including stool microscopy and culture, should always be performed *before* chemical tests are requested whenever an infectious cause of a GI disorder needs to be excluded. We assume here that microbiological causes of intestinal disease have been excluded.

A faecal specimen should be inspected; this may suggest that the patient has steatorrhoea. The specimen should also be tested for occult blood. If the specimen is very loose and watery, the following may be helpful:

1 *Faecal pH*. A pH below 6.0 in the watery supernatant of the stool indicates fermentation of unabsorbed carbohydrate.

2 *Osmotic gap*. This may be measured on the watery supernatant of the stool. It is defined as the observed osmolality minus twice the sum of the supernatant $[Na^+]$ and $[K^+]$. A large osmotic gap indicates the presence of other cations (e.g. Mg^{2+}, due to excessive use of purgatives).

3 *Sodium : potassium ratio*. In general, this ratio is increased in colonic disorders and decreased in small intestinal disorders.

Preliminary chemical investigations on blood specimens should include plasma [albumin], which may indicate the presence of a protein-losing enteropathy, and other 'liver function tests'. Preliminary haematological investigations (haemoglobin, full blood count, vitamin B_{12} and folate) should also be performed.

Further investigations

Radiology (e.g. barium meal, barium enema), endoscopy (e.g. gastroscopy, duodenoscopy, endoscopic retrograde cholangio-pancreatography (ERCP), colonoscopy) and mucosal biopsy (e.g. duodenal biopsy) may be indicated. They may define the site of an anatomical abnormality, and are more reliable in this respect than most of the organ-directed chemical tests considered in this chapter.

Faecal fat (or alternative tests of fat absorption) may be abnormal whenever there is malabsorption. However, in general, severe fat malabsorption is only encountered in pancreatic and small intestinal disease. Several other chemical abnormalities may occur in association with intestinal malabsorption, and require appropriate investigation and treatment. These include:

1 *Defects in calcium absorption* that may cause rickets or osteomalacia.

2 *Malabsorption of iron*. This may cause iron-deficiency anaemia. Mixed deficiencies of vitamin B_{12}, folate and iron may also occur.

3 *Malabsorption of protein*. Reduction in plasma [albumin] most often results, but hypogammaglobulinaemia may be marked.

Carcinoid tumours and the carcinoid syndrome

Carcinoid tumours arise in the gut or in tissues derived from the embryological foregut (e.g. thyroid, bronchus). The commonest sites are the terminal ileum and the ileocaecal region. The tumours produce vasoactive amines which, because of the venous drainage of the tumours, are usually carried directly to the liver and there inactivated. Symptoms are only likely to occur either when the tumour has metastasized to the liver, or when the tumour drains into the systemic circulation (e.g. bronchial adenoma of the carcinoid type).

Most carcinoid tumours secrete large amounts of 5-hydroxytryptamine or serotonin (5-HT); the main urinary metabolite of 5-HT is 5-hydroxyindoleacetic acid (5-HIAA). 'Atypical carcinoids' contain excessive amounts of 5-hydroxytryptophan (5-HTP) and relatively little 5-HT; atypical tumours may also secrete histamine. Normally, only about 1% of dietary tryptophan is metabolized along the 5-hydroxyindole pathway to 5-HTP, 5-HT and 5-HIAA. However, over-production of 5-HT is a constant feature of the carcinoid syndrome, as much as 60% of dietary tryptophan being metabolized to 5-HTP, 5-HT and 5-HIAA in these patients.

The carcinoid syndrome is usually associated with tumours of the terminal ileum and extensive secondary deposits in the liver. The main presenting features include flushing attacks, abdominal colic and diarrhoea, and dyspnoea sometimes associated with asthmatic attacks. Valvular disease of the heart is often present. Carcinoid tumours can give rise to severe hypoproteinaemia and oedema, even in the absence of cardiac complications. There may also be signs of niacin deficiency, due to major diversion of tryptophan metabolism away from the pathway leading to niacin production (p. 237). Some carcinoid tumours produce ACTH or ACTH-like peptides and may cause Cushing's syndrome (p. 271) in the absence of the symptoms commonly associated with the carcinoid syndrome.

Chemical investigation of 5-HT metabolism

Measurement of 5-HIAA excretion in a 24-hour urine specimen is the most widely performed investigation; the output is usually greatly increased. The following points need to be observed before or during the collection of specimens:

1 *Drugs.* Urinary 5-HIAA output should be determined before treatment is started, whenever possible, especially before treatment with drugs that release 5-HT from body stores. If treatment has started, it should have been unchanged for at least 2 weeks before measuring 5-HIAA excretion.

2 *Diet.* Bananas and tomatoes contain large amounts of 5-HT; they should not be eaten the day before or during the urine collection.

3 *Timing of urine collection.* If attacks of symptoms are frequent, the time of starting the collection is unimportant. If attacks are less often than daily, the patient should be instructed to wait and begin the collection when the next attack occurs.

'Atypical carcinoid' tumours in various sites are sometimes associated with abnormal metabolism of tryptophan. They include carcinoma of the stomach and pancreas, islet cell tumour of the pancreas, hepatoma, small cell carcinoma of the bronchus, and medullary carcinoma of the thyroid. It is rare for these tumours to be associated with features of the carcinoid syndrome, although they may contain increased amounts of 5-HT, and urinary excretion of 5-HIAA may be abnormal. More information about the pattern of 5-hydroxyindole metabolites can be obtained from urine chromatography. If increased amounts of 5-HTP are found, this indicates the presence of an 'atypical carcinoid'.

Chapter 11
Disorders of Carbohydrate Metabolism

The liver plays a key role in carbohydrate metabolism and in maintaining blood [glucose]. After a carbohydrate-containing meal, it removes about 70% of the glucose load that is delivered via the portal circulation; some of the glucose is oxidized and some converted to glycogen for use as a fuel under fasting conditions. Glucose in excess of these requirements is partly converted by the liver to fatty acids and triglycerides, which are then incorporated into very low density lipoproteins (VLDL) and transported to adipose tissue stores.

In the fasting state, blood [glucose] is maintained partly by glycogen breakdown in the liver, and partly by gluconeogenesis (from glycerol, lactate and pyruvate and from the gluconeogenic amino acids), occurring mostly in the liver but also in the kidneys. Glucose is spared, under fasting conditions, by the ability of muscle and other tissues to adapt to the oxidation of fatty acids, and by the ability of the brain and some other organs to utilize ketone bodies that are formed under these conditions.

The hormones mainly concerned with regulating glucose metabolism in the fed and fasting states and with blood glucose homeostasis are insulin, glucagon, somatostatin, growth hormone, adrenaline and cortisol. Of these, insulin has the most marked effects in man (Table 11.1), and is the only hormone with a lowering effect on blood [glucose]. Glucagon, growth hormone, adrenaline and cortisol all tend, in general, to antagonize the actions of insulin (Table 11.2).

Insulin secretion

Insulin is synthesized in the β-cells of the islets of Langerhans in the pancreas. It is

Table 11.1 The effects of insulin on cellular metabolism

Tissue	Processes activated by insulin	Processes inhibited by insulin
Liver	Uptake of amino acids and glycerol Production of NADPH Synthesis of glycogen, proteins, triglycerides and VLDL	Glycogenolysis Gluconeogenesis Ketone body formation
Muscle	Uptake of glucose and amino acids Synthesis of glycogen	Triglyceride utilization
Adipose	Uptake of chylomicrons and VLDL and of glucose Utilization of glucose	Lipolysis

Table 11.2 The effects on glucose metabolism of hormones that antagonize the actions of insulin

Tissue and hormone	Effects of the various hormones on glucose metabolism			
	Gluconeogenesis	Glycogenolysis	Glycolysis	Glucose uptake
Liver				
Adrenaline	Increased	Increased	Decreased	
Cortisol	Increased			Decreased
Glucagon	Increased	Increased		
Growth hormone	Increased	Increased	Decreased	
Muscle				
Adrenaline		Increased	Increased	
Cortisol				Decreased
Growth hormone				
(a) Short term			Increased	
(b) Long term			Decreased	
Adipose				
Cortisol			Decreased	

formed as pre-pro-insulin which is rapidly cleaved to pro-insulin. The pro-insulin is packaged into secretory granules in the Golgi apparatus and is subsequently cleaved to insulin and the connecting or C-peptide; insulin and C-peptide are later released into the circulation in equimolar amounts.

A rise in blood [glucose] is the main stimulus for insulin secretion. Some amino acids (e.g. leucine), fatty acids and ketone bodies also promote insulin secretion. By itself, hyperglycaemia is a poor stimulus to insulin release; it appears to require the presence of glucose-dependent insulinotrophic peptide (GIP) or glucagon. GIP is probably the most important factor in the entero-insular axis, the mechanism that accounts for the larger release of insulin that occurs in response to an oral glucose load, as compared with the same dose of glucose given intravenously. Vagal stimulation also promotes insulin release.

The mechanism of action of insulin is not fully understood. An insulin receptor has been identified which is internalized after insulin binding. Within different organs, target enzymes have been identified which serve to explain the known effects of insulin on intermediary metabolism. For instance, activation of glucose transport, induction of hexokinase (or glucokinase) and activation of phospho-fructokinase, pyruvate kinase and pyruvate dehydrogenase in the liver are all consistent with insulin's actions of promoting increased glucose uptake and glycolytic breakdown. Stimulation of glycogen synthase also accords with the known effects of insulin on glycogen formation in the liver.

Blood and plasma glucose

Through the actions of insulin and the hormones with anti-insulin action, blood [glucose] is normally maintained within fairly narrow limits. Blood and plasma [glucose] are usually measured by enzymic methods that employ glucose oxidase or hexokinase, enzymes with a high degree of specificity for glucose. Results with non-enzymic, reductive, methods are less specific and usually yield values 0.3–0.6 mmol/L higher (sometimes as much as 1.0 mmol/L higher) than those obtained by enzymic measurements. Both enzymic and reductive methods can be used satisfactorily for the diagnosis and control of diabetes mellitus, but enzymic methods are essential for the proper investigation and recognition of hypoglycaemia.

In this book, the terms plasma [glucose] and blood [glucose] are used when measurements depend on enzymic methods specific for glucose, whereas plasma [sugar] and blood [sugar] are used when referring to non-enzymic methods that also measure other reducing substances. The corresponding distinction between the terms glycosuria and glucosuria is described on p. 14.

Blood specimens for glucose analysis
Most laboratories measure plasma [glucose], but some still use whole blood. Plasma is to be preferred, as the measurements yield more reliable results. At normal plasma [glucose], there is little difference between results obtained on capillary and venous blood. However, at hyperglycaemic levels, capillary plasma [glucose] may be significantly higher than venous plasma [glucose]. This is important in the interpretation of glucose tolerance tests.

If there is likely to be any delay in measuring [glucose] in blood specimens, it is essential either to separate off the plasma immediately or to inhibit glycolysis in blood by using a sodium fluoride-containing collection tube. This stabilizes the [glucose] for several hours, and allows blood specimens to be sent considerable distances (e.g. by post) to a central laboratory. However, measurements of blood [glucose] that are to be performed by one of the 'side-room' methods that depend on the use of enzyme-impregnated 'sticks' (p. 17) must be carried out without delay on specimens that do not contain sodium fluoride; lithium heparin is a satisfactory anticoagulant for these specimens.

Diabetes mellitus

Diabetes mellitus can be defined as a state of diminished insulin action due to its decreased availability or effectiveness. Chronic hyperglycaemia results, usually accompanied by glucosuria and other biochemical abnormalities, expressed as a wide range of clinical presentations ranging from asymptomatic patients with relatively mild biochemical abnormalities to patients admitted to hospital with severe metabolic decompensation of rapid onset that has led to coma. Long-term clinical sequelae may develop including retinopathy, neuropathy, nephropathy and vascular disease.

The diagnosis of diabetes mellitus may be suggested on the basis of the patient's history or by the results of 'side-room' tests for glucose on urine specimens. However, urine glucose measurements are inadequate by themselves, for diagnostic purposes. Although convenient and sensitive, they yield many false-positive results and, in fasting diabetics, may yield false-negative results. A provisional diagnosis of diabetes mellitus must always be confirmed by glucose measurements on blood specimens.

The criteria for the diagnosis of diabetes mellitus have been laid down by the World Health Organization (WHO). The American Diabetic Association has produced a set of guidelines similar to the WHO criteria, but the two sets are not identical. These criteria are for specific enzymic assays, and separate sets of criteria are described for different types of sample, depending on whether venous or capillary whole blood, or venous or capillary plasma specimens are used.

According to the WHO criteria, a fasting venous plasma [glucose] of 8 mmol/L or more is diagnostic of diabetes mellitus. Alternatively, a random venous plasma [glucose] of 11.1 mmol/L or more establishes the diagnosis.

The oral glucose tolerance test (see below) was, for many years, regarded as the definitive test for confirming or refuting a provisional diagnosis of diabetes mellitus, but it is much less widely used now. Nevertheless, WHO criteria have been established for blood or plasma [glucose] 2 hours after a 75 g load of anhydrous glucose (82.5 g glucose monohydrate), and this test should be carried out if there is any doubt.

Table 11.3 summarizes data for blood and plasma [glucose], for venous and capillary specimens, for three groups of subjects — healthy adults, patients with diabetes mellitus and individuals with impaired glucose tolerance — in the fasting state and 2 hours after a 75 g load of anhydrous glucose (82.5 g glucose monohydrate). The criteria for diagnosing diabetes mellitus and impaired glucose tolerance do not differ between symptomatic and asymptomatic individuals,

Table 11.3 Diagnostic criteria for diabetes mellitus; their dependence on the nature of the specimens collected for analysis (WHO Expert Committee on Diabetes Mellitus)

	Glucose concentration (mmol/L)		
	Fasting		Two hours post-75 g glucose
Normal individuals			
Venous plasma	< 7.8		< 7.8
Capillary plasma	< 7.8		< 7.8
Venous blood	< 6.7		< 6.7
Capillary blood	< 6.7		< 7.8
Diabetes mellitus			
Venous plasma	⩾ 8.0	and/or	⩾ 11.0
Capillary plasma	⩾ 8.0	and/or	⩾ 12.0
Venous blood	⩾ 7.0	and/or	⩾ 10.0
Capillary blood	⩾ 7.0	and/or	⩾ 11.0
Impaired glucose tolerance			
Venous plasma	< 8.0	and	⩾ 8.0 but < 11.0
Capillary plasma	< 8.0	and	⩾ 9.0 but < 12.0
Venous blood	< 7.0	and	⩾ 7.0 but < 10.0
Capillary blood	< 7.0	and	⩾ 8.0 but < 11.0

Note
The data in the table are for glucose measurements performed by an enzymic method specific for glucose. If measurements are made using a reductive method, all figures should be increased by 1.0 mmol/L.

although it is important to confirm the diagnosis in asymptomatic patients by a repeat measurement of a fasting, or 2-hour post-glucose load, blood sample.

Oral glucose tolerance test (GTT) (Fig. 11.1)

The main value of a GTT is that it may help to establish the diagnosis of diabetes mellitus or impaired glucose tolerance at a time when the metabolic abnormality is mild. The GTT is particularly valuable in the diagnosis of impaired glucose tolerance in pregnancy (p. 316). Several precautions must be observed in preparing for and in performing the test.

Before the test

It should not be performed on patients who are suffering from the effects of trauma or recovering from a serious illness. It should also be delayed if the patient has an intercurrent infection. Drugs such as corticosteroids and diuretics may impair glucose tolerance; they should be stopped before the test, if possible.

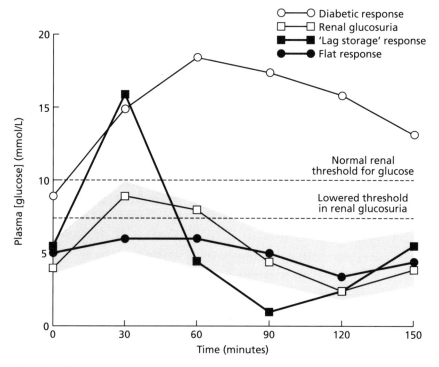

Fig. 11.1 Plasma [glucose] changes in response to an oral glucose tolerance test. The shaded area indicates the approximate limits within which responses to a 75 g load of anhydrous glucose normally fall.

Glucose can be detected in urine specimens collected after the renal threshold for glucose has been exceeded; the normal threshold corresponds to a plasma [glucose] of 10 mmol/L, and the lowered threshold in patients with renal glucosuria to a lower level of plasma [glucose]. The various responses to the glucose tolerance test are described in greater detail in the text.

The patient should have been on an unrestricted diet containing at least 150 g carbohydrate/day for at least 3 days, and should not have indulged in unaccustomed amounts of exercise. The patient must not smoke on the day of the test, either before or during the test, nor eat or drink anything other than as specified below.

Performing the test

A GTT is usually performed after an overnight fast, although a fast of 4–5 hours may be enough. The patient is allowed to drink water during the fast, and may have a cup of unsweetened tea before the test; this helps to reduce any tendency to nausea that might otherwise be caused by the oral glucose drink.

A standard dose of glucose (82.5 g glucose monohydrate or 75 g anhydrous glucose) dissolved in 250–350 mL of water, lemon-flavoured or chilled (or both) to avoid nausea, is given by mouth. Smaller amounts of glucose (1.92 g glucose monohydrate or 1.75 g anhydrous glucose/kg body weight) should be given to children or small adults to a maximum dose of 82.5 g glucose monohydrate or 75 g anhydrous glucose.

During the test the patient should be sitting up, or lying over on the right side so as to facilitate rapid emptying of the stomach, *not* lying flat or over on the left side.

Blood specimens are collected before giving the glucose load, and thereafter (in a full GTT) at 30-minute intervals for 2 hours. In terms of the WHO criteria for tests performed on patients with symptoms, it is only necessary to collect fasting and 2-hour post-glucose specimens. However, having decided to perform the test, it is advisable to collect a full set of blood specimens. They are needed for making the diagnosis of renal glucosuria (see below), and for the recognition of abnormally shaped GTT responses (e.g. 'lag-storage' curve). In cases of suspected reactive hypoglycaemia, it may be worthwhile to prolong the blood collections until 6 hours after the dose of glucose.

Urine specimens should be collected before the test and at 1 and 2 hours after the dose of glucose; they should be tested for glucose by 'side-room' tests (Table 2.2, p. 13). Although the results for these urine measurements are not included among the WHO diagnostic criteria for diabetes mellitus, urine needs to be tested if patients with renal glucosuria are to be recognized.

Abnormal GTT not associated with increased risk of diabetes

'Flat response' to GTT describes the response when the plasma [glucose] fails to rise significantly. If the fasting plasma [glucose] was 5.0 mmol/L, the 30-minute and 60-minute or 60-minute and 90-minute specimens, or all three specimens, would normally have a value of 7.0 mmol/L or more in a GTT. A 'flat response' is often caused by incorrect positioning of the patient during the test, resulting in delayed gastric emptying. It is occasionally due to intestinal malabsorptive disease; it may also occur in hypopituitarism and in adrenal hyposecretory states.

'Lag-storage' response to GTT describes the pattern of results in which there is a sharp rise in plasma [glucose], with the peak value appearing early and sometimes exceeding 11.0 mmol/L. There is also a tendency for the 2-hour value to be much lower than the fasting value. There may be glucosuria. This pattern of response is due to rapid absorption of glucose from the intestine; the tissues, mainly the liver, are unable to attain a sufficiently rapid uptake to match the rapid absorption. It may be seen after gastric surgery (e.g. gastroenterostomy) or in patients with severe liver disease, and is sometimes seen in apparently healthy individuals.

Renal glucosuria is the term applied to patients who exhibit glucosuria at some point in the GTT although the plasma [glucose] at all times remains below 10.0 mmol/L. It is due to a lowered renal threshold for glucose, and usually has no pathological significance. However, it may be associated with other renal tubular defects (e.g. Fanconi syndrome, p. 134).

Classification of diabetes mellitus

Clinically, patients with diabetes mellitus may be classified as idiopathic (primary or essential) or as secondary diabetes. There are other groups of patients in whom abnormalities of glucose tolerance may be detected, but who do not fit into either of these categories (see above).

Idiopathic diabetes

This may be caused by factors in the blood which antagonize or inhibit the action of insulin, or by the production of an abnormal form of insulin, or by inability of the pancreas to produce sufficient insulin from the earliest stages of the disease. It is divided into types I and II.

Insulin-dependent diabetes (type I)

In these patients there is defective insulin secretion. The condition usually presents acutely in young (under 30) non-obese subjects, but it can occur at any age. In addition to polyuria, thirst and glucosuria, there is often marked weight loss and ketoacidosis. In general, insulin is required for treatment. The condition is sometimes subdivided into types Ia and Ib.

Islet cell antibodies that react specifically with the β-cells of the pancreas have been demonstrated in serum from over 90% of patients with newly diagnosed type Ia diabetes; over the subsequent few years, these antibodies usually disappear. They have also sometimes been demonstrated in serum several years before clinical and biochemical features of diabetes develop. Individuals with certain human leucocyte antigens (HLA) have also been shown to have a particularly high risk of developing type Ia diabetes. The importance of these immunological findings is in their application to relatives of diabetic patients. If a sibling has islet cell antibodies, or HLA characteristics identical with the patient's, the sibling is potentially diabetic and has an increased probability of developing impaired glucose tolerance or frank diabetes mellitus.

Type Ib patients show persistent islet cell antibodies and their diabetes mellitus shows a clear association with other forms of auto-immune endocrine disease. The age of presentation is, on average, older than for the type Ia patients.

Non-insulin-dependent diabetes (type II)

This condition may be subdivided into obese and non-obese categories. It generally presents in older (over 40) patients who are obese, a condition that used to be called 'maturity onset' diabetes; it usually presents less acutely than type I diabetes. Rarely, type II diabetes occurs in young patients.

Measurable levels of insulin are normally present, and the metabolic defect appears to lie either in defective insulin secretion or in insulin resistance. Insulin levels tend to be lower in the non-obese type II patient. In general, insulin is not required for the prevention of ketosis as these patients are relatively resistant to its development. However, insulin may be needed to correct abnormalities of blood [glucose].

There appears to be no association between type II diabetes and either the HLA system or the development of auto-immunity. However, there is a strong genetic element to the disorder. For instance, if one identical twin develops type II diabetes, there is a high probability that the other twin will develop it.

Secondary diabetes

This occurs as a consequence of other diseases, either pancreatic or endocrine. With pancreatic diabetes, the secretion of insulin is reduced due to pancreatitis, haemochromatosis or resection of the pancreas. In diabetes secondary to other endocrine disorders, ineffective insulin action is caused by abnormal secretion of hormones with 'diabetogenic' activity. Several drugs adversely affect glucose tolerance and secondary diabetes may also occur in a number of genetic disorders. Table 11.4 summarizes the different causes.

Gestational diabetes mellitus

Impaired glucose tolerance and hyperglycaemia in pregnancy are associated with an increased incidence of fetal macrosomia and neonatal hypoglycaemia. In established diabetic patients who become pregnant, poor blood glucose control is associated with a higher incidence of intra-uterine death and fetal malformation. If a known diabetic patient becomes pregnant, it is very important to maintain close control of blood [glucose].

Gestational diabetes mellitus is the term used to describe the abnormal glucose tolerance or diabetes mellitus that may develop during pregnancy; in the majority of these cases, the response to a GTT reverts to normal after the pregnancy but about 50% of cases go on to develop diabetes mellitus later, within

Table 11.4 Examples of causes of secondary diabetes or of impaired glucose tolerance

Category of cause	Examples
Drugs	Oestrogen-containing oral contraceptives, salbutamol and some other catecholaminergic drugs, thiazide diuretics
Endocrine disorders	Acromegaly, Cushing's syndrome and Cushing's disease, glucagonoma, phaeochromocytoma, prolactinoma, thyrotoxicosis (occasionally)
Insulin receptor abnormalities	Auto-immune insulin receptor antibodies, congenital lipodystrophy
Pancreatic disease	Chronic pancreatitis, haemochromatosis, pancreatectomy

the next 7 years. When investigating a pregnant woman, the normal criteria for interpreting the oral GTT should be used (see above). Mild abnormalities should be reassessed not less than 6 weeks after delivery.

Since the diagnosis of gestational diabetes mellitus is made on the basis of an oral GTT, the question arises as to who should be selected for this investigation. Glucosuria detected at routine antenatal testing may suggest the need for an oral GTT, but it may have no significance since the renal threshold for glucose tends to be lowered in pregnancy. One approach is to select women with appropriate risk factors, such as a family history of diabetes mellitus, a previous large baby, unexplained stillbirth, etc. Also, glucosuria is more significant if detected on the *second* specimen of urine passed after an overnight fast (i.e. the first specimen passed is discarded), and this can be used to select patients. Even normal women tend to show slightly impaired glucose tolerance in pregnancy; this is especially true in the third trimester.

There may be lactosuria late in pregnancy, usually detected by 'side-room' tests for reducing substances (p. 14). It is readily distinguishable from glucosuria, and has no pathological significance.

Monitoring the treatment of diabetic patients

The frequency with which blood or plasma [glucose] needs to be measured depends on each patient's diabetic characteristics. During initial stabilization on insulin in hospital, 5–10 determinations may be required each day. Thereafter, with *type I* diabetics at home, it may be advisable for fasting blood [glucose] to be measured daily, to monitor blood [glucose] before and after each main meal on one mid-week and one weekend day, and to measure one post-prandial blood [glucose] on other days; the closeness of monitoring needed depends on the 'brittleness' of the diabetes. Much less frequent monitoring is needed in *type II* diabetics. Indeed, many older patients may be advised to continue on a urine-testing regime.

The use of simple chemical 'side-room' tests by patients testing their own urine specimens regularly for glucose and ketone bodies (p. 13, Table 2.2), recording the results, and in some cases adjusting their treatment on the basis of the glucose results, had been standard practice for many years before home-monitoring of blood [glucose] was introduced. Proper control of diabetes mellitus is essential if long-term complications are to be avoided or their onset delayed. As a result of developments in methods for blood [glucose] measurement (p. 17), their use in home-monitoring now provides a practical and preferable alternative to urine testing. Nevertheless, many diabetic patients continue to achieve good control using only urine testing to monitor and regulate their treatment.

Out-patient surveillance of diabetic patients

Blood [glucose] measurements made at the clinic have the drawback that they are infrequent and only indicate the [glucose] at that time. They may be adequate for monitoring patients with type II diabetes mellitus, but they are not by themselves sufficient for good control of patients with type I diabetes mellitus, nor can apparently satisfactory records of home-monitoring of blood [glucose] always be relied upon. Measurements of glycated (glycosylated) proteins provide valuable indices of the adequacy of control of longer-term blood [glucose].

Glycated haemoglobin (reference range 4.5–8%)

Glucose reacts spontaneously and non-enzymically with free amino groups on proteins to form covalent glycated proteins. The extent of protein glycation depends on the average [glucose] to which the protein is exposed and on the half-life of the protein. Thus, long-lived structural proteins (e.g. lens protein) may be damaged as a result of the abnormal increase in protein glycation found in diabetics. Indeed, it has been suggested that glycation of structural proteins in arterial walls and elsewhere might be responsible for some of the long-term sequelae of diabetes. Shorter half-life proteins such as haemoglobin may also undergo excessive glycation in diabetics.

Haemoglobin (Hb) normally consists mostly of two components, A and a small amount of A_2. These are the forms found in reticulocytes when released from the bone marrow. Thereafter, in the course of the normal 120-day lifespan of the red cell, a small percentage of the Hb becomes glycated. Glycation of Hb has very little effect on its oxygen-carrying properties.

Several demonstrably different glycated derivatives of Hb exist, derived from the reaction of Hb with glucose, glucose-6-phosphate, etc.; these are collectively known as HbA_1. The principal complex is the one formed with glucose itself, HbA_{1c}; it normally forms about 5% of circulating Hb. Methods of measuring blood [total HbA_1] and [HbA_{1c}] are available but, for technical reasons, [total HbA_1] is the measurement most often performed; results are expressed as a percentage of [total Hb].

Since the half-life of Hb is about 60 days, the HbA_1 value reflects the average level of blood [glucose] over the previous 1–2 months. As a consequence, levels of HbA_1 tend to be higher in diabetics. The extent of the elevation indicates the overall average degree of blood glucose control; in poorly controlled diabetics, it may rise as high as 25%. *In type 1 diabetics*, the percentage of total Hb present as HbA_1 provides doctors with a better out-patient index of diabetic control than blood or plasma [glucose], since it is little affected by short-term fluctuations in blood [glucose].

In diabetic clinics, HbA_1 is mostly used to assess control of insulin-dependent diabetics and to complement home-monitoring of blood [glucose]. Studies have shown that the HbA_1 value correlates well with the mean blood [glucose] over the preceding 1–2 months and with clinical impressions of each patient's state of health. It provides an objective measurement of glycaemic control and can be used to define a treatment goal for both the patient and physician. Results of HbA_1 measurements have an important place in studying the relationship between diabetic control and the longer-term development of diabetic complications, and they are valuable in the assessment of new treatment regimes.

It is unlikely that HbA_1 measurements will ever displace home-monitoring of blood [glucose] as the mainstay of day-to-day control of diabetes by patients themselves, their friends or relatives. Technically, HbA_1 measurements are more time-consuming and much more expensive than glucose measurements.

Glycated plasma proteins

Measurement of glycated plasma proteins, e.g. glycated albumin (the major component of these proteins), can also be used to monitor diabetic control. The short half-life of albumin means that this test reflects control of blood [glucose] over the previous 10–15 days. This has some advantages over HbA_1 measurements, for instance in pregnancy where stringent control is particularly necessary.

The only widely available measure of plasma [glycated proteins] is the so-called *fructosamine assay*. This test is rapid and relatively inexpensive, but has been criticized because it lacks specificity and for other technical reasons.

'Microalbuminuria'

Long-standing diabetes mellitus may give rise to proteinuria, and 'side-room' tests sometimes provide the first indication of the development of diabetic nephropathy. However, measurement of 'microalbuminuria' is more sensitive and is to be preferred for this purpose. The albumin that is lost is normal in size.

'Microalbuminuria' is a term that refers to an excessive and abnormal urinary albumin loss which is, nevertheless, below the lower limit of detection of the 'side-room' tests widely used when testing for the presence of urinary protein. The more sensitive tests required to detect 'microalbuminuria' are performed in the laboratory. Up to 50% of type I diabetics may develop nephropathy and the occurrence of 'microalbuminuria' has been shown in a number of studies to signal an eventual progression to diabetic nephropathy.

Testing for 'microalbuminuria' should only be requested if 'side-room' tests for protein are negative. Although there is no analytical difficulty in measuring these low levels of albumin, there is lack of agreement as to the type of sample to use and how best to express the results. Overnight, timed urine collections are increasingly favoured, rather than random urine samples or 24-hour timed collections. Results are expressed as an albumin excretion rate. Patients with 'microalbuminuria' excrete 20–200 µg albumin/minute.

Metabolic complications of diabetes mellitus

Diabetics can develop severe metabolic derangements, leading to coma or to a comatose state, for several reasons. The metabolic derangements can be classified as follows:

1 Hyperglycaemic coma, with or without ketosis.
2 Lactic acidosis, with or without hyperglycaemia.
3 Hypoglycaemic coma, due to insulin excess (p. 176).
4 Uraemia, e.g. due to diabetic nephropathy.

Hyperglycaemic coma is a term that denotes the condition of patients who develop metabolic decompensation that requires urgent treatment with insulin and electrolyte solutions, irrespective of their state of consciousness. It is a serious medical emergency; despite modern advances in treatment, it still carries an average mortality of about 7% *per episode*.

Ketotic, hyperglycaemic coma

This is the usual presentation of classical, hyperglycaemic coma. The clinical features are dehydration, ketosis and hyperventilation ('air hunger'). The condition is most often seen in patients who develop an intercurrent infection, or suffer trauma, or unusual physical or mental stress.

The consequences of metabolic decompensation are primarily those due to lack of effective insulin action. There is hyperglycaemia, glucosuria and urinary loss of water, Na^+ and K^+, as well usually as ketonaemia, ketonuria, metabolic acidosis and hyperkalaemia. The major metabolic abnormalities result from hyperglycaemia or ketoacidosis, or both. Lactic acidosis and pre-renal uraemia may also be present. The height of the plasma [urea] is a better prognostic guide than the height of the plasma [glucose] in these patients.

Hyperglycaemia causes extracellular hyperosmolality, which in turn leads to intracellular dehydration as well as to an osmotic diuresis. The osmotic diuresis causes loss of water, Na^+, K^+, calcium and other inorganic constituents, and leads to a fall in circulating blood volume. Vomiting may exacerbate all these effects.

Ketoacidosis is due to insulin deficiency, which is accompanied by raised plasma concentrations of the so-called 'diabetogenic' hormones (adrenaline, cortisol, growth hormone and glucagon). The changes in these circulating hormones result in mobilization of free fatty acids from adipose tissue and subsequent greatly increased ketone body production in the liver.

'Ketone bodies'

Acetoacetate, 3-hydroxybutyrate (β-hydroxybutyrate) and acetone are collectively described as the 'ketone bodies' although 3-hydroxybutyrate is not in fact a ketone; they are most commonly found in the blood in excessive amounts in uncontrolled diabetes. Levels also increase in starvation since ketone bodies form an important energy source for many tissues when carbohydrate intake or metabolism is limited; this is called the 'glucose sparing' effect of ketones.

Ketone bodies are synthesized in the liver from acetyl CoA, itself derived from the oxidation of free fatty acids. Some of the acetoacetate may then be reduced to 3-hydroxybutyrate or decarboxylated with the formation of acetone and CO_2. Acetoacetic acid and 3-hydroxybutyric acid production give rise to a metabolic acidosis as the liver and other tissues cannot, in general, completely metabolize the increased amounts of these ketone bodies that are being formed. The acidosis is partly compensated by hyperventilation, with reduction in P_{CO_2}. The acidosis causes H^+ to move into cells and K^+ to move out; increased plasma [K^+] often results from the combined effects of (i) the acidosis and (ii) the lack of insulin action that normally promotes K^+ entry into cells.

Lactic acidosis

If tissue perfusion is affected by extreme dehydration (hyperosmolality), or by the factors which precipitated the original metabolic decompensation (e.g. severe infection, myocardial infarction), tissue anoxia may lead on to lactic acidosis.

Lactate itself is not an acid, and addition of lactate anions to blood does not produce an acidosis. The cause of the acidosis associated with increased plasma [lactate], and of the condition called lactic acidosis, is the net overproduction of

H^+ that occurs when cellular energy requirements are met by anaerobic metabolism. There is no net overproduction of H^+ when glucose is metabolized aerobically to CO_2 and water.

Non-ketotic, hyperglycaemic coma

These patients are usually older than the ketotic group. This difference may relate to poorer renal function in older patients, leading to greater losses of water and electrolytes. Also, insulin deficiency may be less severe, allowing there to be some suppression of ketogenesis by endogenous insulin.

Diagnosis and treatment of hyperglycaemic coma

Diagnosis is usually made initially on the basis of the history, clinical examination and 'side-room' testing of urine for glucose and ketone bodies and 'side-room' measurement of blood [glucose]. Laboratory-based tests on blood are needed to evaluate the nature of the metabolic decompensation and the severity of the condition more precisely, and to monitor progress during treatment. It is rarely necessary, and indeed may be positively dangerous, to wait for laboratory results before starting treatment. However, further emergency treatment should be based upon regular clinical assessment and on chemical measurements in the laboratory.

Initial laboratory assessment

Plasma glucose, urea, Na^+, K^+, and total CO_2 concentrations are usually measured, on samples of venous blood. Plasma $[Na^+]$ may be normal or low initially, except in hyperglycaemia without ketoacidosis, when it is often high. Plasma $[K^+]$ may be increased or normal, but is occasionally decreased. Plasma [total CO_2] is nearly always reduced, often being less than 5 mmol/L in severe cases. Plasma [urea] is usually increased due to dehydration.

Full assessment of acid–base status (arterial blood $[H^+]$, P_{CO_2}, $[HCO_3^-]$ and P_{O_2}) is rarely needed, except when plasma [total CO_2] is very low. Results indicating a severe degree of metabolic acidosis with compensatory reduction in P_{CO_2} are then often found. A lowered P_{O_2} is an indication for oxygen therapy.

Treatment aims to replace fluid and electrolyte deficits, and to correct the metabolic abnormality by injection of insulin. Knowledge of the fluid and electrolyte deficits likely to be present helps in planning appropriate therapy. There may be deficits of as much as 5–10 L of water, 500 mmol of Na^+, 250–800 mmol of K^+ and 300–500 mmol of base (e.g. HCO_3^-) in patients with severe acidosis.

Fluid replacement is usually given initially as 'physiological saline' (150 mmol/L NaCl); K^+ and other electrolytes may be added to the infusion fluid once insulin begins to exert its effects. Infusion of $NaHCO_3$ can be dangerous, as rapid correction of the acidosis augments the K^+ influx into cells and can precipitate dangerous hypokalaemia. By shifting the O_2-dissociation curve to the left, $NaHCO_3$ may interfere with O_2 delivery to the tissues, already compromised by the hypovolaemia; it may also cause CSF $[H^+]$ to rise rather than fall, due to the diffusion of CO_2 more rapidly than HCO_3^- into the CSF. In severe acidosis (arterial blood $[H^+]$ over 100 nmol/L or pH below 7.0), $NaHCO_3$ should be given provided other fluid replacement has begun to restore the circulation.

Further laboratory assessment during treatment of diabetic coma
The frequency and timing of repeat analyses depends on the clinician's experience, on the severity and nature of the coma, and on the method of treatment. For most patients, it is advisable to repeat some of the initial analyses, particularly plasma $[K^+]$, after 1 hour and thereafter at longer intervals (e.g. 2-hourly) if treatment is progressing satisfactorily. The following investigations are likely to be the most valuable for monitoring treatment of patients with *ketotic, hyperglycaemic coma*:

1 *Plasma [glucose]*. Insulin therapy is usually based on the response shown by the plasma [glucose]. When this is between 10 and 15 mmol/L, glucose should be administered intravenously together with insulin. Not only does this provide fuel to cells which have been starved of glucose, but it helps to reduce the development of cerebral oedema.

2 *Plasma [K$^+$]*. In many centres potassium replacement is started within a few minutes of the initial dose of insulin, in the knowledge that: (i) the patient has almost certainly developed a large K^+ deficit; (ii) insulin will rapidly cause K^+ to enter the cells from the ECF; and (iii) serious hypokalaemia is likely to develop fairly quickly in the absence of early corrective action.

3 *Plasma [total CO$_2$]*. This provides an index of the continuing degree of acid–base disturbance.

It generally proves possible to manage patients with blood analyses performed less often than every 2 hours once the plasma [glucose] has fallen satisfactorily, the plasma $[K^+]$ is fairly stable and the plasma [total CO_2] has risen considerably. As convalescence proceeds, dependence on laboratory investigations becomes less as ward-based and, in due course, patient-performed measurements regain their usefulness.

Treatment of patients with *non-ketotic, hyperglycaemic coma* is similar to the treatment of ketotic, hyperglycaemic patients, except that *hypotonic* fluid replacement may be required initially if plasma $[Na^+]$ is normal, and especially if it is raised. Less K^+ replacement is needed, and $NaHCO_3$ infusion is not indicated. There is an increased risk of thrombotic episodes in these patients and treatment with anticoagulants is generally considered advisable.

Hypoglycaemia

The plasma [glucose] at which hypoglycaemic symptoms appear is very variable, often related more to the rate of fall of blood [glucose] than to the absolute value observed. Arbitrarily, a venous plasma [glucose] below 2.2 mmol/L is the biochemical definition of hypoglycaemia. This is open to criticism, particularly when interpreting plasma [glucose] in a specimen collected 2–4 hours after meals; some reduction of venous plasma [glucose] normally occurs during this period, i.e. when the insulin secreted in response to glucose absorption may produce large arterio-venous differences in plasma [glucose]. However, the definition has been widely accepted since, even in the post-prandial state, venous plasma [glucose] seldom falls below 2.2 mmol/L.

It is convenient to distinguish between the hypoglycaemia that occurs in response to fasting and the hypoglycaemia that is due to some other stimulus

---

Case 11.1

A 31-year-old civil servant was found by his wife in a drowsy and uncooperative state. When the general practitioner arrived, she told him that her husband had seemed unusually thirsty for the past 1–2 months, and she thought he had lost weight. Recently, he had been complaining of abdominal pain and discomfort. The patient was admitted to hospital as an emergency, where chemical investigations on blood specimens gave the following results:

Blood or plasma analysis	Result	Reference range	Units
Venous [Urea]	37.5	2.5–6.6	mmol/L
[Na^+]	128	132–144	mmol/L
[K^+]	6.9	3.3–4.7	mmol/L
[Glucose]	35		mmol/L
Arterial [H^+]	82	36–44	nmol/L
P_{CO_2}	3.9	4.4–6.1	kPa
[HCO_3^-]	9.0	21.0–27.5	mmol/L
P_{O_2}	16	12–15	kPa

What is the probable diagnosis and how would you confirm this quickly? What principles would guide your treatment of this patient? He is discussed on p. 180.

(stimulative hypoglycaemia). *The finding of hypoglycaemia, by itself, is never diagnostic.* It has to be related to other information about the illness, and may only be one of the first in a series of investigations.

Stimulative (reactive) hypoglycaemia

This may be due to drugs (e.g. insulin overdose, accidental or deliberate) or poisons (e.g. some toadstools), inborn errors of metabolism (e.g. galactosaemia, hereditary fructose intolerance) or previous gastrectomy. It may be brought about by excess alcohol intake or be idiopathic in origin.

Essential reactive hypoglycaemia, which includes the idiopathic group, is probably due to an exaggeration of the normal insulin response to carbohydrate ingestion. Demonstration of a plasma [glucose] less than 2.2 mmol/L within 6 hours (usually 2–4 hours) after a meal, or after an oral load of 75 g anhydrous glucose (82.5 g glucose monohydrate) is required in order to diagnose essential reactive hypoglycaemia.

Fasting hypoglycaemia

Severe starvation and malnutrition may be accompanied by failure to maintain a normal blood [glucose]. Under these conditions, glycogen reserves become exhausted, and there is enhanced utilization of glucose (produced by hepatic gluconeogenesis) by the tissues. Failure to maintain a normal blood [glucose] is also a feature of some inborn errors of metabolism that give rise to neonatal and

Table 11.5 Fasting hypoglycaemia

Cause	Examples
Enhanced glucose utilization	
Endogenous over-production of insulin	Hyperinsulinism of childhood (nesidioblastosis), insulinoma, pancreatitis, pancreatic tumours (as part of MEN I syndrome)
Defective glucose production	
Endocrine disorders	Adrenocortical insufficiency and hypothyroidism (in both cases, primary and secondary), growth hormone deficiency
Liver disease	Severe portal cirrhosis, acute hepatic necrosis, hepatic tumours
Renal disease	End-stage renal failure
Miscellaneous	Severe malnutrition, starvation, inherited metabolic disorders (e.g. glycogen storage disease type I)

childhood hypoglycaemia (p. 331). Other causes of fasting hypoglycaemia are summarized in Table 11.5, subdivided into causes of enhanced glucose utilization and defective glucose production.

Insulinoma

This is usually a small, solitary, benign adenoma of the pancreatic islets that secretes inappropriate amounts of insulin. Occasionally, multiple pancreatic adenomas may be associated with adenomas in other endocrine organs as part of the multiple endocrine neoplasia (MEN I) syndrome (p. 205). The symptoms may be bizarre and laboratory investigations play a major part in diagnosis.

Most patients develop symptomatic hypoglycaemia after a fast of 24–36 hours, but in a few the fast may have to last for up to 72 hours before hypoglycaemia develops. Rarely, hypoglycaemia does not develop at all. A blood specimen is collected when hypoglycaemic symptoms develop, or at the end of the fast, for measurement of plasma [glucose]. A specimen should also be collected for determining plasma [insulin] when the patient has hypoglycaemic symptoms; this must be carefully stored prior to analysis.

Plasma [insulin] is measured after the occurrence of fasting hypoglycaemia has been confirmed. The diagnostic finding in patients suspected of having an insulinoma is a fasting plasma [insulin] that is *inappropriately high* in relation to the low plasma [glucose].

It can be difficult to demonstrate fasting hypoglycaemia satisfactorily in some patients. In these, it may still be possible to obtain support for a diagnosis of insulinoma by measuring plasma [C-peptide] during an infusion of exogenous insulin sufficient to induce hypoglycaemia. Exogenous insulin contains little or no C-peptide and failure to detect a fall in plasma [C-peptide] shows that endogenous insulin release is not switching off, as it should do, in response to hypoglycaemia. This finding is strongly suggestive of insulinoma.

Therapeutic insulin preparations contain little or no C-peptide. Accidental or deliberate overdose of insulin, giving rise to hypoglycaemia, can therefore be distinguished from insulinoma by measuring both plasma [insulin] and plasma [C-peptide].

Other causes of fasting hypoglycaemia

Some non-pancreatic tumours are associated with hypoglycaemia, mainly in patients with advanced malignant disease. Large sarcomas, especially retroperitoneal or pleural, may cause fasting hypoglycaemia, as may primary hepatomas, adrenal carcinomas and carcinoid tumours. Some of the larger tumours may consume excessive amounts of glucose, but there is also evidence for the production of hormonal insulin-like substances (NSILA or non-suppressible insulin-like activity).

Inherited metabolic disorders

Glycogen storage diseases

Glycogen is a polysaccharide composed of straight chains of glucose molecules joined by α-1,4-glucosidic links, and with branching points connecting these chains by α-1,6-glucosidic links. It can be synthesized by most tissues. It is stored mainly in liver and muscle, for use later by these tissues in metabolism. Glycogen synthesis and breakdown involve several enzymes (Fig. 11.2). The glycogen storage diseases are rare inborn errors of carbohydrate metabolism due to deficiency or reduced activity of one or more of the many enzymes involved.

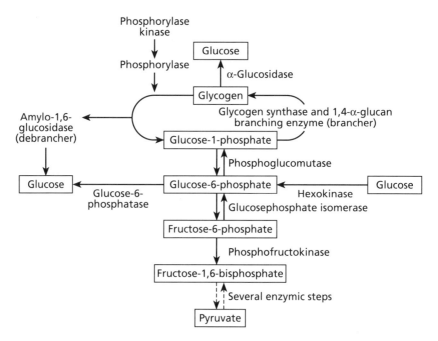

Fig. 11.2 Glycogen synthesis and breakdown. Deficiencies of most of the enzymes named in the figure have been shown to occur in one or more of the many forms of glycogen storage disease. In gluconeogenesis, the hydrolysis of fructose-1,6-bisphosphate by fructose-1,6-bisphosphatase is not shown.

The common feature in this complex group of conditions is an abnormality in the storage of glycogen, usually in increased amount and sometimes with an abnormal structure. As secondary features, there may be hypoglycaemia, abnormalities of blood lipids, hyperuricaemia, lactic acidosis, etc. These secondary features, and other indirect forms of testing, are no substitute for tissue enzyme assays; these sometimes need to be supplemented by carbohydrate structural studies. Some types of the disease have been recognized *in utero*, by culture of amniotic fluid cells, where there has previously been an index case.

Von Gierke's disease (Cori type I) is the best known of the glycogen storage diseases; it is due to deficiency of glucose-6-phosphatase and the glycogen that accumulates (mainly in the liver, kidney and intestine) has normal structure. Fasting hypoglycaemia may be very marked in von Gierke's disease. The least uncommon type of glycogen storage disease is Cori type VI(A), which is due to deficiency of phosphorylase kinase; liver and muscle are the main sites where glycogen that has normal structure accumulates in this disease.

Galactosaemia

The liver is the principal site for the conversion of galactose into glucose. Three separately identifiable defects have been described, due to deficiency of galactose-1-phosphate uridylyltransferase (Gal-1-PUT) or galactokinase or UDP-galactose epimerase (Fig. 11.3). They all interfere with the normal metabolism of galactose, and galactose gives rise to positive results in neonates if urinary 'side-room' tests for reducing substances (p. 14) are performed, unless milk intake is inadequate or vomiting is severe.

Galactosaemia is rare (Table 21.2, p. 322). The commonest and most severe enzymic defect is due to *Gal-1-PUT deficiency*. This usually manifests itself in the neonatal period or early in infancy, giving rise to vomiting and being accompanied by hypoglycaemia. If galactose-containing foods are given to the child, plasma [galactose] rises and galactose can be identified in the urine by chromatography. The precise diagnosis is established by measuring Gal-1-PUT activity in erythrocytes. Although all neonates in some countries (e.g. Scotland) are screened for defective galactose metabolism as an extension of the screening programme for phenylketonuria (p. 329), the response time is usually too slow for this rapidly

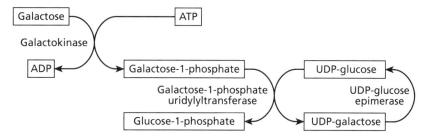

Fig. 11.3 The enzymic conversion of galactose to glucose. Galactosaemia may be caused by deficiency of any of these three enzymes, but the most common of the three causes is deficiency of galactose-1-phosphate uridylyltransferase. UDP, uridine diphosphate.

fatal condition and diagnosis is nearly always made following clinical presentation, except in the case of infants born into a family where an index case has been previously identified. Treatment is controlled by measurements of blood [galactose-1-phosphate]. *Galactokinase deficiency* may not present clinically in the neonatal period, and may escape detection until cataracts develop unless 'side-room' tests for reducing substances are routinely performed.

Those infants that have positive tests for reducing substances in urine, but normal erythrocyte Gal-1-PUT activity, should have a urine specimen examined by chromatography. If galactose is identified, blood [galactose] and [galactose-1-phosphate] should be measured; both are increased if there is deficiency of UDP-galactose epimerase, but only blood [galactose] is increased if galactokinase is deficient. Confirmation of the diagnosis is obtained by measuring erythrocyte enzyme activities. It is important to note that erythrocyte studies are only valid if the infant has not been transfused.

Miscellaneous causes of glycosuria

Several conditions give rise to glycosuria due to the presence of substances other than glucose in the urine:

Hereditary fructose intolerance. The liver is the principal site for the conversion of fructose into glucose and this condition, which is due to deficiency of fructose-1-phosphate aldolase, causes intracellular accumulation of fructose-1-phosphate. Vomiting and hypoglycaemia occur after ingestion of fructose-containing foods, usually the disaccharide sucrose. The age of presentation depends on feeding patterns and on the severity of the defect; most patients develop a strong aversion to sucrose. Investigation can be by means of either an oral or an intravenous fructose tolerance test. Patients with the deficiency show marked and prolonged falls in plasma [glucose] and plasma [phosphate] following fructose administration, as well as fructosuria. Urine chromatography confirms the presence of fructose.

Essential fructosuria is a benign condition, caused by fructokinase deficiency. Its importance lies in the need to distinguish it from other causes of glycosuria.

Essential pentosuria is a benign inborn error of metabolism in which the sugar L-xylulose is excreted in the urine in excess, due to a defect in NADP-linked xylitol dehydrogenase, one of the enzymes in the glucuronic acid oxidation pathway.

Lactosuria is of no pathological significance. It often occurs in the later stages of pregnancy and while lactation continues after delivery. Its importance stems from the need to distinguish lactosuria from glucosuria.

Comments on Case 11.1 (p. 176)

The patient almost certainly had diabetic ketoacidosis. This was confirmed by testing a urine specimen for ketone bodies, but if he had been too dehydrated to produce urine a drop of plasma could have been used instead (note that only some people can smell acetone in patients' breath). Strictly speaking, it was not necessary to perform blood-gas analysis (total CO_2 would have sufficed).

The mainstays of treatment of patients with diabetic ketoacidosis are:

1   Insulin infusion, usually starting at a rate of 6 units/hour.

2 Fluid and electrolyte replacement, starting with 'physiological' saline (150 mmol/L NaCl) and containing added potassium chloride (40 mmol/L), usually as a standard regime (e.g., 1 L in the first 30 minutes, a second litre in the next hour and a third litre in the following 2 hours, etc.).

3 Frequent monitoring of the patient's plasma [glucose] and $[K^+]$, and monitoring of the central venous pressure. As the treatment takes effect, plasma $[K^+]$ is liable to fall rapidly, due to the large whole-body K^+ deficit, despite the initially raised plasma $[K^+]$.

Chapter 12
Disorders of Plasma Lipids
and Lipoproteins

The main classes of lipids in plasma are cholesterol esters, triglycerides and phospholipids. These are all esters of long-chain fatty acids, which are also present in plasma in the free form, and are transported in plasma as complexes with protein, the *lipoproteins*. In order to understand the abnormalities of plasma lipids in disease, it is necessary to outline some aspects of their physiology.

Lipids

Lipids act as energy stores and as important structural components of cells. They also have specialized functions (e.g. as hormones). To fulfil these functions, they have to be transported in plasma between tissues.

Cholesterol is present in the diet in small amounts (1 g/day). It can be synthesized by all nucleated cells, but most is synthesized in the liver and small intestine. Some is incorporated into lipoproteins and carried in plasma to the peripheral tissues where it is a major component of cell membranes. It acts as the substrate for steroid hormone formation in the adrenals and the gonads and for the synthesis of 7-dehydrocholesterol (pro-vitamin D_3) in the skin. The body cannot break down the sterol nucleus, so cholesterol is either excreted unchanged in bile or converted to bile acids and then excreted; cholesterol and bile acids both undergo an enterohepatic circulation.

Triglycerides are the main lipid component of the diet, their daily intake usually being between 100 g and 200 g. Dietary triglycerides are broken down in the small intestine to a mixture of monoglycerides, fatty acids and glycerol. These products are absorbed and triglycerides resynthesized from them in the mucosal cell. Most of these *exogenous* triglycerides are incorporated into *chylomicrons* and transported into the intestinal lymph, and thence to the systemic circulation via the thoracic duct.

The liver is the major site of *endogenous* triglyceride synthesis, from fatty acids and glycerol. The triglycerides so synthesized are transported as *very low density lipoproteins* (VLDL) in plasma to sites of fat storage, mainly adipose tissue, and energy utilization.

Fatty acids, in man, are mostly straight-chain monocarboxylic acids with an even number of carbon atoms, between 12 and 24, mainly derived from dietary triglycerides. The body is also able to synthesize most fatty acids, apart from certain polyunsaturated (essential) fatty acids, which must be provided in the diet. Fatty acids act as an alternative or additional energy source to glucose.

Phospholipids have a structure which is related to, but more complex than, triglycerides. One of the three fatty acid components is replaced by a polar group (e.g. phosphorylcholine). The presence of both polar and non-polar (fatty acid) groups gives the phospholipids their characteristic detergent properties. Phospholipids are mainly synthesized in the liver and small intestine; they are important constituents of cells, and are always present in cell membranes.

Lipoproteins (Table 12.1)

Cholesterol and its esters, triglycerides and phospholipids are all transported in plasma as lipoprotein particles. Fatty acids are transported bound to albumin.

Lipoprotein particles comprise a peripheral envelope, consisting mainly of phospholipids and free cholesterol (which have both water-soluble polar and lipid-soluble non-polar groups) with some *apolipoproteins*, and a central non-polar core. The molecules in the envelope are distributed in a single layer in such a way that the polar groups face out towards the surrounding plasma while the non-polar groups face inwards towards the lipid core in which the insoluble lipids are carried. *Most lipoproteins are assembled in the liver or small intestine.* Five main types of lipoprotein particle can be recognized:

1 *Chylomicrons* are the principal form in which dietary triglycerides are carried to the tissues.

2 *Very low density lipoproteins (VLDL)* are triglyceride-rich particles which form the major route whereby endogenous triglycerides are carried to the tissues from the liver and, to a lesser extent, from the small intestine.

Table 12.1 Properties of the five main classes of lipoproteins

Property	Chylomicrons	VLDL	IDL	LDL	HDL
Physical properties					
Diameter (nm)	100–500	30–80	25–30	20–35	5–10
Density (kg/L)	< 0.95	< 1.006	1.006–1.019	1.019–1.063	> 1.063
Electrophoresis	Stay at origin	Pre-β	β	β	α$_1$
Lipoprotein composition (approximate percentages)					
Triglyceride	90	65	35	10	5
Cholesterol	5	20	40	50	35
Phospholipid	5	10	15	20	35
Protein	1	5	10	20	25
*Apolipoprotein composition**	C,B,E,(A)	C,B,E,(A)	B,(C,E,A)	B	A,C,E,(B)

* The main apolipoprotein components are listed in descending order of amount (trace components in parentheses).

In summary, although an oversimplification, this table shows the following:

1 The largest particles (the chylomicrons) have the lowest density, the highest content of triglycerides and the lowest content of protein.

2 The smallest particles (HDL) are the most dense, have the lowest content of triglycerides and the highest content of protein.

3 Between these extremes, as the particles become smaller (VLDL, IDL and then LDL), their relative contents of triglyceride fall while their relative contents of cholesterol and protein both rise. These changes are accompanied by progressively increasing density.

3 *Intermediate density lipoproteins (IDL or 'VLDL remnants')* are particles formed by the removal of triglycerides from VLDL, during the transition from VLDL to LDL.

4 *Low density lipoproteins (LDL)* are cholesterol-rich particles, formed from IDL by the removal of more triglyceride and apolipoprotein.

5 *High density lipoproteins* are of two main types, HDL_2 and HDL_3. They probably act as a means whereby cholesterol can be transported from peripheral cells to the liver, prior to excretion.

A sixth type of lipoprotein particle, *Lp(a)*, is synthesized in the liver and has about the same lipid composition as LDL but is probably not derived from VLDL. The physiological role of Lp(a) is not known but it has been shown to compete with plasminogen for tissue plasminogen receptors.

The above classification of the lipoprotein particles has replaced the one that was based on electrophoretic mobility in which, for instance, the α-lipoproteins corresponded approximately to HDL, the β-lipoproteins to LDL and the pre-β-lipoproteins to VLDL. The electrophoretic nomenclature is still used in relation to the primary hypolipoproteinaemias (p. 192).

The apolipoproteins

The protein components of the lipoproteins, the apolipoproteins, are a complex family of polypeptides. The roles of the apolipoproteins are:

1 *Physical.* They promote the solubility of lipids in plasma and enhance the stability of the lipoprotein particles.

2 *Regulatory.* They have a role in controlling lipid metabolism, e.g. by activating key enzymes of lipid metabolism.

3 *Tissue binding.* Some apolipoproteins attach to specific binding sites in tissues, thus helping to regulate tissue uptake.

The apolipoproteins are separable into four main groups (apoA, B, C and E), two minor groups (apoD and apoF) and apo(a). Some of the apolipoprotein groups can be further subdivided into apoA-I, apoA-II, etc.

ApoA. This group of proteins is synthesized in the intestine and the liver. Both of its two main components, apoA-I and apoA-II, are initially present in chylomicrons in lymph, but they rapidly transfer to HDL.

ApoB is present in plasma in two forms, $apoB_{100}$ and $apoB_{48}$. $ApoB_{100}$ is the protein component of LDL and is also present in chylomicrons, VLDL and IDL. $ApoB_{48}$ (the N-terminal half of $apoB_{100}$) is only found in chylomicrons. $ApoB_{100}$ is recognized by specific receptors in peripheral tissues (see below).

ApoC. This family of three proteins (apoC-I, apoC-II and apoC-III) is synthesized in the liver and incorporated into HDL.

ApoE is synthesized in the liver, incorporated into HDL, and transferred in the circulation to chylomicrons and VLDL. There are three major isoforms (apoE2, apoE3 and apoE4) at a single genetic locus, giving rise to several genotypes (E3/3, E2/3, E2/4, etc.). ApoE is probably mainly involved in the hepatic uptake of chylomicron remnants and IDL; it binds to apoB receptors in the tissues.

Apo(a) is present in equimolar amounts to $apoB_{100}$, in Lp(a). It has a high carbohydrate content and has a similar amino acid sequence to plasminogen.

Enzymes involved in lipid transport

Five enzymes of relevance to clinical disorders need to be described:

1   *Lecithin cholesterol acyltransferase (LCAT)* transfers an acyl group (fatty acid residue) from lecithin to cholesterol, forming a cholesterol ester. In plasma, this reaction probably takes place exclusively on HDL, and may be stimulated by apoA-I.

2   *Lipoprotein lipase* splits triglycerides, present in chylomicrons and VLDL, to glycerol and free fatty acids. It is attached to the capillary endothelium in adipose, muscle and other tissues. Its activity increases after a meal, partly as a result of activation by apoC-II, present on the surface of triglyceride-bearing lipoproteins.

3   *Hepatic lipase* has an action similar to lipoprotein lipase. It seems to be more effective in hydrolysing triglycerides in smaller particles ('VLDL remnants' or IDL) than the triglycerides contained in chylomicrons.

4   *Mobilizing lipase*, present in adipose tissue cells, controls the release of fatty acids from adipose tissue into plasma. It is activated by catecholamines, growth hormone and glucocorticoids (e.g. cortisol) and inhibited by glucose and by insulin.

5   β-*Hydroxy-*β-*methylglutaryl-coenzyme A (HMG CoA) reductase* catalyses the rate-limiting step in cholesterol synthesis. Its activity is regulated by the amount of cholesterol in cells which, in turn, largely depends on cholesterol uptake from the bloodstream.

Metabolism of plasma lipoproteins

The above description of the lipoproteins and apolipoproteins is an over-simplification, and the following points should be emphasized:

1   *Plasma lipids and apolipoproteins exist in a dynamic state.* There is interchange of both (i) between different lipoprotein particles and (ii) with tissues.

2   *There is considerable variation in size and composition* of individual lipoprotein particles within each lipoprotein class.

Chylomicron metabolism

Chylomicrons are formed in the intestinal mucosa, in response to fat-containing meals, and reach the systemic circulation via the thoracic duct. After entering the bloodstream, they transfer apoA to HDL and acquire apoC and apoE from HDL. The apoC-II then activates lipoprotein lipase and triglycerides are progressively removed from the chylomicrons.

As triglycerides are removed from the hydrophobic core of the chylomicrons, the surface area of the particles decreases and the more hydrophilic surface components (apoC, unesterified cholesterol and phospholipid) transfer to HDL. The triglyceride-poor chylomicron remnants (now consisting mainly of cholesterol esters, apoB and apoE) are taken up by the liver, where they are catabolized.

VLDL and IDL metabolism

Most VLDL are secreted into plasma by the hepatocytes ('endogenous' VLDL) but some originate from the intestinal mucosa ('exogenous' VLDL). Hepatic synthesis is increased whenever there is increased hepatic triglyceride synthesis, e.g. when there is increased transport of fatty acids to the liver.

When first produced, VLDL consist mainly of triglycerides and some unesterified cholesterol, with $apoB_{100}$ and lesser amounts of apoE. ApoC-II is then acquired, mainly from HDL, and triglycerides are removed from the VLDL 'core' in a manner analogous to that for chylomicrons. The residual particles are known as 'VLDL remnants', or IDL.

IDL are normally present in the circulation only in low concentration; they are either rapidly converted to LDL or removed from the circulation. It seems that the liver plays the major role in both processes, possibly through recognition of IDL-apoE.

LDL metabolism

Probably all LDL arise from VLDL metabolism in man. There is a one-for-one relationship between the particles, i.e. each LDL derives from a single VLDL particle. The LDL particles are rich in cholesterol esters, probably derived from HDL; $apoB_{100}$ is the only apolipoprotein in these particles.

LDL are removed from the circulation by two processes; one is regulated by the cholesterol requirements of individual tissues, the other is unregulated.

The *regulated mechanism* involves the binding of LDL to *specific $apoB_{100}$ receptors* present on 'surface pits' of hepatocytes and other peripheral tissue cells. The entire LDL particle is incorporated into the cell, by invagination of the cell membrane; inside the cell, the particle fuses with lysosomes. ApoB is then broken down and the cholesterol esters are hydrolysed, thereby making unesterified cholesterol available to the cell. The size of the intracellular cholesterol pool regulates:

1   The rate of cholesterol synthesis in the cell, through the effect of cholesterol on HMG CoA reductase.
2   The number of LDL-apoB receptors on the cell surface.

The *unregulated mechanism* involves *receptor-independent mechanisms* of cholesterol uptake by cells; these are present particularly in macrophages. These mechanisms are brought into operation especially when plasma [cholesterol] is increased.

HDL metabolism

This heterogeneous group of particles (HDL_2, HDL_3, etc.) is formed in the liver and intestinal mucosa. The HDL particles then undergo fairly complex exchanges of lipid and protein with other plasma lipoproteins. However, the main point to note is that HDL is responsible for the uptake, and subsequent esterification by LCAT, of free cholesterol from tissues. Most of the cholesterol esters derived from HDL are returned to the liver by means of LDL uptake, since the liver is the major 'peripheral tissue' capable of LDL uptake on to apoB receptors. Thus, HDL forms the principal route whereby cholesterol can return from other peripheral tissues to the liver.

Investigation of plasma lipid abnormalities

Most laboratories measure plasma [cholesterol] and [triglycerides]. Further tests to characterize the lipoprotein abnormalities may be indicated if these initial investigations are abnormal or if the patient has clinical features suggestive of hyperlipidaemia.

Plasma [lipids] vary in health with age, sex, diet, drug therapy (e.g. oral contraceptives) and other factors which must be taken into account when interpreting results.

Plasma cholesterol

Plasma [cholesterol] is affected by both within-individual and between-individual factors:

1 *Within-individual factors* include *diet* (considered below), *age*, and *exercise*. In adults in industrial societies, plasma [cholesterol] rises with age, tending to increase by about 0.2 mmol/L per decade. Exercise, especially when regular, tends to cause a fall in plasma [total cholesterol] with a rise in plasma [HDL-cholesterol].

2 *Between-individual variation* may be due to *race, sex* and other *genetic factors*, most of which have not been fully identified. The effects of race are difficult to distinguish from those of diet but, in general, values are particularly high in North European countries such as the UK. In pre-menopausal women, plasma total [cholesterol] and [LDL-cholesterol] are lower than in men, whereas plasma [HDL-cholesterol] is higher, but these differences disappear after the menopause.

The major *dietary factor* affecting plasma [cholesterol] is the amount and composition of the dietary fat. Fats contain polyunsaturated (P) and saturated (S) fatty acids in different proportions, often referred to as the P : S ratio. Meat and dairy products have a low P : S ratio whereas most fish and vegetable oils have a relatively high P : S ratio. In general, intake of *saturated fats*, with a low P : S ratio, *raises* the plasma [cholesterol] whereas intake of *mono- and polyunsaturated fats* causes plasma [cholesterol] to *fall. Dietary fibre* may have a small effect in lowering plasma [cholesterol]. The consumption of about two units of *alcohol* per day causes a significant rise in plasma [HDL-cholesterol], which may have a moderate protective effect against the development of ischaemic heart disease. Dietary cholesterol intake has relatively little effect on plasma [cholesterol].

Numerous studies have shown that the incidence of ischaemic heart disease is directly correlated with plasma [cholesterol] (Fig. 12.1) *even within the 'reference range'*. There is no clear cut-off between values for normal risk and increased risk although risk rises particularly rapidly above about 6.5 mmol/L. Because of this association, we think it is *inappropriate to employ reference ranges* for plasma [cholesterol] in the usual way, as these imply health without increased risk of disease. Instead, it seems more appropriate to define a *desirable* concentration (e.g. below 5.2 mmol/L), and another, higher concentration (e.g. 6.5 mmol/L) above which active therapeutic measures should be considered.

Although the above discussion has been couched in terms of plasma [total cholesterol], mainly because this is the simple test that is generally available, this is a rather unsatisfactory measurement since it represents the sum of the various ways in which cholesterol is transported in plasma. In fact, whereas *raised plasma [LDL-cholesterol]* is associated with *increased* risk of ischaemic heart disease, *raised plasma [HDL-cholesterol]* is associated with a *decreased* risk of ischaemic

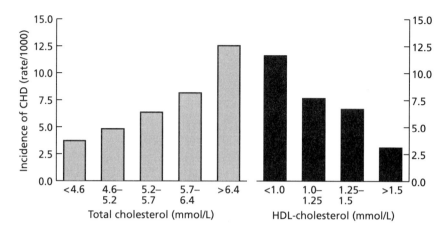

Fig. 12.1 The variation in incidence of coronary heart disease (CHD) with the plasma concentrations of cholesterol (histograms drawn from data in Martin *et al.*, 1986) and HDL-cholesterol (histograms drawn from data in Castelli *et al.*, 1986).

heart disease and seems to have a protective effect. As analytical methods improve, it is likely that separate measurements of plasma [LDL-cholesterol] and [HDL-cholesterol] will be made as a routine.

Plasma triglycerides

Plasma [triglycerides] also show variations with age and sex, but more especially with diet. There is, in addition, a very considerable within-individual variation which makes interpretation of a single result difficult.

Specimen collection

It is very important to collect specimens for plasma lipid and lipoprotein studies under the appropriate, standardized conditions:

1 The patient should have been leading a normal life in terms of diet (including alcohol consumption) and exercise, for at least the previous fortnight.

2 Blood specimens should be collected after an overnight fast of 10–14 hours, if triglyceride measurements are to be performed.

3 Venous stasis should be minimal.

Routine investigations

Certain investigations should be performed as a routine, for diagnostic purposes, in all cases of suspected hyperlipidaemia *before* treatment is started. We recommend the following measurements or observations:

1 Plasma [cholesterol].

2 Plasma [fasting triglycerides].

3 Inspection of plasma that has been stored at 4°C, undisturbed, for 12–18 hours, if the patient has hyperlipidaemia.

4 Plasma [HDL-cholesterol], if plasma [cholesterol] is raised or if additional risk factors are present.

Helpful information about the nature of the lipoproteins giving rise to hyper-triglyceridaemia can be obtained by the inspection of stored plasma. Triglyceride-rich particles (chylomicrons and VLDL) cause plasma turbidity, whereas triglyceride-poor particles do not. Also, chylomicrons (but not VLDL) float to the surface if the specimen is left *undisturbed* for several hours (usually overnight).

Measurement of plasma [HDL-cholesterol] helps to define the risk of ischaemic heart disease in patients with raised [total cholesterol]. It is also needed for the diagnosis of hyper-α-lipoproteinaemia.

Specialized investigations

Occasionally, further and more specialized investigations may be indicated, on the basis of clinical features and the results of the preliminary, routine investigations.

Patients with a mixed hyperlipidaemia may require to be investigated by *ultracentrifuge studies* in order to confirm a diagnosis of WHO type III hyper-lipoproteinaemia, or the diagnosis can be supported (though less satisfactorily) by *lipoprotein electrophoresis*, which reveals a broad β-band in this treatable condition.

Measurement of plasma *lipoprotein lipase* activity, following an intravenous injection of heparin to release the enzyme, may be needed to establish the diagnosis in some patients in whom there is chylomicronaemia.

Cautionary note

Results of plasma lipid and lipoprotein investigations can be misleading, often showing hypertriglyceridaemia and sometimes reduced plasma [cholesterol], in specimens collected during or within a few weeks after a serious illness (e.g. a myocardial infarction or a major operation).

The primary hyperlipoproteinaemias

These conditions have been classified in several ways. One classification, based principally on the nature of the plasma abnormalities, was introduced by WHO. The WHO terminology was widely accepted, but is now little used to describe patterns of lipoprotein abnormality because more has become known about the nature of the defects in some of the genetic hyperlipoproteinaemias, and about their modes of inheritance. The description given here is based on the genetic classification (Table 12.2) and other factors. *Increased plasma lipid concentrations may be:*

1 Due to purely genetic factors.
2 Due to a combination of genetic and environmental factors.
3 Secondary to other diseases.

Primary hypercholesterolaemia (WHO types IIa, IIb)

In about 95% of patients with primary hypercholesterolaemia, the abnormality is due to a combination of dietary factors and a number of so far unidentified genetic abnormalities in handling cholesterol. Both the genetic predisposition and the increased cholesterol load are necessary before the condition develops.

Table 12.2 The primary hyperlipoproteinaemias (genetic classification)

| Hyperlipoproteinaemia | Concentrations in plasma | | Lipoproteins mainly affected |
	Cholesterol	Trigylcerides (fasting)	
Familial hypercholesterolaemia	↑↑	N (or ↑)	LDL
Familial hypertriglyceridaemia	↑ or N	↑↑	VLDL (and chylo)
Familial combined hyperlipidaemia	↑ or N	↑ or N	LDL and/or VLDL
Remnant hyperlipoproteinaemia	↑	↑	IDL and chylo remnants
Lipoprotein lipase deficiency (or apoC-II deficiency)	↑ or N	↑↑	Chylo and VLDL

chylo, chylomicrons; N, normal; ↑, increased; ↑↑, much increased.

In the remaining 5%, patients who have *familial hypercholesterolaemia*, there is a specific genetic defect in the production or nature of high-affinity tissue apoB$_{100}$ receptors; heterozygotes have about 50% of normal receptor activity and homozygotes have no receptor activity. Many heterozygotes have *tendon xanthomas* and over 50% will have symptoms of coronary artery disease by the fourth or fifth decade. In homozygotes, heart disease often presents in the second decade. Plasma [cholesterol] is usually raised to 8–15 mmol/L in heterozygotes, and is even higher in homozygotes.

Familial hypertriglyceridaemia (WHO types IV, V)

This comprises a group of conditions associated with defects either in the production or in the catabolism of VLDL. Plasma [triglycerides] and [VLDL] are increased but, whereas plasma [cholesterol] is often also moderately increased, plasma [LDL] and [HDL] are often reduced. Patients have an increased risk of ischaemic heart disease.

In patients with the type V phenotype, there is chylomicronaemia in addition to increased plasma [VLDL]. This pattern may be brought on by alcohol excess and is also seen in diabetics. These patients may have eruptive xanthomas and attacks of acute pancreatitis.

Familial combined hyperlipidaemia

This disorder is difficult to classify and the method of inheritance is unclear. Even in the same family, the gene does not always express itself in the same way as there may be increased plasma [LDL] only (WHO type IIa phenotype), increased plasma [VLDL] only (WHO type IV phenotype) or increases in both (WHO type IIb phenotype). The incidence of ischaemic heart disease is three to four times greater than in the general population.

Remnant hyperlipoproteinaemia (WHO type III)

This is an uncommon disorder characterized clinically by cutaneous xanthomas and a high risk of premature ischaemic heart disease. In the plasma, there is an increase in cholesterol-rich but otherwise VLDL-like particles; these are probably IDL (i.e. 'VLDL remnants'). On electrophoresis, they give rise to a characteristic broad β-band. Both plasma [cholesterol] and [triglycerides] are increased; plasma [LDL] is decreased.

This disorder is probably due to a combination of factors. There is abnormal conversion of VLDL to LDL. This is usually associated with the apoE2/2 genotype. However, since as many as 1% of normal individuals have this genotype whereas the incidence of remnant hyperlipoproteinaemia is only about one in 5000, an additional factor must be present.

Remnant hyperlipoproteinaemia responds well to treatment with fibric acid derivatives (e.g. gemfibrozil) so its recognition is important. Ultracentrifuge studies provide the definitive means of confirming the diagnosis.

Lipoprotein lipase deficiency (WHO type I)

This is a rare autosomal recessive disorder causing hypertriglyceridaemia and chylomicronaemia. The incidence of ischaemic heart disease and acute pancreatitis is increased; eruptive xanthomas often occur. The primary defect is deficiency of either *lipoprotein lipase* or its activator, *apoC-II*.

Treatment involves restriction of normal dietary fat and replacement by means of triglycerides containing fatty acids of medium chain length (C_8-C_{11}); these are less prone to lead to chylomicron formation.

Other inherited defects

Hyper-α-lipoproteinaemia is an inherited abnormality, giving rise to increased plasma [HDL] and mildly increased plasma [cholesterol]. Patients have a *reduced* incidence of ischaemic heart disease. The only importance of hyper-α-lipoproteinaemia is that treatment for the raised plasma [cholesterol] should *not* be given.

Secondary hyperlipidaemia

Probably less than 20% of cases of hyperlipidaemia are secondary to other disease. Patterns of abnormality tend to vary, even within a single disease; plasma [cholesterol] or [triglycerides], or both, may be affected.

Hypercholesterolaemia is often a marked feature of hypothyroidism and of the nephrotic syndrome; in these two disorders, there is increased plasma [LDL]. It also occurs in cholestatic jaundice, but in this condition there is accumulation of abnormal discoid particles rich in phospholipid and unesterified cholesterol, and lipoprotein X is detectable (p. 117). Coronary artery disease tends to develop in those patients with secondary hyperlipidaemia who have had increased plasma [LDL] for a considerable time.

Hypertriglyceridaemia, secondary to other disease, is most commonly due to diabetes mellitus or to alcoholism. It may also occur in chronic renal disease and in patients on oestrogen therapy, including women taking oestrogen-containing oral contraceptives.

The effects of alcohol on plasma lipids are complex. Regular drinking of small amounts increases plasma [HDL] without affecting other lipoprotein particles. Some heavy drinkers develop hypertriglyceridaemia due to increased plasma [VLDL], possibly as a result of increased direction of fatty acid metabolism into triglyceride synthesis in the liver.

The hyperlipidaemia secondary to diabetes mellitus is also complex. Increased plasma [VLDL] is the usual finding, but plasma [LDL] is often increased also whereas plasma [HDL] is reduced.

The primary hypolipoproteinaemias

Three rare familial diseases require brief mention. Their recognition has helped with the understanding of normal lipoprotein metabolism.

Tangier disease is due to an increased rate of apoA-I catabolism causing α-lipoprotein deficiency. Only traces of HDL are detectable in plasma, and plasma [LDL-cholesterol] is also reduced. Cholesterol esters accumulate in the lympho-reticular system, probably due to excessive phagocytosis of the abnormal chylomicrons and VLDL remnants that result from the apoA-I deficiency.

Abetalipoproteinaemia is associated with a complete absence of apoB. The lipoproteins that normally contain apoB in significant amounts (i.e. chylomicrons, VLDL, IDL and LDL) are *absent* from plasma. Plasma [cholesterol] and [triglycerides] are very low.

Hypobetalipoproteinaemia is due to decreased synthesis of apoB. Plasma [VLDL] and [LDL], although reduced, are not absent.

Secondary hypolipidaemia

Greatly reduced plasma [cholesterol] occurs whenever hepatic protein synthesis is depressed, as in protein-energy malnutrition (e.g. kwashiorkor in children), severe malabsorption or some forms of chronic liver disease.

Hyperlipidaemia and arterial disease

The following associations are now clearly established:

1 Increased plasma [LDL-cholesterol] is *positively* correlated with the incidence of ischaemic heart disease. This association *usually* also holds for plasma [total cholesterol], most of which consists of LDL-cholesterol.

2 Increased plasma [HDL-cholesterol] is *negatively* correlated with the incidence of ischaemic heart disease. This is presumably explained by the role of HDL in transporting cholesterol from the peripheral tissues to the liver.

3 Increased plasma [triglycerides] is *positively* correlated with the incidence of ischaemic heart disease but the association is much weaker than that with plasma [cholesterol].

4 Plasma [Lp(a)] is *positively* associated with the incidence of ischaemic heart disease independently of other lipoprotein fractions. The effect may be due to competition between Lp(a) and plasminogen for endothelial cell receptors, thereby inhibiting thrombolysis.

Plasma [cholesterol], hypertension and cigarette smoking are the major risk factors for ischaemic heart disease. It is essential to recognize that the separate effects of each risk factor are *multiplicative* rather than additive, so it is especially important to treat patients who have more than one risk factor.

Screening for hypercholesterolaemia

In populations with a high incidence of hypercholesterolaemia, the simplest and most cost-effective strategy to reduce the incidence of ischaemic heart disease is a widely based publicity campaign to reduce plasma [cholesterol] in the population at large, by encouraging an appropriate diet. An additional approach would be to *target* treatment to those at highest risk, identified by *screening* for raised plasma [cholesterol].

At present, the optimal screening strategy is not clear but it might involve, for example, measuring plasma [cholesterol] in all patients aged between 40 and 65 years attending a general practice surgery for any complaint, whether or not related to heart disease. Patients, on the basis of their plasma [cholesterol] and the presence of other risk factors, would receive counselling on diet, smoking habits, etc. They might also require drug treatment and regular follow-up. Although this 'opportunistic' policy does not encompass the whole population, it is relatively easy and cheap to administer.

Screening strategies whereby members of the general public are encouraged, sometimes by commercial interests, to arrange for their own plasma cholesterol measurements to be performed (e.g. in supermarkets or other retail outlets) may be less satisfactory unless there are stringent safeguards (p. 18). These would require the quality of the results to be monitored regularly and appropriate counselling about diet, the implications of the result, etc., to accompany every cholesterol result. Without this advice, the screening process is largely valueless and may lead to inappropriate action or unwarranted anxiety on the part of the patient.

Treatment of hyperlipidaemia

It is possible to lower plasma [LDL-cholesterol] by dietary or other means, but little is known about ways of modifying plasma [HDL]. Both primary and secondary prevention trials have shown that reduction in plasma [cholesterol] is accompanied by a significant reduction in the overall rate of *non-fatal myocardial infarction*; no statistically significant change in the rate of fatal infarction has been demonstrated. In all patients, treatment with diet must precede drug therapy and, in many cases, will be the only measure required.

Patients with mild hyperlipidaemia

It is usually only necessary to alter the diet. Reduction in fat intake and substitution of much of its saturated fat content by poly- and mono-unsaturated fats will usually result in a lowering of plasma [cholesterol] by 10–20%. Reduction of plasma [triglycerides] is more likely to be achieved by restricting dietary carbohydrate intake.

Patients with more severe hyperlipidaemia

More aggressive treatment is indicated, especially of hypercholesterolaemia. Drug therapy may be aimed at increasing cholesterol excretion or at decreasing its synthesis.

Cholesterol excretion can be increased by the oral administration of *bile acid-binding resins*, e.g. *cholestyramine*, which bind bile acids in the intestine thereby interrupting their enterohepatic circulation. They may lower plasma [cholesterol] by about 20% but are not very acceptable to patients since they cause constipation.

Synthesis of cholesterol can be reduced by drugs which *inhibit HMG CoA reductase (statins)*, thereby reducing the intracellular cholesterol pool and stimulating production of tissue $apoB_{100}$ receptors, except in patients with homozygous familial hypercholesterolaemia. These drugs cause plasma [cholesterol] to fall by 30–40%; they are well tolerated by patients but have not been in use long enough to be sure of their long-term safety.

Nicotinic acid may be used to treat patients with mixed hyperlipidaemia, as it reduces both plasma [cholesterol] and [triglycerides]. *Fibric acid derivatives* are also effective in mixed hyperlipidaemias and in remnant hyperlipoproteinaemia.

Patients with severe hypercholesterolaemia

These patients (e.g. familial hypercholesterolaemia) are sometimes treated by means of an *ileal by-pass operation*. This acts like the bile acid sequestrants by interrupting the enterohepatic circulation. In homozygous familial hypercholesterolaemia, *plasma exchange* (at weekly or fortnightly intervals) may be the only effective treatment.

Chapter 13
Disorders of Calcium, Phosphate and Magnesium Metabolism

Calcium[1] is the most abundant mineral in the body, there being about 25 mol (1 kg) in a 70 kg adult. About 99% of the body's calcium is present in bone, in which the inorganic material consists mainly of hydroxyapatite, $3\ Ca_3(PO_4)_2$, $Ca(OH)_2$. On purely physicochemical considerations, calcium and phosphate would precipitate spontaneously from the ECF as their solubility product is greatly exceeded. Deposition of bone salt, however, is not simply a passive process but is markedly influenced by the hormonal environment. Mineralization may also depend upon the removal of inhibitors of this process; pyrophosphate, the breakdown of which is catalysed by alkaline phosphatase, may be one such inhibitor.

Calcium salts in bone have a mechanical role, but are not metabolically inert. There is a constant state of turnover in the skeleton associated with deposition of calcium in sites of bone formation and release at sites of bone resorption. Calcium in bone acts as a reservoir which helps to stabilize ECF $[Ca^{2+}]$.

In adults, calcium intake and output are normally in balance. In infancy and childhood there is normally a positive balance, especially at times of active skeletal growth. In older age, calcium output may exceed input and a state of negative balance then exists; this negative external balance is particularly marked in women after the menopause, and is important in the development of post-menopausal osteoporosis.

The normal dietary intake of calcium in the UK is about 25 mmol/day (1 g/ day); the minimum daily requirement in adults is about 0.5 g. Significant amounts (over 3 mmol/day) are normally contained in GI secretions. Absorption of calcium occurs from the small intestine, a process dependent upon the availability of 1 : 25-dihydroxycholecalciferol (1 : 25-DHCC or calcitriol); it is sometimes impaired if the diet contains large quantities of inorganic phosphates, or organic phosphates (e.g. phytate, present in cereals). The efficiency of calcium absorption tends to decrease with age, and an increased dietary intake may be needed in the elderly. Faecal calcium excretion is normally in the range 5–15 mmol/day. In women, the mother loses calcium to the fetus during pregnancy, and by lactation.

External balance is largely achieved through the body normally matching net absorption over 24 hours closely with the corresponding 24-hour urinary

[1]In this book, 'calcium' is used as a composite term that embraces ionized calcium $[Ca^{2+}]$, protein-bound calcium and complexed calcium, whereas Ca^{2+} means that only calcium ions are being considered. The total concentration of calcium in plasma or urine is shown as plasma or urine [calcium], whereas plasma $[Ca^{2+}]$ refers specifically and solely to the concentration of ionized calcium.

excretion; this varies with the diet, but the relationship is not a simple linear one. On a normal diet, urinary calcium excretion in healthy adults may overlap with the output in some patients who are stone-formers. On a restricted diet, even if dietary calcium intake is severely restricted (i.e. to less than 150 mg/day for at least 7 days), urinary calcium does not normally fall below 2.5 mmol/24 h (100 mg/24 h).

Hormonal control of plasma calcium concentration

Calcium is present in plasma in three forms (Table 13.1), in equilibrium with one another. Plasma $[Ca^{2+}]$ is the physiologically important component and is closely regulated in man by parathyroid hormone (PTH) and 1 : 25-DHCC; these both act to increase plasma $[Ca^{2+}]$ and hence plasma [calcium]. The body's responses to a fall in plasma $[Ca^{2+}]$, in terms of changes in PTH and 1 : 25-DHCC production, are shown in Fig. 13.1. Growth hormone, glucocorticoids (e.g. cortisol), oestrogens, testosterone and thyroid hormones (T4 and T3) also exert minor influences on calcium metabolism.

Table 13.1 The components of calcium in plasma

Calcium component	Percentage of plasma [calcium]
Ionized calcium, Ca^{++}	50–65
Calcium bound to plasma proteins	30–45
Calcium complexed with citrate, etc.	5–10

Parathyroid hormone (PTH)

Parathyroid hormone is initially synthesized in the parathyroid glands as pre-pro-PTH (115 amino acids). After the loss of leader sequences, the active hormone (84 amino acids) is secreted in response to a fall in plasma $[Ca^{2+}]$; a rise in plasma $[Ca^{2+}]$ suppresses PTH secretion. The biological activity of PTH lies in its 30 N-terminal amino acids. Its principal action is to elevate plasma $[Ca^{2+}]$. It does this through the following:

1 *A direct effect on bone*; PTH probably stimulates bone turnover, i.e. bone formation and resorption are both increased. However, resorption exceeds formation so there is a net loss of calcium from bone (i.e. increased matrix breakdown).

2 *A direct effect on the renal tubules*; PTH increases the reabsorption of calcium.

3 *An indirect effect on the small intestine*; PTH stimulates the formation of 1 : 25-DHCC in the kidney. In turn, 1 : 25-DHCC increases the absorption of calcium from the small intestine.

Biochemical measures of both increased osteoblast activity (e.g. increased plasma alkaline phosphatase) and increased osteoclast activity (e.g. raised urinary hydroxyproline excretion) may be evident if PTH activity is increased. Bone fibrous tissue may increase and, in more extreme cases, the radiological changes of osteitis fibrosa cystica may develop.

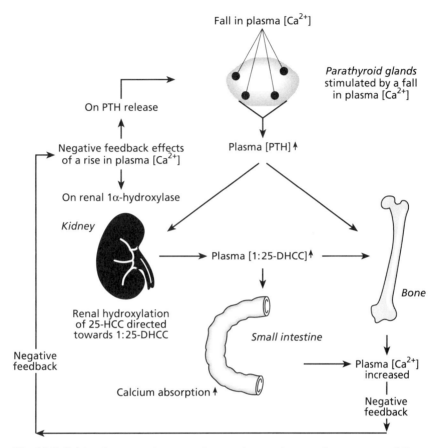

Fig. 13.1 Calcium homeostasis in man, showing the main hormonal responses to a fall in plasma $[Ca^{2+}]$, and indicating the places where the negative feedback mechanism operates if plasma $[Ca^{2+}]$ becomes high. The effect of PTH on the renal tubules, causing increased reabsorption of calcium, is not shown.

In the kidney, in addition to increasing the reabsorption of calcium, PTH reduces the reabsorption of phosphate and HCO_3^-. Hence, when plasma [PTH] is increased, whether pathologically or in response to low plasma $[Ca^{2+}]$, plasma [phosphate] tends to be low provided renal function is normal. Likewise, a mild metabolic acidosis may be present as a result of the renal loss of HCO_3^-.

In the presence of hypercalcaemia due to the effects of raised plasma [PTH], there may be increased renal excretion of calcium. This is because the hypercalcaemia increases the amount of calcium filtered at the glomerulus, and this effect may then predominate over the tubular reabsorption effect of PTH. Nevertheless, where a high plasma $[Ca^{2+}]$ is due to a raised plasma [PTH], the urinary calcium excretion at a given level of plasma $[Ca^{2+}]$ is lower than where a non-PTH cause is the reason for the increased plasma $[Ca^{2+}]$.

1 : 25-Dihydroxycholecalciferol (1 : 25-DHCC or calcitriol)

There is more than one active form of vitamin D and more than one source (i.e. *in vivo* synthesis and dietary intake). In man, cholecalciferol (vitamin D_3) is normally the principal form of the vitamin, synthesized *in vivo* from cholesterol via 7-dehydrocholesterol (a minor metabolite of cholesterol), provided that the skin is exposed to UV light (Fig. 13.2). Vitamin D_3 is also normally present in the diet.

Endogenous synthesis of vitamin D_3 is important. Vitamin D deficiency can develop if exposure to sunlight is inadequate, or because of inadequate dietary intake, but usually it arises as a result of the combined effects of these two factors. In the body, vitamin D_3 and vitamin D_2 (ergosterol) undergo two hydroxylation steps before attaining full physiological activity. These are described for vitamin D_3 (Fig. 13.2).

25-Hydroxylation. This takes place in the liver, with the production of 25-hydroxycholecalciferol (25-HCC or calcidiol). This process is regulated by the amount of 25-HCC in the liver. The main form of vitamin D circulating in the plasma is 25-HCC, bound to a specific transport protein; it is carried to the kidney for further metabolism. Plasma [25-HCC] shows marked seasonal variation, with levels highest in summer.

1α-Hydroxylation of 25-HCC. This takes place in the kidney, with the production of 1 : 25-DHCC, biologically the most active naturally occurring derivative of vitamin D.

The kidney contains other hydroxylases, e.g. 24-hydroxylase which converts 25-HCC to 24 : 25-dihydroxycholecalciferol (24 : 25-DHCC). *The pathway for*

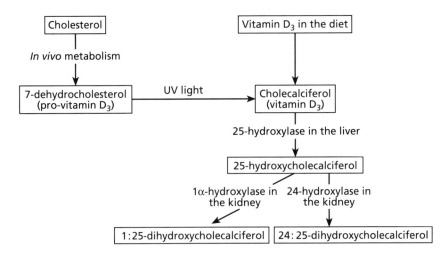

Fig. 13.2 The formation of 1 : 25-dihydroxycholecalciferol (1 : 25-DHCC), the most active form of vitamin D_3, from pro-vitamin D_3 (normally the main source of the vitamin in man) and from dietary vitamin D_3. Vitamin D_2 (ergosterol) undergoes similar hydroxylations. By the action of ultraviolet (UV) light, pro-vitamin D_3 is converted in the dermis into pre-vitamin D_3 (not shown) in which the B-ring of the steroid skeleton has been opened; pre-vitamin D_3 then rearranges spontaneously to give vitamin D_3. The factors that influence the hydroxylation of 25-HCC in the direction of 1 : 25-DHCC or 24 : 25-DHCC are described in the text.

further metabolism of 25-HCC in the kidney is determined by the body's requirement for calcium. If there is a tendency to hypocalcaemia, whatever the cause (e.g. vitamin D deficiency, low calcium diet), metabolism of 25-HCC is directed by PTH towards the formation of 1 : 25-DHCC. If plasma [calcium] is normal, or in the presence of hypercalcaemia, metabolism of 25-HCC is directed towards the formation of 24 : 25-DHCC; this is a much less potent stimulant of intestinal uptake of calcium than 1 : 25-DHCC. The activity of renal 1α-hydroxylase is stimulated by growth hormone and is affected by the renal [1 : 25-DHCC], which exerts a local negative feedback effect.

1 : 25-DHCC induces the synthesis of a Ca^{2+}-binding protein in the intestinal epithelial cell; this protein is involved in the absorption of calcium from the small intestine. In bone, if 1 : 25-DHCC is deficient, there is defective mineralization. It is uncertain whether 1 : 25-DHCC directly stimulates mineralization, and it is possible that its function in helping to maintain both ECF [Ca^{2+}] and ECF [phosphate] is the key factor in normal mineralization. At higher concentrations, 1 : 25-DHCC promotes bone resorption, but it is not known whether it exerts this effect at more physiological concentrations.

Osteocalcin is a vitamin K-dependent Ca^{2+}-binding protein present in bone matrix that depends on 1 : 25-DHCC for its synthesis. It may regulate calcification of osteoid, and plasma [osteocalcin] has been used as a measure of bone turnover (p. 212).

Calcitonin

The importance of calcitonin in the physiological regulation of plasma [Ca^{2+}] in man is uncertain. Its role is at most minor by comparison with PTH and with 1 : 25-DHCC. Its use as a tumour marker is discussed elsewhere (p. 264).

Intracellular calcium

The ECF [Ca^{2+}] is about 1 mmol/L (10^{-3}M); cytosolic or intracellular [Ca^{2+}] is much lower, about 100 nmol/L (10^{-7}M). Cells possess a number of transport mechanisms for Ca^{2+} that allow maintenance of this large gradient across the cell membrane.

An increase in cytosolic [Ca^{2+}] serves as a signal for several cell processes which include cell shape change, cell motility, metabolic changes, secretory activity and cell division. Many intercellular signals, including several hormones, bring about an increase in cytosolic [Ca^{2+}] by opening plasma membrane Ca^{2+} channels, or by releasing intracellular stores of Ca^{2+}, or by a combination of these effects.

Release of intracellular Ca^{2+} is closely linked to breakdown of membrane phospholipids, the polyphosphoinositides, hydrolysis of which yields diacylglycerol and an inositol trisphosphate. Inositol trisphosphate then releases Ca^{2+} from an intracellular Ca^{2+} store and diacylglycerol activates a multifunctional protein kinase, protein kinase C.

There are indications that derangements in these intracellular metabolic events may underlie various disease processes, including essential hypertension, cystic fibrosis and possibly some types of malignancy.

Investigation of abnormal calcium metabolism

A standard group of widely available chemical measurements is commonly performed when investigating possible abnormalities of calcium metabolism. The group consists of plasma calcium and albumin, inorganic phosphate and alkaline phosphatase measurements.

Plasma calcium (reference range, 2.12–2.62 mmol/L)

Most laboratories only measure plasma [calcium], as a routine, even though the physiologically important fraction is plasma $[Ca^{2+}]$. Measurements of plasma [calcium] can be misleading in the investigation of disorders of calcium metabolism since the results may be abnormal at times when plasma $[Ca^{2+}]$ is normal, and vice versa. It would be preferable to measure plasma $[Ca^{2+}]$ rather than plasma [calcium], and thereby circumvent these problems. However, for reasons related to specimen collection and analytical technique, measurements of plasma $[Ca^{2+}]$ on the large numbers of specimens on which determinations of plasma [calcium] are requested would not be practicable. Measurements of plasma $[Ca^{2+}]$ are, in general, reserved for the investigation of those few patients in whom the presence of an abnormal plasma $[Ca^{2+}]$ is suspected, but in whom difficulty has arisen over the interpretation of other much more readily available investigations of calcium metabolism.

Most of the pitfalls in the interpretation of results for plasma calcium measurements concern the effects of changes in plasma [albumin] or $[H^+]$ on the equilibrium between protein-bound calcium and free (i.e. ionized) calcium.

Effects of plasma albumin

Changes in plasma [albumin], in general, cause parallel changes in plasma [calcium], while plasma [PTH] maintains plasma $[Ca^{2+}]$ constant (Fig. 13.3).

1 *Low plasma [albumin]*, with *low* plasma [calcium] and *normal* plasma $[Ca^{2+}]$, may be due to diminished albumin synthesis (e.g. protein malnutrition, intestinal malabsorption, chronic liver disease), albumin loss (e.g. nephrotic syndrome) or increased protein breakdown (e.g. hypercatabolic states associated with trauma, sepsis, major surgery, burns or malignant disease).

2 *High plasma [albumin]*, with *high* plasma [calcium] and *normal* plasma $[Ca^{2+}]$, may result from dehydration or albumin infusion or be caused by poor technique, i.e. excessive venous stasis during specimen collection, by specimen collection from ambulant patients rather than from patients who have been sitting or lying down for a few minutes beforehand.

'Correction' factors have been described that seek to adjust the observed plasma [calcium] so as to take account of the plasma [albumin] in the specimen. This approach is subject to considerable error, but the following is an example of a 'correction factor':

1 *For each g/L that plasma [albumin] is above 40 g/L, 0.02 mmol/L should be subtracted from the plasma [calcium] observed in the same specimen.*

2 *For each g/L that plasma [albumin] is below 40 g/L, 0.02 mmol/L should be added to the plasma [calcium] observed in the same specimen.*

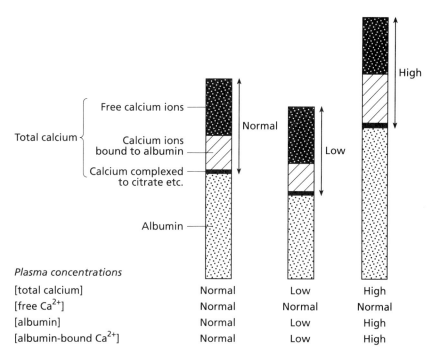

Fig. 13.3 The effects of changes in plasma [albumin] on the distribution of calcium between free and albumin-bound calcium ions, and the consequent effects on plasma [total calcium]; plasma [free Ca^{2+}] is unaltered. 50–65% of calcium in plasma is normally present in the free, ionized, form and 30–45% bound to albumin, with the remaining 5–10% consisting of calcium complexed with organic ions (e.g. citrate).

Effects of plasma H^+

Plasma [H^+] influences the position of the equilibrium between protein-bound and ionized calcium. The action of [H^+] can best be explained as competing with Ca^{2+} for the binding sites on albumin. A high plasma [H^+] displaces bound calcium from its binding to albumin, leading to an increase in plasma [Ca^{2+}] whereas a low plasma [H^+] means that more calcium binds to albumin, with a consequent reduction in plasma [Ca^{2+}]. In neither case is there a change in plasma [calcium].

In chronic states of acidosis or alkalosis, PTH acts to readjust the plasma [Ca^{2+}] back to normal. The effects of changes in plasma [H^+] on plasma [Ca^{2+}] may be much more evident in acute acidosis or alkalosis, e.g. tetany (p. 207).

Plasma phosphate (reference range, 0.8–1.4 mmol/L)

Phosphate compounds, inorganic and organic, are present in both the ECF and ICF. In the cell, phosphate is largely organic, as a component of phospholipids, phosphoproteins, nucleic acids and nucleotides (e.g. ATP). In the ECF, phosphate is mostly inorganic, as a mixture of HPO_4^{2-} and $H_2PO_4^-$ at physiological pH. Plasma [phosphate] shows considerable diurnal variation, especially following meals; the reference range relates to the fasting state. Different ranges should be used for different age-groups.

Hypophosphataemia may be caused by the effects of PTH on renal tubular phosphate handling (p. 197), and by insulin which increases the uptake of phosphate into liver and muscle, thereby altering the distribution of phosphate between the ECF and ICF. Hypophosphataemia may also be due to decreased intake.

Hyperphosphataemia may be due to decreased renal excretion, altered distribution between the ECF and ICF, or increased intake.

Alkaline phosphatase (local reference range, 40–125 IU/L)

Reference ranges for plasma alkaline phosphatase activity are very method-dependent. There are also considerable variations in this enzyme's activity, for physiological reasons, in childhood and adolescence (p. 79).

The bone isoenzyme of alkaline phosphatase activity is increased in plasma from patients with diseases in which there is increased osteoblastic activity, e.g. hyperparathyroidism, Paget's disease, rickets and osteomalacia, and carcinoma with osteoblastic metastases.

Hypercalcaemia

Increased ECF $[Ca^{2+}]$ directly damages the kidneys and, if prolonged, is liable to cause tubular malfunction. In particular, distal tubular damage may lead to impaired ability to produce a concentrated urine. Dehydration may result, thereby aggravating the condition. More often, pathological hypercalcaemia of long duration causes irreversible nephrocalcinosis; increased clearance of calcium predisposes to renal stone formation. Patients may also complain of generalized muscle weakness, or nausea and vomiting, or constipation.

The apparent incidence of hypercalcaemia has been rising, mainly as a result of unselective (screening) requests. The commonest cause of hypercalcaemia depends on the population screened. In hospitals, where screening of patients on first attendance or when admitted is widely practised, the commonest cause is malignant disease, but when hypercalcaemia is detected by well-population screening (p. 2) this is more likely to be due to primary hyperparathyroidism.

The causes of hypercalcaemia are summarized in Table 13.2. Potentially misleading hypercalcaemia, in which plasma $[Ca^{2+}]$ is normal, often results from abnormal calcium binding, due to raised plasma [albumin]. If this can be excluded, the hypercalcaemia must be pathological and reflects the presence of an abnormally high ECF $[Ca^{2+}]$; this may have serious implications.

Hypercalcaemia of malignancy

Several factors are responsible for the hypercalcaemia of malignancy. These vary, depending on the type of tumour and on whether or not there are bone metastases:

1 *Solid tumours that have metastasized to bone* may cause hypercalcaemia by paracrine activation of osteoclasts, e.g. the local release into bone of prostaglan-

Table 13.2 The causes of hypercalcaemia

Category	Examples
Parathyroid disease	Hyperparathyroidism, primary and tertiary; multiple endocrine neoplasia syndromes, MEN I and MEN IIa
Malignant disease	Carcinoma, with osteolytic deposits; multiple myeloma; humoral hypercalcaemia of malignancy
Excessive absorption of calcium	Vitamin D overdose (including self-medication); excessive dietary calcium; milk-alkali syndrome
Bone disease	Osteoporosis and Paget's disease (rare in both, and usually only if the patient is immobilized)
Drug-induced	Thiazide diuretics
Miscellaneous causes (mostly rare or uncommon causes of hypercalcaemia)	Familial hypocalciuric hypercalcaemia, alone or as part of MEN I or MEN IIa syndromes Hypercalcaemia in childhood (p. 338) Ectopic production of PTH by tumours Cushing's syndrome and Cushing's disease Sarcoidosis Thyrotoxicosis Hypercalcaemic periostitis
Artefact	Poor venepuncture technique (excessive venous stasis)

dins of the E series has been implicated in the hypercalcaemia frequently observed with metastatic breast carcinoma. The tumour cells may also increase bone resorption directly.

2 *Some solid tumours, in the absence of bony metastases*, may give rise to hypercalcaemia as a result of the release of humoral factors (e.g. carcinoma of the lung, head and neck, pancreas). Several factors have been implicated in this *humoral hypercalcaemia of malignancy*. They include transforming growth factors α and β, platelet-derived growth factor, and PTH-related protein (PTHrP). There is marked sequence homology between PTHrP and the first 13 N-terminal amino acids of PTH; eight of the 13 residues are identical. Acting through the PTH receptor, PTHrP can cause hypercalcaemia, hypophosphataemia and increased urinary cyclic AMP formation. True ectopic production of PTH appears to be rare.

3 *In multiple myeloma*, hypercalcaemia appears to result from the release of osteoclast-activating factors (OAF) which promote local bone resorption. These factors may include tumour-necrosing factor and lymphotoxin. Lymphomas also produce OAF, but may in addition synthesize and release 1 : 25-DHCC.

Primary hyperparathyroidism

This is usually caused by a parathyroid adenoma and less often by multiple adenomas, diffuse hyperplasia or carcinoma. Classically, patients used to present with renal calculi or with metabolic bone disease. However, many patients found

Table 13.3 'First-line' chemical tests for investigating suspected hyperparathyroidism

Plasma or serum	Comments
Calcium*	If increased [calcium], supports the diagnosis
Albumin*	Should be performed as a check on plasma [calcium]
Phosphate (fasting)	If decreased [phosphate], supports the diagnosis
Alkaline phosphatase	If enzymic activity increased, supports the diagnosis
Creatinine and/or urea	Simple tests of renal function, needed in all patients with suspected abnormalities of calcium metabolism

*The only essential 'first-line' investigations are measurements of plasma [calcium] and [albumin], which may need to be repeated on several occasions. The others listed are all widely available and have been included either because they may provide useful supporting evidence or because they are often performed as part of a 'calcium screen' or 'bone screen'.

by screening to have primary hyperparathyroidism may be asymptomatic when the diagnosis is first made.

Tests to be performed as part of the *initial or 'first-line' investigation* of suspected primary hyperparathyroidism are listed in Table 13.3. The finding of the *combination* of an increased plasma [calcium], decreased fasting plasma [phosphate] and increased plasma alkaline phosphatase activity strongly supports a diagnosis of primary hyperparathyroidism. It may be necessary to measure plasma [calcium] and [albumin] on two or more occasions before hypercalcaemia is detected since hypercalcaemia can be intermittent. It is not possible to place reliance on the finding of a low plasma [phosphate], by itself, since this is not a constant feature of primary hyperparathyroidism.

Patients with primary hyperparathyroidism often have a mild metabolic acidosis, as a consequence of the urinary HCO_3^- excretion in response to the raised plasma [PTH]. This is reflected in a low plasma [total CO_2]. Other causes of hypercalcaemia are usually associated with a low plasma [PTH], mild metabolic alkalosis and increased total plasma [total CO_2].

Urine excretion studies of calcium and phosphate output are rarely performed nowadays in the investigation of hyperparathyroidism. Most laboratories, if reporting the results of urine calcium measurements, relate these to urinary creatinine and some express the results as a calcium : creatinine clearance ratio in an attempt to improve the discriminating power of the test. Other indices (e.g. phosphate excretion index) have also been used, but these time-consuming and relatively indirect tests of PTH activity have largely been rendered obsolete by the availability of serum [PTH] measurements.

Serum intact PTH (reference range, 10–55 ng/L)

The definitive diagnosis depends largely on finding hypercalcaemia accompanied by a high or normal (i.e. unsuppressed) serum [PTH]. However, measurement of serum [PTH] should only be requested *after* the results of initial investigations (Table 13.3), if necessary repeated several times, have been considered and on the basis of a reasonably high probability that this 'first-line' information supports the diagnosis.

Modern immunometric assays for PTH are sensitive and are specifically designed to measure only the intact PTH molecule. However, these methods are expensive and this means that the definitive measurement of serum [PTH] must be requested selectively. Earlier assays for PTH were less sensitive, and had the serious added disadvantage that they measured both PTH and biologically inactive fragments of PTH.

Chemical tests to help locate a parathyroid tumour are not normally performed prior to surgery. However, if a parathyroid adenoma or other parathyroid abnormality is not found in any of the usual sites, blood can be collected from veins draining other regions before completing the operation, if the evidence in support of the diagnosis of primary hyperparathyroidism is sufficiently strong. Measurement of serum [PTH] in these regional blood specimens may help in planning further surgery.

Management of primary hyperparathyroidism

In view of the technical difficulty often associated with parathyroid surgery, it is not unusual for operation to be deferred in patients with asymptomatic hyperparathyroidism if their plasma [calcium] is less than 3.00 mmol/L. As symptoms may develop insidiously, these patients must be followed up with regular further measurements of plasma [calcium] and careful clinical reassessment. It is advisable to proceed to parathyroidectomy early rather than late.

After parathyroidectomy, plasma [calcium] falls rapidly, and it should be measured several times on the first post-operative day and at least daily for the next few days. If the plasma [calcium] falls below normal, calcium gluconate should be given and treatment with 1 : 25-DHCC or 1α-hydroxycholecalciferol (1α-HCC) started.

Multiple endocrine neoplasia (MEN) syndromes

Three types of MEN syndrome have been described, all of them familial. Patients with these syndromes have adenomas of several endocrine tissues, and sometimes hypersecretion of the hormones they produce. The MEN I group (Werner's syndrome) is the commonest of the three groups; its form of presentation and pattern of investigation depend on the endocrine glands involved.

Primary hyperparathyroidism is the commonest abnormality in MEN I, being present in up to 85% of patients. About 70% of patients have tumours in two glands, and sometimes three or more are involved. In addition to the parathyroid gland, the other tissues most commonly affected in the MEN I syndrome are the pancreatic islet cells (up to 80%) and the anterior pituitary (up to 65%). The pancreatic tumours may secrete insulin, gastrin, VIP and various other peptide hormones (e.g. ACTH, glucagon, somatostatin). Overproduction of ACTH, growth hormone and prolactin by the pituitary tumours has been reported.

Hyperparathyroidism is present in about 20% of patients with MEN IIa

(MEN 2), but is not a feature of MEN IIb (MEN 3). The MEN II syndromes are discussed elsewhere (p. 265).

Other causes of hypercalcaemia

The history of the patient's illness, the findings on clinical examination, and various investigations as suggested by the provisional diagnosis will usually mean that the other conditions (Table 13.3) can be recognized. They will be briefly considered.

Vitamin D excess. Increased plasma [1 : 25-DHCC] can produce hypercalcaemia. This can occur if vitamin D intake is excessive or if overdosage with 25-HCC, 1α-HCC or 1 : 25-DHCC occurs. Measurement of serum [25-HCC] or [1 : 25-DHCC] confirms the diagnosis.

Sarcoidosis. About 10–20% of patients with sarcoidosis may have mild hypercalcaemia, often only intermittently. Much more often, they have hypercalciuria. Plasma [1 : 25-DHCC] is sometimes increased, leading to enhanced absorption of calcium from the intestine, hypercalciuria and sometimes hyper-

---

Case 13.1

A 47-year-old secretary was admitted as an emergency with left-sided ureteric colic. She had had one similar episode 3 years before, when she had passed a small calculus spontaneously. She had also been being treated with cimetidine for the previous 6 months, for dyspepsia. Physical examination only revealed slight tenderness in the left loin and on palpating the abdomen. 'Side-room' tests showed that there was a trace of blood in her urine, and a plain X-ray of the abdomen detected a small opacity in the line of the left ureter. Chemical investigations on blood gave the following results:

Analysis	Result	Reference range	Units
[Creatinine]	150	55–120	μmol/L
[Urea]	8.1	2.5–6.6	mmol/L
[Na$^+$]	141	132–144	mmol/L
[K$^+$]	4.2	3.3–4.7	mmol/L
[Total Co$_2$]	20	24–30	mmol/L
[Calcium]	3.29	2.12–2.62	mmol/L
[Albumin]	40	36–47	g/L
[Phosphate]	0.6	0.8–1.4	mmol/L
Alkaline phosphatase activity	160	40–125	IU/L

What was the most likely cause of the patient's urinary calculi? What further investigations would you request in order to confirm your diagnosis? Would you consider it appropriate to treat this patient medically, and if so how, while awaiting the results of any further investigations? The patient is discussed on p. 214.

calcaemia. There may be excessive conversion of 25-HCC to 1 : 25-DHCC by sarcoid tissue.

Milk–alkali syndrome. Milk consumption may be excessive in patients with symptoms of peptic ulceration; calcium intake is correspondingly increased. If this is accompanied by excessive intake of alkali (e.g. $NaHCO_3$), as an antacid, hypercalcaemia may develop. The alkali is thought to reduce urinary calcium excretion and to be important in the pathogenesis of the condition.

Tertiary hyperparathyroidism. This description refers to the development of a functioning parathyroid adenoma as a complication of previously existing secondary hyperparathyroidism (p. 138). This diagnosis needs to be considered in patients with renal failure or intestinal malabsorption, if they develop hypercalcaemia that is not attributable to treatment with vitamin D or one of its hydroxylated derivatives (usually 1α-HCC or 1 : 25-DHCC). Plasma [calcium] is almost always increased and serum [PTH] always increased. Unlike primary hyperparathyroidism, however, fasting plasma [phosphate] may be increased, especially if tertiary hyperparathyroidism develops in a patient with renal failure.

Other bone-related causes. Causes, other than malignant disease, include Paget's disease in which there is an increase in bone turnover that is occasionally accompanied by hypercalcaemia. Prolonged immobilization can also sometimes lead to hypercalcaemia, especially during adolescence when bone turnover is increased.

Endocrine disorders. Hypercalcaemia has been reported occasionally in association with acromegaly, Cushing's syndrome, hypoadrenalism, phaeochromocytoma and thyrotoxicosis.

Drugs. A mild degree of hypercalcaemia may develop during treatment with thiazide diuretics; these interfere with renal calcium excretion. Long-term lithium therapy may also be a cause, possibly by stimulating PTH secretion.

Familial hypocalciuric hypercalcaemia (FHH). This uncommon disorder is transmitted by an autosomal dominant gene. Patients with FHH mostly have lifelong hypercalcaemia, but unaccompanied by the hypercalciuria that would normally be expected under these circumstances. This is one of the few conditions in which it is important to measure urinary calcium excretion.

Hypocalcaemia

The causes are listed in Table 13.4. If potentially misleading hypocalcaemia due to decreased plasma [albumin] is first excluded, the hypocalcaemia must be pathological and must result from a decrease in plasma $[Ca^{2+}]$.

Tetany is the symptom that classically suggests the presence of a low plasma $[Ca^{2+}]$. Occasionally it is due to a low plasma $[Mg^{2+}]$ in the absence of low plasma $[Ca^{2+}]$ and rarely it is due to low plasma $[K^+]$. Neuropsychiatric symptoms and cataract are other possible consequences of hypocalcaemia.

Tetany may occur in any of the conditions listed in Table 13.4. It may also be caused by the rapid fall in plasma $[H^+]$ that can occur in the acute respiratory alkalosis produced by hyperventilation or as a result of the intravenous infusion of $NaHCO_3$.

Table 13.4 The causes of hypocalcaemia

Category	Examples
Hypoproteinaemia	Low plasma [albumin] (p. 89)
Renal disease	Hydroxylation of 25-HCC impaired, acidosis
Inadequate intake of calcium	Dietary deficiency of calcium or vitamin D, or of both; intestinal malabsorption (p. 160)
Hypoparathyroidism	Acquired or idiopathic PTH deficiency
Pseudohypoparathyroidism	Target organ resistance to PTH
Neonatal hypocalcaemia	p. 332
Acute pancreatitis	Calcium soaps in the abdominal cavity?

Vitamin D deficiency

The commonest pathological cause of hypocalcaemia is defective calcium absorption due to inadequate plasma levels of 1 : 25-DHCC. In malnutrition, the effects of vitamin D deficiency are accentuated by inadequate dietary calcium. Deficiency of 1 : 25-DHCC may result from lack of vitamin D or failure at any stage in its conversion to 1 : 25-DHCC (Fig. 13.2); rarely the action of 1 : 25-DHCC is defective at the receptor level.

Plasma [calcium] is low, unless the increased PTH secretion that occurs in response to the low ECF $[Ca^{2+}]$ is sufficient to compensate for the impaired absorption of calcium. The elevated serum [PTH] is secondary to the low ECF $[Ca^{2+}]$; it is physiologically appropriate and is termed *secondary hyperparathyroidism*. Plasma [phosphate] is often low, partly through impaired absorption but also as a result of the secondary hyperparathyroidism, except in those renal tubular diseases where phosphate retention occurs. Plasma alkaline phosphatase activity is often increased, reflecting increased osteoblastic activity. However, its measurement is of limited diagnostic value in childhood because of the marked physiological variations in activity that normally occur in this age-group (Fig. 6.2, p. 79). Urinary calcium excretion is nearly always low or very low.

Confirmation of the diagnosis of vitamin D deficiency depends on measurement of serum [25-HCC] or, less widely available, serum [1 : 25-DHCC]. Serum [25-HCC] assays provide a reasonable indication of the overall vitamin D status of the patient, if renal function is normal and renal 1α-hydroxylase activity can be assumed to be normal. There is a seasonal variation in serum [25-HCC] that can make interpretation of single results difficult. Measurement of serum [25-HCC] is also of value in monitoring patients who are being treated for vitamin D deficiency by dietary supplementation.

The main causes of hypocalcaemia due to lack of vitamin D or to disturbances of its metabolism (Fig. 13.2) will be briefly considered:

1 *Nutritional deficiency of vitamin D.* Poor diet, inadequate exposure to sunlight, or a combination of these can lead to vitamin D deficiency; calcium absorption is reduced. Dietary deficiency of vitamin D is usually accompanied by dietary calcium deficiency. The elderly are particularly at risk as they are often confined indoors and often have a poor diet. Cultural and geographical factors are

probably important in the susceptibility to vitamin D deficiency of the immigrant Asian community in Northern Europe.

2 *Malabsorption of vitamin D.* This may be due to coeliac disease, or may occur as a result of fat malabsorption due to pancreatic disease or biliary obstruction, or as a complication of gastric or intestinal surgery (e.g. intestinal by-pass or resection).

3 *Liver disease.* This may be the cause of reduced 25-hydroxylation of vitamin D. However, altered enterohepatic circulation of bile salts is more likely to lead to 1 : 25-DHCC deficiency.

4 *Renal disease.* Destruction of the renal parenchyma leads to loss of 1α-hydroxylase activity, reduced formation of 1 : 25-DHCC and consequent malabsorption of calcium. Plasma [phosphate] is likely to be high in renal failure, and this may interfere with the 1α-hydroxylation step. Specific deficiency of 1α-hydroxylase may be the cause of hypocalcaemia in vitamin D-resistant rickets, type I, a rare inherited disorder.

5 *End-organ unresponsiveness to 1 : 25-DHCC.* This may be the cause of hypocalcaemia in vitamin D-resistant rickets, type II, another rare inherited disorder.

Rickets and osteomalacia

Patients who have vitamin D deficiency or disturbed metabolism of vitamin D are all liable to suffer from osteomalacia or, in children, from rickets. These patients have bone pain, with local tenderness, and may have a proximal myopathy. Skeletal deformity may be present, particularly in rickets. Mineralization of osteoid is defective, with absence of the calcification front.

Other causes of rickets or osteomalacia, unrelated to vitamin D deficiency or defects in its metabolism, have also been described. An inherited defect in the tubular reabsorption of phosphate, hypophosphataemic vitamin D-resistant rickets, leads to similar bone deformities but without muscle weakness; there is a low plasma [phosphate] and phosphaturia. In the Fanconi syndrome, tubular phosphate loss may also lead to low plasma [phosphate] associated with rickets or osteomalacia.

Hypophosphatasia is a hereditary disease in which vitamin D-resistant rickets is the most prominent finding. Tissue and plasma alkaline phosphatase activities are usually low, and excessive amounts of phosphoryl-ethanolamine are present in the urine.

Hypoparathyroidism

Primary hypoparathyroidism is rare. The combination of a reduced plasma [calcium] and an increased [phosphate] in a patient who does not have renal disease suggests the diagnosis of hypoparathyroidism; plasma alkaline phosphatase activity is usually normal in these patients. Measurement of serum [PTH] confirms the diagnosis; it is reduced to below 10 ng/L, and is sometimes undetectable even by the most sensitive assays.

Failure to secrete PTH may be a complication of surgery, or it may be familial or sporadic in origin. Also, the parathyroid glands may be destroyed by an autoimmune process or as a result of infiltration by carcinoma of the thyroid or other neoplasms. Occasionally, the parathyroid glands are suppressed as a result of magnesium deficiency; normal magnesium levels are necessary for PTH release.

Pseudohypoparathyroidism

This is a rare inborn error of metabolism in which the end-organ receptors in the bone and the kidneys fail to respond normally to PTH; sometimes only one of these two sets of receptors is affected. The diagnosis is suggested by the family history and by the presence of characteristic skeletal abnormalities. As in patients with idiopathic and acquired hypoparathyroidism, there is reduced plasma [calcium] and increased fasting plasma [phosphate]. However, patients with pseudohypoparathyroidism have *increased* serum [PTH].

Nephrogenic cyclic AMP excretion is increased in states of PTH excess since PTH exerts its renal effects through activation of adenylate cyclase. Measurement of urinary cyclic AMP is of value in the diagnosis of the end-organ unresponsiveness to PTH in pseudohypoparathyroidism.

Other causes of hypocalcaemia

Surgical removal of or serious damage to the parathyroid glands can lead to hypoparathyroidism and hypocalcaemia. Treatment with anticonvulsant drugs (e.g. phenytoin) or diphosphonates (used in the treatment of Paget's disease and some metabolic bone disorders) is another iatrogenic cause of hypocalcaemia; these drugs appear to antagonize the peripheral actions of 1 : 25-DHCC. Treatment with corticosteroids may also cause hypocalcaemia.

Large transfusions of citrated blood can lead to complex formation between Ca^{2+} and the citrate anion, thereby lowering plasma $[Ca^{2+}]$. Hypocalcaemia in the neonatal period is discussed elsewhere (p. 332).

Metabolic bone diseases

Generalized defects in bone mineralization, frequently associated with abnormal calcium or phosphate metabolism, are sometimes grouped together under the term metabolic bone diseases. The most common are rickets and osteomalacia, hyperparathyroidism and osteoporosis.

In many examples of metabolic bone disease, patients show features of two or more of these conditions, and it can be difficult to define the pathological process fully, even with the aid of radiological examination and bone biopsy. Results of chemical investigations (Table 13.5) must be interpreted in relation to all the available evidence. For example, in renal osteodystrophy, a combination of osteomalacia, hyperparathyroidism and other metabolic abnormalities contributes to the metabolic bone disease. Various other conditions, often rare, may produce generalized bone disease, with or without biochemical changes.

Osteoporosis

This is a very common disorder. However, it is not usually diagnosed with certainty until there is a marked loss in bone density, revealed by X-ray investigations. Results of routine chemical investigations are usually all normal. Careful

Table 13.5 Metablic bone disease: chemical investigations on blood specimens

Diagnosis	Calcium	Phosphate (fasting)	PTH	Alkaline phosphatase	Ca^{++}
Hyperparathyroidism					
Primary	↑ (or N)	↓ or N	↑ or N*	N or ↑	↑ (or N)
Secondary	↓ or N	↑ or N	↑	↑ or N	N
Tertiary	↑ or N	↑ or N	↑	↑ or N	↑
Rickets and osteomalacia					
Deficient intake	↓ or N	↓ or N	↑ (or N)	↑	N (or ↓)
Renal failure	↓ or N	↑ or N	↑	↑	N
Fanconi syndrome†	↓ or N	↓ or N	N	↑	N
Osteoporosis	N	N	N	N	N
Paget's disease	N (or ↑)	N	N	↑	N

N, normal; ↑, increased; ↓, decreased. N* indicates that, with sensitive PTH assays, plasma [PTH] is sometimes within the reference range, i.e. it is inappropriately high in primary hyperparathyroidism and not suppressed, as would normally be expected in the presence of hypercalcaemia. With less sensitive PTH assays, plasma [PTH] may be below the reference range or even undetectable in the presence of hypercalcaemia due to primary hyperparathyroidism. † Included as an example of proximal renal tubular defects.

metabolic balance studies are demanding but, if performed, sometimes reveal a negative calcium balance, especially during active stages of the disease.

The diagnosis may have to depend on finding *skeletal rarefaction in a patient who does not have* hyperparathyroidism, osteomalacia, carcinoma, multiple myeloma, etc., and in whom plasma calcium, albumin and phosphate concentrations and alkaline phosphatase activity and other commonly performed chemical tests are all normal.

As an index of osteoblastic activity, plasma [osteocalcin] can be used to categorize patients with osteoporosis as having high turnover, low turnover or normal turnover of calcium in bone. Although there have been reports that osteocalcin can be used as a marker in the diagnosis of osteoporosis, its value is still being assessed.

Paget's disease

This is a common disorder of bone, affecting about 5% of the UK population over 55 years old. It occurs in osteosclerotic and osteolytic forms. Plasma [calcium] and [phosphate] are usually normal though hypercalcaemia can develop, especially as a result of immobilization. It is a common cause of markedly increased plasma alkaline phosphatase activity in this age group. Some would not classify Paget's disease as a metabolic bone disease because it is often local rather than general in its manifestations.

Renal osteodystrophy

The pathophysiology of renal osteodystrophy is complex. The bone changes in it

---

Case 13.2

A 64-year-old retired shop assistant with Crohn's disease had been well controlled by means of oral prednisolone until 2–3 months before attending for her regular follow-up appointment. Latterly, however, she had had severe pain in the back and radiological examination showed a compression fracture of the fourth lumbar vertebra. Chemical investigations on blood gave the following results:

Analysis	Result	Reference range	Units
[Creatinine]	110	55–120	µmol/L
[Urea]	5.8	2.5–6.6	mmol/L
[Na$^+$]	136	132–144	mmol/L
[K$^+$]	3.5	3.3–4.7	mmol/L
[Total CO$_2$]	21	24–30	mmol/L
[Calcium]	1.72	2.12–2.62	mmol/L
[Albumin]	26	36–47	g/L
[Phosphate, fasting]	0.8	0.8–1.4	mmol/L
Alkaline phosphatase activity	170	40–125	IU/L

How would you interpret these results, and what further investigations might be indicated in the light of these findings? The patient is discussed on p. 215.

---

are varied, and derive from one or more of the following mechanisms:

1 *Vitamin D metabolism.* There is ineffective conversion of 25-HCC to 1 : 25-DHCC due to loss of renal 1α-hydroxylase. This causes defective calcium absorption and osteomalacia in adults, or rickets in children. It may be corrected by treatment with 1α-HCC or 1 : 25-DHCC.

2 *Phosphate retention.* There is increased plasma [phosphate], and this, by complexing with Ca^{2+}, tends to make plasma [Ca^{2+}] fall. This leads to hyperactivity of the parathyroid glands (secondary hyperparathyroidism) which tends to restore plasma [phosphate] and [Ca^{2+}], and therefore plasma [calcium], towards normal. Osteitis fibrosa, if it develops, may require parathyroidectomy.

3 *Phosphate binders.* Failure of the secondary hyperparathyroidism to maintain normal plasma [phosphate] as renal disease progresses leads to treatment of patients with oral phosphate binders, usually aluminium hydroxide. Excess absorption of aluminium may cause osteomalacia and dialysis dementia. Plasma [aluminium] should be measured periodically.

4 *Dialysis fluid composition.* The fluid [calcium] must be carefully controlled; if it is too low, osteoporosis often develops. If fluid [calcium] is too high, extraskeletal calcification may occur. Care is also needed to ensure that dialysis fluid [aluminium] is sufficiently low.

In order to control and treat these various abnormalities, all patients with chronic renal failure require biochemical monitoring. Plasma creatinine, urea, Na^+, K^+, total CO_2, albumin, calcium and phosphate concentrations and alkaline phosphatase activity should all be measured regularly. The main object of treatment with 1α-HCC or $1:25$-DHCC is to increase plasma [calcium] to normal and to reverse bone disease due to parathyroid overactivity. If treatment is successful, plasma alkaline phosphatase activity falls to normal. When treatment is first started, it may be difficult to adjust the dose of 1α-HCC or $1:25$-DHCC satisfactorily and hypercalcaemia, possibly with extra-skeletal calcium deposition, may occur if too much is given.

Magnesium metabolism

Magnesium is the second most abundant intracellular cation. It is essential for the activity of many enzymes, including the phosphotransferases. Bone contains about 50% of the body's magnesium; a small proportion of the body's content is in the ECF.

Dietary intake of magnesium is normally about 10 mmol (250 mg) daily. Significant amounts are contained in gastric and biliary secretions. Factors concerned with the control of magnesium absorption have not been defined, but may involve active transport across the intestinal mucosa by a process involving a specific binding protein. Renal conservation of magnesium is at least partly controlled by PTH and aldosterone. When the dietary intake is restricted, renal conservation mechanisms are normally so efficient that depletion, if it develops at all, only comes on very slowly.

Plasma magnesium (reference range, 0.7–1.0 mmol/L)

Plasma [magnesium] is normally kept within narrow limits, which implies close homeostatic control. Marked alterations in the body's content can occur with little or no change detectable in plasma [magnesium]. In this respect, magnesium is very like potassium. The plasma [magnesium] may be normal although a state of intracellular depletion exists.

Hypomagnesaemia and magnesium deficiency

Magnesium deficiency (Table 13.6) rarely occurs as an isolated phenomenon. Usually it is accompanied by disorders of potassium, calcium and phosphate metabolism. It may, therefore, be difficult to identify signs and symptoms that can be specifically attributed to magnesium deficiency. However, muscular weakness, sometimes accompanied by tetany, cardiac arrhythmias and CNS abnormalities (e.g. convulsions), may be due to magnesium deficiency.

Magnesium deficiency should be suspected in patients with hypocalcaemia or hypokalaemia, and who fail to respond to treatment of these abnormalities. Plasma [magnesium] is usually below 0.5 mmol/L in patients with symptoms directly attributable to magnesium deficiency; its level should be measured before treatment with magnesium salts is instituted.

Plasma [magnesium] may not reflect the true state of the body's reserves, particularly in chronic disorders. Other tests have been advocated (e.g. erythro-

Table 13.6 Magnesium deficiency

Causes	Examples
Abnormal losses	
GI tract	Prolonged aspiration, persistent diarrhoea, malabsorptive disease, fistula, jejuno-ileal by-pass, small bowel resection
Urinary tract	
Renal disease	Renal tubular acidosis, chronic pyelonephritis, hydronephrosis
Extra-renal causes	Conditions that modify renal function (e.g. primary and secondary hyperaldosteronism, diuretics, osmotic diuresis) Conditions affecting transfer of magnesium from cells to bone (e.g. primary and tertiary hyperparathyroidism, ketoacidosis)
Lactation	Only if lactation is excessive
Reduced intake	If severe and prolonged (e.g. kwashiorkor, marasmus)
Mixed aetiology	Chronic alcoholism, hepatic cirrhosis

cyte [magnesium], muscle [magnesium], magnesium loading tests), but there is no general agreement on the best test to use. Urinary excretion of magnesium is relatively easy to measure and is useful in distinguishing renal losses of magnesium from the other causes of hypomagnesaemia and magnesium deficiency. Renal excretion of magnesium often falls below 0.5 mmol/24 h when there is a non-renal cause of magnesium deficiency.

Hypermagnesaemia

This is most often due to acute renal failure or the advanced stages of chronic renal failure. Its presence is readily confirmed by measuring plasma [magnesium]. There may be no symptoms. However, if plasma [magnesium] exceeds 2.5 mmol/L, nausea and vomiting, weakness and impaired consciousness may then develop, but these symptoms may not necessarily be caused solely by the hypermagnesaemia.

Other rarer causes of hypermagnesaemia include haemodialysis against hard water, which has a high [magnesium], and intravenous injection of magnesium salts. Adrenocortical hypofunction may cause a slight increase in plasma [magnesium].

Comments on Case 13.1 (p. 206)

The most likely diagnosis is primary hyperparathyroidism; the history of recurrent renal calculi and peptic ulceration is highly suggestive, and strongly supported by the results for the plasma calcium, phosphate and alkaline phosphatase measurements, and by the presence of a mild metabolic acidosis.

The diagnosis in this patient was confirmed by measuring serum [PTH]; results for this analysis are most readily interpreted if the blood specimen is collected at a time when the plasma [calcium] is increased, i.e. before any calcium-lowering treatment is instituted. This patient's plasma [calcium] was so high that it warranted urgent attempts to lower it, after performing an intravenous urogram to make sure that the calculus was not causing obstruction. Urgent treatment then consisted of fluids to correct dehydration and a loop diuretic (frusemide).

Comments on Case 13.2 (p. 212)

The plasma [calcium] is low, and lower than can be accounted for in terms of the low plasma [albumin]. The combination of a low plasma [calcium] with a low-normal plasma [phosphate] and elevated alkaline phosphatase activity is consistent with a diagnosis of osteomalacia. The low plasma [total protein] and [albumin] and the low plasma [total CO_2] are indicative of a mild metabolic acidosis, and suggest that chronic diarrhoea with intestinal malabsorption could be the cause of the osteomalacia.

A diagnosis of osteomalacia is best confirmed by bone biopsy. However, this is seldom required if the history is suggestive and the results of chemical investigations and radiological examination (generalized rarefaction of bones, Looser's zones) are characteristic. If available, measurement of vitamin D metabolites in plasma might be considered worthwhile. Responses to a therapeutic trial of vitamin D may be helpful, as a means of making a diagnosis of osteomalacia retrospectively.

Chapter 14
Disorders of Iron and Porphyrin Metabolism

Iron[1] and porphyrins are both important in haem formation, but disorders affecting their metabolism otherwise have little in common with one another. The haemoglobinopathies and the thalassaemias are usually investigated in haematology departments, as also are red cell enzyme abnormalities (e.g. glucose-6-phosphate dehydrogenase deficiency, pyruvate kinase deficiency). However, abnormal derivatives of haemoglobin (e.g. methaemoglobin) will be considered here, as they are usually investigated in clinical biochemistry departments.

Iron metabolism

The body contains about 70 mmol (4 g) of iron of which about 70% is in Hb, up to 25% in iron stores (mainly in liver, spleen, bone marrow) and 5–10% in other haem proteins (e.g. myoglobin, cytochromes). About 0.1% of total body iron is present in plasma. Iron balance is regulated by alterations in intestinal absorption of iron. There is only limited capacity to increase or decrease the body's rate of loss of iron.

Dietary iron and iron absorption

The normal intake of iron is about 0.2–0.4 mmol/day (10–20 mg/day). Normally, about 5–10% of this is absorbed. *The rate of absorption is controlled* by physiological factors:

1 *State of iron stores* in the body. Absorption is increased in iron deficiency, and decreased when there is iron overload.

2 *Rate of erythropoiesis.* When this rate is increased, absorption may be increased even though the iron stores are adequate or overloaded.

The rate of absorption is influenced by the contents of the diet and by the nature of GI secretions, as follows:

1 *Contents of diet.* Substances that form soluble complexes with iron (e.g. ascorbic acid) facilitate absorption. Substances which form insoluble complexes (e.g. phytate) inhibit absorption.

2 *The chemical state of the iron.* Iron in the diet does not usually become available for absorption unless released during digestion. This depends, at least partly, on gastric acid production; Fe^{2+} is more readily absorbed than Fe^{3+}, and the presence of H^+ helps to keep iron in the Fe^{2+} form. Iron in haem (in meat products) can be absorbed while still contained in the haem molecule.

[1]In this book, 'iron' is used to refer collectively to all forms of iron, organic and inorganic. The symbols Fe^{2+} and Fe^{3+} refer specifically to the inorganic ions, ferrous and ferric, respectively.

Iron transport, storage and utilization

After being taken up by the intestinal mucosa, iron may be transported across the mucosal cells directly to the plasma, where it is carried, mainly combined with transferrin, which binds two Fe^{3+} ions reversibly. Binding sites on transferrin are normally about 30–50% saturated; the total iron circulating bound to transferrin is normally about 50–70 µmol (3–4 mg). Exogenous iron is also retained in the mucosal cells, incorporated into ferritin; this iron is later lost when mucosal cells slough into the intestinal lumen.

In bone marrow and other sites (e.g. liver, spleen), iron is chelated with protoporphyrin IXα to form haem and is then incorporated into haem proteins. Excess iron is stored as ferritin or as haemosiderin.

Ferritin is made up from an iron-free protein, apoferritin, that consists of a number of polypeptide subunits encircling a central core in which is contained a variable amount of iron. Haemosiderin is a less well-defined protein, probably formed by condensation of several molecules of ferritin, which are then partly catabolized.

Iron released by the breakdown of Hb, at the end of the erythrocyte's life, is normally efficiently conserved and later reused.

Iron excretion and sources of loss

Iron excreted in the faeces is principally *exogenous*, i.e. dietary iron that has not been absorbed by the mucosal cells and transported into the circulation.

In males there is an average loss of *endogenous* iron of about 20 µmol/day (1 mg/day) in cells desquamated from the skin and the intestinal mucosa. To a small extent, intestinal losses of *endogenous* iron can be varied according to the state of the body's iron stores, being approximately doubled in iron overload and halved in iron depletion. In females there may be additional losses due to menstruation or pregnancy. Urine contains negligible amounts of iron.

Chemical investigation of disorders of iron metabolism

Haematological investigations are of primary importance in many disorders of iron metabolism. However, only chemical tests are considered here.

Plasma iron (reference ranges, see Table 14.1)

The plasma iron pool turns over several times each day. As a result, small changes in the rate of input to or output from the pool cause large fluctuations in plasma [iron]; this may vary from half to double the value first observed over a few days. Much of this variation appears to be random, but some specific causes can be recognized:

1 *Diurnal variation*, with higher values in the morning.

2 *Menstrual cycle*, with low values just before and during the menstrual period.

3 *Oral contraceptives*, which cause increased plasma [iron].

4 *Pregnancy*, which tends to cause increased plasma [iron]. However, it is often accompanied by iron deficiency.

Plasma [iron] is low in iron deficiency and is raised in iron overload; these changes occur relatively late in the progress of the disorders, when iron stores

Table 14.1 Plasma iron, ferritin and total iron-binding capacity

	Iron (μmol/L)	Ferritin (μg/L)	TIBC (μmol/L)	TIBC saturation (%)
Reference ranges				
Males	14–32	15–350*	45–72	30–50
Females	10–28	8–300*	45–72	30–50
Physiological changes				
Pre-menstrual	↓	N	N	↓
Steroid contraceptives	↑	N	↑	N
Pregnancy	N or ↓†	↓	↑	↓
Disease states				
Iron deficiency	↓	↓	↑	< 30
Iron overload	↑	↑	N or ↓	Up to 100
Infections, neoplasms	↓	↑ or N	↓	N
Hypoplastic anaemia	↑	↑ or N	N or ↓	> 40

N, normal; ↑, increased; ↓, decreased.
* A plasma [ferritin] below 20 μg/L suggests that the body's iron stores are depleted.
† Plasma [iron] is often reduced in pregnancy due to the associated iron deficiency.

have already become either completely depleted or seriously overloaded.

Plasma [iron] also alters in conditions not associated with changes in iron stores. Acute infections or trauma precipitate a rapid fall in plasma [iron], and chronic inflammatory disorders (e.g. rheumatoid arthritis) and malignant diseases are also associated with low levels.

Measurements of plasma [iron] do *not* provide an adequate index of iron status. They are nowadays only required, for diagnostic purposes, for a few conditions, e.g. in suspected cases of acute iron poisoning and in the assessment of individuals with an increased risk of haemochromatosis.

Plasma ferritin (reference ranges, see Table 14.1)

Plasma [ferritin] is closely related to body iron stores, whether these be decreased, normal or increased, whereas plasma [iron] only becomes abnormal in the presence of gross abnormalities of iron storage. A low plasma [ferritin], less than 20 μg/L, indicates the presence of depleted iron stores. Values in the lower part of the reference range may also be compatible with depleted iron stores, since ferritin is one of the acute phase reactants (p. 92) and, as such, may increase in infections or other acute disorders; in these patients, ferritin measurements should be repeated after recovery from the acute stress.

Increased plasma [ferritin] is found in iron overload, irrespective of the cause, and in many patients with liver disease or cancer. A normal plasma [ferritin] virtually excludes untreated iron overload.

Determination of plasma [ferritin] currently provides the most useful measure of iron status widely available on a routine basis.

Plasma total iron-binding capacity (TIBC) (reference ranges, see Table 14.1)

This is a measure of the total amount of iron with which plasma can combine. Normally, *nearly all the binding capacity is due to transferrin* and about 40% of its binding sites are occupied by iron. Transferrin has a much longer half-life in plasma than iron, and plasma [transferrin] shows fewer short-term fluctuations.

Plasma TIBC is usually raised in iron deficiency. It is normal or even low in iron overload. In these conditions, it alters in the opposite direction to plasma [iron] (Table 14.1). This effect is particularly marked in haemochromatosis, in which saturation of the iron-binding capacity usually rises above 60% fairly early in the disorder, or equivalent changes are seen in the plasma iron : transferrin ratio. Plasma TIBC falls in protein-losing states, infections and neoplastic disease.

As with plasma [iron], there is little place for determining plasma [transferrin] or TIBC as a routine measure of iron status. However, in the detection of early or latent haemochromatosis, plasma [transferrin] or TIBC should be measured. Also, in patients being treated with erythropoietin for the anaemia of chronic renal failure, the percentage saturation of the plasma TIBC is a better index of available iron than is plasma [ferritin] and a better guide to the need to give iron treatment.

The percentage saturation of plasma TIBC is helpful in determining the significance of very high plasma [ferritin] in patients with disordered liver function of unknown cause, where the differential diagnosis may be between haemochromatosis and malignancy. The finding of a high plasma [ferritin] in the absence of an increased percentage saturation of TIBC indicates that cancer is more likely to be the diagnosis.

Iron deficiency

This common condition is often first suspected on the basis of routine haematological investigations revealing a microcytic, hypochromic anaemia. The main groups of causes are deficient intake, impaired absorption (e.g. intestinal malabsorptive disease, abdominal surgery) and excessive loss (e.g. menstrual loss, GI bleeding). Measurement of plasma [ferritin] may be indicated if other causes of the hypochromic anaemia seem more likely. Tests for the presence of occult blood in faeces (p. 15) should be performed if no source of blood loss is apparent.

In patients who develop iron deficiency, (i) plasma [ferritin] falls, then (ii) plasma [transferrin] or TIBC increases, after which (iii) plasma [iron] falls, and finally (iv) anaemia becomes evident. In general, plasma [ferritin] is the best diagnostic test for iron deficiency (renal failure is one of the few exceptions), but in monitoring iron replacement therapy the percentage saturation of the plasma TIBC is a more sensitive test and can be useful in assessing compliance.

Iron overload

This is much less common than iron deficiency. Diagnosis is not usually difficult, once the possibility has been considered. Increased plasma [iron] and [ferritin], often to more than 1000 µg/L, and TIBC that is up to 100% saturated are characteristic of iron overload, whatever the cause. The following are the causes:

1 Increased intake and absorption, which may be acute or chronic.

2 Parenteral administration of iron, including repeated blood transfusions.

3 Primary (idiopathic) haemochromatosis.

Abnormally large amounts of iron are occasionally ingested and absorbed and can cause severe iron intoxication. This may occur acutely in children who have accidentally ingested iron tablets. A more chronic state of overload can occur when the diet contains excess absorbable iron (e.g. an acid-containing diet and with this food cooked in iron pots). Under these conditions, there is a slow progressive build-up of iron deposits in the body (e.g. in liver, spleen, myocardium) and hepatic fibrosis may develop.

Primary (idiopathic) haemochromatosis

This hereditary disorder is probably due to increased absorption of dietary iron caused by a defect in the mechanism controlling its absorption. Excessive deposits build up as haemosiderin in the liver, causing cirrhosis, and in the pancreas, leading to fibrosis with the development of diabetes mellitus. Myocardial damage may also occur.

Primary haemochromatosis can be detected at the preclinical stage in affected members of a family in which an index case has occurred. The haemochromatosis gene is closely linked with the genes that determine HLA antigens. In families at risk, apparently unaffected members with a susceptible HLA genotype should have regular (e.g. twice-yearly) measurements of plasma [iron], [ferritin] and TIBC. The first abnormalities to appear in plasma are increased [ferritin] and percentage saturation of TIBC; if either of these becomes abnormal, liver biopsy is indicated. Case-finding for affected relatives is important; treatment by phlebotomy can prevent the disease from progressing.

Porphyrin metabolism

Porphyrins are tetrapyrroles, some of which are intermediates in the formation of haem. Most cells can synthesize haem but bone marrow and liver are the most active, and are the sites most often affected by disorders of porphyrin metabolism. To understand the place of chemical tests in investigating porphyrias, stages in the synthesis of haem need to be reviewed (Fig. 14.1).

All the porphyrinogens (uro-, copro- and proto-isomers) are unstable and readily oxidized to their corresponding porphyrins in tissues, in urine and in faeces. In addition, porphobilinogen (PBG) is unstable and forms porphyrins spontaneously.

The porphyrias

The underlying defect in all the porphyrias is a partial deficiency of one or more of the enzymes in the pathway leading to the synthesis of haem (Fig. 14.1, Table 14.2). As one result, due to the removal of product inhibition of the rate-limiting enzyme, 5-aminolaevulinate (ALA) synthase, there is overproduction of porphyrins or their precursors. *The activity of ALA synthase is increased in all the porphyrias.*

Most of the porphyrias are at least partly genetically determined. Different stages in haem synthesis are affected in each disease and many different symptoms

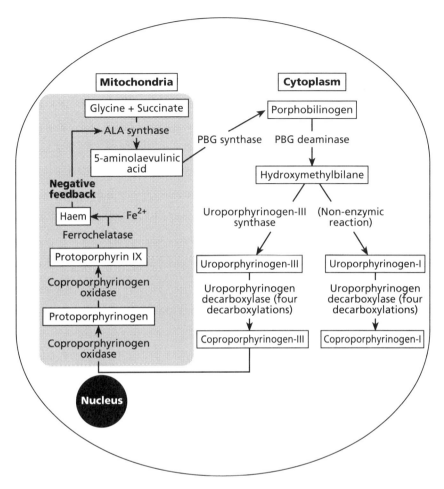

Fig. 14.1 The intracellular distribution of the enzymic steps in the synthesis of haem. In the presence of uroporphyrinogen-III synthase, the formation of porphyrins from PBG (via hydroxymethylbilane, an unstable intermediate) is mainly directed along the series III pathway and thence onwards towards haem.

may be present. However, two main groups of manifestations can be recognized, depending on the nature of the enzyme deficiency:

1 *Photosensitivity* is often a feature of those porphyrias in which there are excessive amounts of uro-, copro- or protoporphyrin in tissues. In practice, photosensitivity may be present in all the porphyrias except the acute intermittent type. The symptom is explicable in terms of the strong absorption of light of 400 nm wavelength by porphyrins present in the upper epidermis. This causes the porphyrin molecule to become activated, and the consequent release of free radicals may cause local lysosomal damage and release of lysosomal enzymes.

2 *Acute abdominal and neurological symptoms* tend to occur in those porphyrias in which there is overproduction of ALA and PBG, both of which probably

Table 14.2 Enzymic defects in the haem-synthetic pathway

Enzymic defect	Porphyria in which activity reduced
Porphobilinogen (PBG) synthase	PBG synthase deficiency (very rare), lead poisoning
PBG deaminase	Acute intermittent porphyria, variegate porphyria (sometimes), Chester porphyria
Uroporphyrinogen-III synthase	Congenital erythropoietic porphyria
Uroporphyrinogen decarboxylase	Porphyria cutanea tarda, toxic porphyria
Coproporphyrinogen oxidase	Hereditary coproporphyria, lead poisoning, harderoporphyria
Protoporphyrinogen oxidase	Variegate porphyria, Chester porphyria
Ferrochelatase	Protoporphyria, lead poisoning

have direct neurotoxic effects. This overproduction can be attributed to the combined effect of *increased ALA synthase activity and decreased PBG deaminase activity*, which only occurs in acute porphyrias. In those porphyrias where acute symptoms do *not* occur, there is usually *increased* PBG deaminase activity.

The porphyrias can be subdivided initially into two groups, depending on whether erythrocyte [porphyrins] are increased or normal. In the latter group, the main site of porphyrin overproduction is the liver, and these diseases are collectively designated as the hepatic porphyrias.

Erythrocyte [porphyrins] increased

As well as the congenital diseases discussed below, there are some acquired disorders in which erythrocyte [porphyrins] are increased, such as lead poisoning (p. 226) and iron deficiency. Over 90% of red cell porphyrins is normally present as zinc-protoporphyrin.

Congenital erythropoietic porphyria is a very rare, recessively-inherited disorder that presents in infancy. Exposed areas of skin (hands, head) are affected by severe blistering due to photosensitivity. Teeth are stained pink and there may be splenomegaly and haemolytic anaemia. It is due to deficiency of uroporphyrinogen-III synthase.

There is overproduction of series I porphyrins, and the erythrocytes and their precursors contain excessive amounts of these. The large amounts of uroporphyrin I (and to a lesser extent coproporphyrin I) excreted in urine cause it to become a pink to red colour. Faecal coproporphyrin I (and uroporphyrin I) excretion is also increased. Congenital erythropoietic porphyria can be treated long-term by repeated blood transfusions, which presumably act by inhibiting porphyrin synthesis.

Protoporphyria is a rare disorder, dominantly inherited. It usually presents with photosensitivity but blistering does not occur. This disease is less severe than congenital erythropoietic porphyria; it is associated with a partial deficiency of ferrochelatase. The diagnosis can be established by measuring red cell [protoporphyrin], which is increased. Urinary porphyrins are normal but faecal protoporphyrin excretion may be increased.

Erythrocyte [porphyrins] normal

The hepatic porphyrias are more common and more important clinically than the two conditions described above. They are largely genetically determined, but environmental factors may precipitate clinical manifestations. The hepatic porphyrias may mimic several other diseases. Four forms are usually distinguished, but others continue to be described:

1 Porphyria cutanea tarda (PCT) or symptomatic cutaneous porphyria.
2 Acute intermittent porphyria (Swedish type).
3 Variegate porphyria (South African type).
4 Hereditary coproporphyria.

Porphyria cutanea tarda (PCT)

This is the commonest type of porphyria. Photosensitivity is the principal symptom. Bullous lesions develop on skin exposed to sunlight. It is usually due to a combination of a genetic deficiency of uroporphyrinogen decarboxylase and acquired hepatic disease; the relative contributions of these vary from patient to patient.

Alcoholic liver disease is present in most patients with PCT in Europe, North America and other 'Western' countries, but occasionally hepatic tumours or other forms of liver disease may cause the symptom complex. Oestrogen therapy, including oral contraceptives, may also cause PCT as may toxic damage to the liver. The best-known example of toxic damage causing PCT occurred in Turkey, in 1957, where a seed wheat had been treated with the fungicide hexachlorobenzene.

The pattern of porphyrin excretion in PCT is complex. There is excessive excretion of a variety of porphyrins in both urine and faeces. Biochemical and clinical remission can usually be achieved by venesection, which probably acts by reducing hepatic iron stores although the precise mechanism is not clear.

Acute intermittent porphyria

This usually takes the form of a series of acute episodes of severe abdominal pain. Intermittent neuromuscular and psychiatric disturbances are frequent, but skin manifestations do not occur. Attacks are commonly precipitated by drugs (e.g. barbiturates, alcohol), changes of hormonal balance (e.g. pregnancy, oral contraceptives, steroid treatment) or by infections.

The basic defect is a deficiency of PBG deaminase. There is also a deficiency of hepatic steroid 5α-reductase; this allows certain steroids, known to be potent inducers of ALA synthase, to accumulate. The steroid 5α-reductase defect could explain the known relationship between acute attacks of porphyria and hormonal imbalance.

During acute attacks, large amounts of ALA and PBG are always present in the urine. Urinary porphyrins are also increased but this may often be due to spontaneous condensation of PBG in the bladder. These abnormalities can usually be detected between attacks, but are then less marked. It is particularly important for the laboratory to be provided with a fresh specimen of urine to test for PBG in patients with symptoms that might be attributable to acute porphyria; 'side-room' tests are not sufficiently reliable. Faecal excretion of porphyrins is usually normal.

Variegate porphyria

This disorder may present acutely, with symptoms similar to those of acute intermittent porphyria. In other patients, photosensitivity is the most marked feature. The two types of symptoms may co-exist.

The basic biochemical defect is deficiency of protoporphyrinogen oxidase. There may, additionally, be impaired activity of steroid 5α-reductase or of PBG deaminase.

Faeces contain excess porphyrins, both during and between attacks, but urinary porphyrin excretion may only be increased during an attack. Urinary ALA and PBG output are often only increased during acute attacks.

Hereditary coproporphyria

This is a rare disease in which the usual features are acute attacks of the type seen in acute intermittent porphyria. It is probably due to a deficiency of coproporphyrinogen oxidase. Excess coproporphyrin III is present in faeces and urine, but urinary porphyrin excretion may be normal between attacks. Excess ALA and PBG are excreted in urine, but only during acute attacks.

Chemical investigation of the porphyrias (Table 14.3)

It is important to recognize that only a proportion, 10–20%, of patients with the enzyme defects of the hereditary porphyrias ever develop symptoms. In the remainder, the disorder remains latent, i.e. the disorder is subclinical. Biochemical manifestations may not be so marked in patients with latent disease, although they are usually present.

Because of the protean manifestations of the porphyrias, the diagnosis is likely to be suspected much more often than it is present. For this reason diagnosis is best considered as a two-stage process. First, the presence or absence of porphyria should be established by relatively simple screening tests which can be done in most laboratories and then, if any of these are positive, complex tests to establish the nature of the defect can be performed in specialist laboratories.

In the following outline we only detail those tests that are likely to be available in non-specialist laboratories. It is important to note that a fresh specimen of urine should be provided for urine tests, rather than a 24-hour specimen, since some of the porphyrins and precursors are unstable.

1   *Urinary porphobilinogen.* A qualitative test with Ehrlich's reagent is carried out first. If positive, quantitative tests for PBG (and possibly ALA) should be performed to exclude false positives (e.g. due to drugs).
2   *Total urinary and faecal porphyrins.* If either of these is increased, the nature of the porphyrins should be determined, by high-performance liquid chromatography or thin layer chromatography, in a specialist laboratory.
3   *Whole blood [total porphyrins].* If these are increased, the proportion of free protoporphyrin should then be measured to enable a diagnosis of protoporphyria to be made.

Clinical indications for performing porphyrin investigations

There are several well-defined clinical circumstances in which the investigation of a patient for porphyria may be indicated:

Table 14.3 Abnormal results of chemical investigations in the porphyrias

Porphyria	ALA Urine	PBG Urine	Increased porphyrins in		
			Urine	Faeces	Red cells
Erythrocyte porphyrins normal					
Porphyria cutanea tarda			Uro I and III, hepta	Isocopro, hepta	
Acute intermittent porphyria	↑ or N	↑↑↑	PBG poly		
Variegate porphyria	↑	↑↑	Copro III, PBG poly	Copro III, Proto IX, X-porphyrin	
Hereditary coproporphyria	↑ or N	↑↑	Copro III, PBG poly	Copro III	
Erythrocyte porphyrins increased					
Lead poisoning	↑↑	↑ or N	Copro III		Zinc proto
PBG synthase deficiency	↑↑	↑ or N	Copro III		Zinc proto
Congenital erythropoietic porphyria			Uro I, Copro I	Copro I	Copro I, Proto IX, Zinc proto
Protoporphyria				Proto IX	Proto IX

N, normal; ↑, ↑↑ and ↑↑↑, increasing degrees of abnormality.
ALA, 5-aminolaevulinic acid; copro, coproporphyrin (of series I and III); hepta, 7-carboxylporphyrins; isocopro, isocoproporphyrin; PBG, porphobilinogen; PBG poly, polymers of porphobilinogen; proto, protoporphyrin; uro, uroporphyrin (of series I or III).

1   In suspected *acute porphyria*, e.g. in a patient with *acute abdominal pain*, a qualitative test for urinary PBG should be performed first. If this is negative, acute intermittent porphyria, variegate porphyria and coproporphyria can *all* be excluded. If positive, results of faecal porphyrin tests (Table 14.3) may indicate the type of acute porphyria.
2   Investigation of *latent porphyria* is more difficult. The patient may be in remission between attacks, or may be a relative of a known sufferer from acute porphyria. In either case, *urinary PBG* may be normal or raised in all forms, and so is not by itself a sufficient test. *Faecal porphyrin* measurements may help make the diagnosis since they are often increased in latent variegate porphyria. However, in many cases it is necessary to perform appropriate tissue enzyme studies (e.g. PBG deaminase in acute intermittent porphyria) or even genetic analysis. These investigations must be performed in a specialist laboratory.
3   If *photosensitivity* is present, e.g. due to *porphyria cutanea tarda* or *protoporphyria*, blood [total porphyrins] should be measured first, to exclude protoporphyria. If these are increased, the ratio of free protoporphyrin to zinc-protoporphyrin should be measured since it is the *free* form that is increased in protoporphyria. The skin lesions of porphyria cutanea tarda can usually be recognized clinically, and the diagnosis can usually be confirmed by measuring

total urinary and faecal porphyrins, but more precise characterization requires measurement of individual porphyrins in urine and faeces.

Lead poisoning

After absorption from the lungs or intestine, lead is carried in the blood mainly on the surface of red cells and is usually stored in bone. Its main toxic effects are peripheral neuropathy, abdominal pain, anaemia and encephalopathy. Three types of diagnostic and public health problems need to be considered:

1 *Patients with symptoms or signs* that may be explained by a diagnosis of lead poisoning. If the diagnosis is correct, biochemical findings are usually grossly abnormal.

2 *Occupational hazard*, where healthy workers may be exposed to increased risk of poisoning. Screening those at risk, by sensitive tests, is required.

3 *Exposure to lead in the general population*, e.g. lead in water, food and petrol.

Lead inhibits many enzyme systems, but most of its effects can be attributed to inhibition of several stages of porphyrin synthesis. Lead poisoning can be regarded as a form of acquired porphyria; it inhibits PBG synthase, ferrochelatase and, to a lesser extent, coproporphyrinogen oxidase (Fig. 14.1). The metabolic consequences include increased erythrocyte [zinc protoporphyrin], increased urinary excretion of ALA and coproporphyrin III, and sometimes a slight increase in urinary PBG.

The following tests may be useful when investigating the possibility of lead poisoning:

1 *Tests demonstrating the presence of excess lead*:
   (a) Blood [lead].
   (b) Chelatable lead excretion in urine after giving EDTA, calcium salt.

2 *Tests demonstrating the toxic effects of lead*:
   (a) PBG synthase activity in erythrocytes.
   (b) Urinary ALA excretion.
   (c) Erythrocyte [zinc protoporphyrin].

Blood [lead] has several drawbacks as the sole measure of either lead poisoning or overexposure. Although it correlates significantly with other biological indices of lead poisoning, there are variations in individual susceptibility to a given blood [lead]. Partly for this reason, it has proved difficult to establish 'acceptable' blood lead levels in a healthy population. Also, the measurement of blood [lead] is technically demanding.

Chelatable lead excretion is a measure of the amount of lead excreted in the 24-hour period after a 60-minute intravenous infusion of 1 g calcium EDTA. The test is an excellent index of lead overexposure but is rather tedious and is unsuitable for screening purposes.

PBG synthase activity, measured in erythrocyte haemolysates, is probably the most sensitive index of exposure to lead. However, this enzyme's activity is subject to genetic variation. In addition, differences in methods between laboratories can render interpretation of results difficult.

Urinary ALA excretion, another sensitive index of lead overexposure, is especially suitable for screening workers exposed to lead. Timed urine collections are required.

Erythrocyte [zinc protoporphyrin] is the most practical routine measure of overexposure to lead. Simple screening methods are available, as well as more complex and specific techniques. This test is to be preferred to urinary ALA excretion when screening children for suspected exposure to lead, since timed urine collections in children are often very unreliable.

Abnormal derivatives of haemoglobin

These all reduce the oxygen-carrying capacity of the blood. The abnormal derivatives of Hb can all be identified by means of their characteristic absorption spectra, and it is possible to measure the various derivatives quantitatively if present in sufficient amount.

Methaemoglobin

This is oxidized haemoglobin (Hb), the Fe^{2+} normally present in haem being replaced by Fe^{3+}; the ability to act as an O_2-carrier is lost. The normal erythrocyte contains small amounts of methaemoglobin, formed by spontaneous oxidation of Hb.

Methaemoglobin is normally reconverted to Hb by reducing systems in the red cells, the most important of which is NADH-methaemoglobin reductase.

Excess methaemoglobin may be present in the blood because of increased production or diminished ability to convert it back to Hb. If there is more than 20 g/L of methaemoglobin, cyanosis develops.

Both genetically determined and acquired conditions can cause methaemoglobinaemia; the acquired group is much the commoner. Haemolysis sometimes occurs in cases of methaemoglobinaemia, and methaemoglobin then appears in the urine, giving it a brownish colour.

Genetic causes of methaemoglobinaemia include the following groups of conditions:

1 A group of haemoglobinopathies, collectively called Hb-M.
2 A group having a deficiency of NADH-methaemoglobin reductase (cytochrome b_5 reductase) or, very rarely, deficiency of cytochrome b_5.

Patients with Hb-M are heterozygous for a gene that codes for a structurally abnormal Hb having an amino acid substitution in the vicinity of the portion of the molecule that stabilizes the haem in the Fe^{3+} form. About 40% of the Hb is present as methaemoglobin. Treatment with reducing agents (e.g. methylene blue, ascorbic acid) is *ineffective* in reducing methaemoglobin to Hb.

Deficiency of NADH-methaemoglobin reductase leads to an accumulation of methaemoglobin that usually amounts to 20–50% of the total Hb. Treatment with reducing agents is *effective* in converting methaemoglobin back to Hb in these patients.

Acquired methaemoglobinaemia usually arises following the ingestion of large amounts of drugs, e.g. phenacetin or the sulphonamides; excess of nitrites or certain oxidizing agents present in the diet may also cause it. Treatment with reducing agents is *effective* in reversing acquired methaemoglobinaemia.

Haematin

This is a protein-free Fe^{3+} complex of protoporphyrin. It may be released from erythrocytes in patients with methaemoglobinaemia, or it may be formed following intravascular haemolysis. In the plasma, it combines with albumin to form *methaemalbumin*, thereby making the plasma brown in colour. Methaemalbumin also sometimes occurs in patients with acute pancreatitis.

Sulphaemoglobin

This is formed when Hb is acted upon by the same substances as cause acquired methaemoglobinaemia, if they act in the presence of sulphur-containing compounds such as hydrogen sulphide which may arise from bacterial action in the intestine. Sulphaemoglobin and methaemoglobin are often present at the same time in these patients.

Sulphaemoglobin cannot act as an O_2-carrier nor can it be converted back to Hb. Because of its spectroscopic characteristics, patients with even a mild degree of sulphaemoglobinaemia are cyanosed.

Carboxyhaemoglobin (COHb)

Carbon monoxide combines at the same position in the Hb molecule as O_2, but with an affinity about 200 times greater than oxygen. As a result, even small quantities of CO in the inspired air cause the formation of relatively large amounts of COHb, with a corresponding reduction in the O_2-carrying capacity of the blood. This is due not only to the blocking effect of CO on O_2-binding sites but also to a shift to the left of the oxygen dissociation curve (Fig. 5.1, p. 67), which occurs even when only one of the four O_2-binding sites on Hb is occupied by CO.

Small amounts of COHb (up to 10%) may be present under 'normal' conditions in city-dwellers. Concentrations above 40% usually result in unconsciousness, and may be fatal. Accurate methods for measuring the amount of COHb in blood are widely available.

Chapter 15
Nutrition

In worldwide terms, nutritional disorders are responsible for much morbidity and mortality. The three main categories of nutritional disorder are *undernutrition*, (which is dominated by insufficient food energy), producing the features of starvation in adults and marasmus in children; *malnutrition*, which is deficiency of one or more of the essential nutrients; and *obesity*, which is excessive positive energy balance.

Principal dietary constituents

The body's requirements for the principal dietary constituents (carbohydrate, fat and protein) will be briefly considered. Its requirements for water and the major inorganic constituents (Na^+, K^+, Ca^{2+}, etc.) are discussed elsewhere. Most of this section is concerned with trace elements and vitamins.

Carbohydrates

The major source of dietary energy is normally provided by carbohydrate. In developed countries, this is in the form of sugars (e.g. sucrose) or digestible polysaccharides; the major food polysaccharide is starch, found in cereals, root vegetables and legumes. Non-digestible polysaccharides do not affect nutritional status but contribute to dietary fibre. Carbohydrates are not essential nutrients, but insufficient carbohydrate intake leads to ketosis.

Fats

Dietary fat consists largely of triglycerides, with small amounts of other constituents (e.g. cholesterol). In Britain it has been reported that, on average, 42% of total energy is taken in as fat, 46% as carbohydrate and 12% as protein. Since the energy content of fat is much greater than that of carbohydrate (about 9 kcal/g, compared with 4 kcal/g for protein and for carbohydrate), the *weight* of dietary fat is substantially less than for carbohydrate on this diet.

Triglycerides contain saturated or unsaturated fatty acids, or both. Saturated fats, especially those containing palmitic and myristic acids, elevate plasma [total cholesterol] and [LDL-cholesterol] whereas unsaturated fats tend to reduce both these concentrations. Monounsaturated fatty acids (e.g. oleic acid) may exert favourable effects on lipoprotein metabolism, and may have the added beneficial effect of increasing plasma [HDL-cholesterol]. Some long-chain, highly unsaturated fatty acids, (e.g. eicosapentaenoic acid, present in fatty fish) may also be cardioprotective, reducing plasma [VLDL] and inhibiting thrombosis.

Linoleic, linolenic and arachidonic acids comprise the 'essential' free fatty acids. They cannot be synthesized by man and are required for membrane synthesis and as precursors of the prostaglandins.

Proteins

Dietary protein from both animal and plant sources normally provides about 11–14% of total calories (70–100 g protein) on a 'Western' diet; the minimum requirement is 40 g of protein of good biological value (i.e. containing all the essential amino acids). Vegetable protein may be deficient in one or more of the essential amino acids, but this deficiency can be overcome by complementation whereby a combination of cereals and legumes together provides protein of good biological value.

Trace elements

Twenty-two elements are known to be essential in animal nutrition. Of these, seven are 'bulk' elements (Na, K, Ca, Mg, Cl, S and P), and 15 are trace elements, present in tissues at less than 50 mg/kg. Six of these (nickel, arsenic, vanadium, tin, silicon and fluorine) have not been shown to be associated with specific deficiency states in man, and will not be further considered. Table 15.1 lists some data about the nine that are known to be *essential* trace elements.

The clinical importance of iron, iodine and cobalt (in cobalamin) is well established. Clinical syndromes associated with deficiency of copper, selenium, zinc, chromium, manganese and molybdenum have all been described and these six elements will be considered here. The effects of iron deficiency are described elsewhere (p. 219). Deficiency of *inorganic* cobalt has not been reported in man.

Table 15.1 Trace elements essential to man

Essential trace element	Approximate total adult body content	Daily oral intake (recommended for adults)*	Plasma concentration
Chromium	< 6 mg	0.1 mg	< 20 nmol/L
Cobalt	1 mg	As vitamin B_{12}	< 10 nmol/L
Copper	100 mg	3 mg	12–26 µmol/L
Iodine	10–20 mg	0.15 mg	< 5 nmol/L†
Iron	4–5 g	Males: 10 mg	14–32 µmol/L
		Females: 10–50 mg‡	10–28 µmol/L
Manganese	10–20 mg	3 mg	<20 nmol/L
Molybdenum	10 mg	0.2 mg	< 15 nmol/L
Selenium	15 mg	0.1 mg	< 4 nmol/L
Zinc	1–2 g	15 mg	10–20 µmol/L

* Much smaller amounts of inorganic trace elements are required if these are being provided as part of TPN.
† The total concentration in iodine-containing compounds in plasma, mainly contained in the thyroid hormones, is 250–600 nmol/L; only 5 nmol/L is present as inorganic iodide.
‡ 10–20 mg/day in the reproductive period; 20–50 mg/day during pregnancy.

Deficiencies of essential trace elements usually arise in association with protein-energy malnutrition or with other abnormal nutritional states (e.g. total parenteral nutrition, neonatal feeds, synthetic diets). Specific inherited disorders in trace element handling are rare. Excessive losses, especially in association with severe and chronic GI diseases, may also cause deficiency.

Methods of assessing essential trace element deficiency are mostly inadequate at present; they mainly depend on blood measurements (e.g. atomic absorption spectroscopy). Plasma levels, if very low, may be useful in diagnosis and management, but smaller changes are of less significance as they may be due to changes in concentration of the plasma proteins which bind the metals. Diagnosis is often only made retrospectively on the basis of there being a clinical condition likely to have given rise to deficiency, occurring in association with clinical symptoms that can be attributed to trace element lack, and which respond to treatment with the appropriate supplementation.

Copper

Copper-containing metalloproteins include ceruloplasmin, dopamine hydroxylase, tyrosinase, cytochrome C oxidase, and superoxide dismutase. Human deficiency has been reported in infants fed exclusively on cow's milk; it is characterized by an iron-resistant anaemia, neutropenia and evidence of intestinal malabsorption with diarrhoea. Copper circulates in plasma over 90% bound to ceruloplasmin (p. 92); the rest is mainly bound to albumin. Wilson's disease (p. 120) and Menkes' disease are inherited metabolic disorders of copper transport.

Menkes' disease is a fatal, sex-linked recessive disorder in which there are cerebral and cerebellar degeneration, connective tissue abnormalities and 'kinky hair'. Both serum [copper] and [ceruloplasmin] are low, and the copper content of the liver is very low. Absorption of copper from the intestine is grossly impaired, but treatment with parenteral copper has not proved successful.

Selenium

Selenium is a component of glutathione peroxidase, which has a cellular antioxidant function. It is also an essential part of iodothyronine deiodinase (type I), the enzyme which converts thyroxine to tri-iodothyronine. For both enzymes, the coding regions of the genomic DNA contain a unique triplet which specifically codes for the insertion of selenocysteine into the primary amino acid sequence of the newly synthesized enzyme.

Selenium deficiency can be investigated by measuring plasma [selenium] or erythrocyte glutathione peroxidase activity. Difficulties in interpretation may occur because reference ranges for plasma [selenium] vary both with age and with geographical location; there is also a marked reduction (about 30%) in pregnancy. Glutathione peroxidase activity in leucocytes, measured before and after selenium supplementation, provides an alternative diagnostic test, but measurement of urinary selenium excretion has not proved helpful. The content of selenium in hair has been shown to be very low in selenium deficiency in children.

Selenium deficiency is the cause of *Keshan disease*, a cardiomyopathy affecting children and young women in parts of China. This hitherto fatal condition has been almost eliminated by prophylactic dietary supplements of selenium. A similar cardiomyopathy has been reported in a few patients on long-term total parenteral nutrition, and in other patients a skeletal muscle myopathy developed; both types of myopathy respond to treatment with selenium supplements.

Zinc

Absorption of zinc from the intestine appears to be controlled in a manner similar to iron (p. 216), with sequestration of zinc in enterocytes and transfer of some of this to the plasma; the rest is lost when the enterocytes are sloughed. Zinc is mostly transported bound to albumin, α_2-macroglobulin and transferrin. Specimens of blood for zinc measurement need to be collected *before* a meal and without venous stasis; plasma [zinc] may fall by as much as 20% after meals. The body does not store zinc to any appreciable extent in any organ; urinary excretion is fairly constant at 10 μmol/24 h, with re-excretion into the gut being the main route for adjusting the amount excreted.

Over 70 enzymes have been shown to contain zinc, including carbonic anhydrase and PBG synthase. It is difficult, therefore, to relate reduction in an individual enzyme's activity to particular effects of zinc deficiency.

Nutritional deficiency has been described in infants, especially in the absence of zinc supplementation, and in patients receiving total parenteral nutrition. Pregnancy, lactation, old age and alcoholism have all been reported as being associated with an increased incidence of zinc deficiency. Alcohol causes an increased loss of zinc in urine, and plasma [zinc] is lower in chronic alcoholics than in normal individuals. Zinc deficiency may also be caused by diuretics, chelating agents and anti-cancer drug treatment. Severe zinc deficiency can lead to a pustular skin rash, loss of body hair, diarrhoea and mood changes.

Marked deficiency of zinc occurs in *acrodermatitis enteropathica*, in which there is an inherited defect of zinc absorption that causes low plasma [zinc] and reduced total body content of zinc. Infants develop skin rashes and chronic diarrhoea and intestinal malabsorption. Several secondary deficiencies occur. The condition responds rapidly to oral zinc supplements, which must be continued for life.

Injury, surgery, infection and a variety of acute illnesses are often accompanied by a fall in plasma [zinc] due to the stimulation of hepatic metallothionein synthesis; this is one of the many components of the acute phase response (p. 92). The catabolism of skeletal muscle protein after injury can also lead to increased urinary loss of zinc.

Chromium

The biologically active form of chromium, Cr^{3+}, is absorbed with low efficiency from the diet. Although its significance in metabolism is not known, chromium is involved in glucose homeostasis; a chromium complex present in brewer's yeast ('glucose tolerance factor') is able to improve glucose tolerance in some diabetics.

Malnourished infants may develop severe glucose intolerance that improves with chromium supplementation. In adults, a syndrome comprising weight loss, peripheral neuropathy, and marked insulin-insensitive glucose intolerance has been described that improves with chromium supplementation. Chromium supplements may also be needed in patients on prolonged parenteral nutrition.

Manganese

Manganese is a component of certain metallo-enzymes and manganese ions activate a large number of other enzymes, e.g. those involved in the synthesis of glycosaminoglycans, cholesterol and prothrombin. Despite this extensive range of enzyme requirements for manganese, true deficiency in man appears to be very rare.

Molybdenum

This is a component of xanthine oxidase and some other metallo-enzymes. Deficiency has been reported to cause xanthinuria, with low plasma [urate] and low urinary uric acid output.

Vitamins

Vitamins are all organic compounds which, as originally defined, cannot be synthesized by man and must be provided in the diet. They are essential for the normal processes of metabolism, including growth and maintenance of health. It is now known that man is able to produce part or even all of his requirements for some of the vitamins, e.g. vitamin D from cholesterol and niacin from tryptophan. Table 15.2 summarizes some data concerning both water-soluble and fat-soluble vitamins.

There are five main groups of causes of a vitamin-deficiency state. These are inadequate diet, impaired absorption, insufficient utilization, increased requirement, and increased rate of excretion. Vitamin deficiency develops in stages:

1 *Subclinical deficiency,* in which there is depletion of body stores. These are normally relatively large in the case of fat-soluble vitamins (e.g. A and D), but small in the case of the water-soluble vitamins except for vitamin B_{12}.

2 *Overt deficiency,* which is usually accompanied by other evidence of malnutrition (e.g. protein-energy malnutrition).

Chemical investigations help to confirm the diagnosis of some overt vitamin-deficiency diseases and may enable the diagnosis to be made at an earlier stage. Several types of chemical tests can be listed, only some of which will be applicable for the investigation of suspected deficiency of a particular vitamin:

1 Direct measurement of [vitamin] in whole blood, plasma, erythrocytes, leucocytes or tissue biopsy specimens.

2 Direct measurement of the vitamin or one of its major metabolites in urine.

3 Measurement in blood or urine of a metabolite that accumulates as a result of a partial or complete blockage of a metabolic pathway involving an enzyme which requires the vitamin (or derivative) as a co-factor or prosthetic group.

4 Measurements as in (3), after the pathway has been stressed by means of a loading test.

5 Enzyme co-factor saturation tests, in which the activity of the enzyme is measured *in vitro* before and after the addition of the enzyme's cofactor or prosthetic group.

Table 15.2 The vitamins

Vitamin	Outline of the principal functions	Recommended daily amounts	Some effects of deficiency
Fat-soluble vitamins			
Vitamin A (retinol)	Vision, epithelial cell function	1.0 mg (males) 0.8 mg (females)	Night blindness, keratomalacia
Vitamin D (cholecalciferol)	Intestinal absorption of calcium, bone formation	10 μg for children 5 μg for adults	Rickets and osteomalacia
Vitamin E (tocopherols)	Antioxidant, membrane stability	4–8 mg, as α-tocopherol	Haemolytic anaemia
Vitamin K (phytomenadione)	Hepatic synthesis of prothrombin	150 μg	Coagulation defects
Water-soluble vitamins			
Thiamin (vitamin B_1)	All the vitamins that comprise the group of B vitamins act as coenzymes or prosthetic groups for various enzymes that are important in intermediary metabolism	0.5 mg/1000 kcal or 1 mg (whichever is the greater)	Beri-beri, cardiac myopathy
Riboflavin (vitamin B_2)		0.6 mg/1000 kcal or 1.2 mg (as for vitamin B_1)	Cheilosis, stomatitis
Niacin		6.6 mg/1000 kcal or 13 mg (as for vitamin B_1)	Pellagra
Pyridoxine (vitamin B_6)	See above	2.2 mg (males) 2.0 mg (females)	Dermatitis, stomatitis, CNS symptoms
Biotin	See above	15 μg/1000 kcal (50 μg/1000 kcal in children)	Anorexia, dermatitis
Folic acid	See above	400 μg	Megaloblastic anaemia
Cyanocobalamin (vitamin B_{12})	See above	3 μg	Megaloblastic anaemia
Vitamin C (ascorbic acid)	Collagen formation	30–60 mg	Scurvy, anaemia

6   Saturation tests, in which the patient's intake of the vitamin that is thought to be deficient is increased; the effects of the increased intake are then monitored.

It is important to note that plasma concentrations of vitamins do not necessarily reflect the vitamin status of the body. Measurements of vitamins in cells (e.g. erythrocytes, leucocytes or tissue biopsy specimens) generally give a much better indication of the body's vitamin status. Plasma levels usually fall before cellular and tissue levels fall, but low or undetectable plasma levels can occur in the absence of deficiency. Conversely, recent dietary intake can cause the plasma concentrations of vitamins to fluctuate markedly, even in severe deficiency. However, a sustained high plasma [vitamin] usually excludes a deficiency state.

For those vitamins or their metabolites that can be measured in urine, there may be low output despite the presence of adequate tissue reserves. However, a high level of urinary excretion means that deficiency is improbable.

Deficiency of fat-soiuble vitamins

Vitamin A

This vitamin is present in the diet as retinol or as β-carotene, which is hydrolysed in the intestine to form retinol. After absorption, followed by esterification in the mucosal cells, the ester is transported in the blood by retinol-binding protein (pre-albumin, p. 91). Specific binding proteins on cell membranes are involved in the uptake of vitamin A ester from plasma into the tissues. The vitamin is stored in the liver, mainly as its ester.

The active form of vitamin A, 11-cis-retinal, is necessary for rod vision and deficiency can cause night blindness. It is also involved in mucopolysaccharide synthesis; xeroderma and xerophthalmia are related to defects in mucopolysaccharide formation. Low plasma [vitamin A] has been shown to be associated with an increased risk of developing cancer.

Plasma [vitamin A] may be decreased in states of severe protein deficiency, due to lack of its carrier protein, and may then increase if the protein deficiency is corrected. Reduced urinary excretion of sulphated mucopolysaccharides has been reported in children with signs of vitamin A deficiency.

The laboratory measurement most frequently carried out is determination of plasma [vitamin A]. If the concentration is less than 0.5 μmol/L (approximately 0.5 IU/L), this supports a diagnosis of vitamin A deficiency, but provides only limited information about the state of the tissue stores.

Vitamin A absorption tests, based on measurements of plasma [vitamin A] before and 5 hours after a large oral dose of vitamin A (50 μmol/kg), have found limited use as a test of intestinal absorptive function.

Vitamin D

The formation and metabolism of vitamin D are considered on p. 198. Rickets in infancy and childhood and osteomalacia in adults are the main forms in which deficiency of vitamin D presents (p. 208).

Vitamin E

Several tocopherols possess vitamin E activity; they have anti-oxidant properties and may protect hepatic stores of vitamin A and vitamin D. They also act like selenium in helping to remove free radicals, superoxides, etc.

Vitamin E deficiency is a rare complication of prolonged and severe steatorrhoea, and of prolonged parenteral nutrition. Altered red cell membrane stability can lead to haemolytic anaemia in children, whilst skeletal muscle breakdown may be responsible for the creatinuria observed in both adults and children. Neurological consequences have also been described. Deficiency is investigated by measuring plasma [vitamin E].

Vitamin K

This vitamin is necessary for the post-translational modification in proteins of side-chains of glutamate by gamma-carboxylation. The presence of a second carboxyl group on the glutamate side-chain confers Ca^{2+}-binding properties on the modified protein. The bone matrix protein, osteocalcin, requires vitamin K for post-translational gamma-carboxylation.

Vitamin K is needed for hepatic synthesis of prothrombin and factors VII, IX and X, all of which require Ca^{2+} for activation. Vitamin K deficiency is most often due to treatment with anticoagulants (e.g. phenindione); it leads to reduced levels of the vitamin K-dependent coagulation factors and, hence, to haemorrhage. Tests to assess vitamin K status include the prothrombin time, an important test in the investigation and management of jaundiced patients (p. 113).

Deficiency of water-soluble vitamins

Thiamin (vitamin B_1)

Dietary thiamin is readily absorbed and phosphorylated to its active form in the liver. As its derivative, thiamin pyrophosphate (TPP), thiamin is important as a coenzyme in carbohydrate metabolism, being necessary for oxidative decarboxylation reactions (e.g. conversion of pyruvate to acetyl CoA) and transketolation reactions. Deficiency can lead to mood changes (depression, irritability), defective memory, peripheral neuropathy and, in more extreme cases, to beri-beri with cardiac failure. A clinical diagnosis of thiamin deficiency can be investigated by measuring erythrocyte transketolase activity or urinary thiamin excretion.

Erythrocyte transketolase provides a specific and sensitive index of tissue [thiamin] and is the chemical measurement of choice for investigating possible thiamin deficiency. Enzyme activity is measured in red cell haemolysates before and after addition of TPP. The increase in enzymic activity produced by adding TPP (the TPP effect) gives a direct indication of the degree of thiamin deficiency.

Urinary thiamin measurements have been extensively used in nutritional surveys; they provide a useful index of deficiency. However, thiamin excretion is considerably influenced by recent dietary intake and by the adequacy of renal function.

Riboflavin (vitamin B_2)

The nucleotides of riboflavin are the prosthetic groups of many enzymes involved in electron transport and riboflavin is essential for normal oxidative metabolism. Specific deficiency of riboflavin is characterized by angular stomatitis, cheilosis and skin and eye lesions. Deficiency usually occurs as part of a mixed state involving several vitamins of the B complex, often including thiamin as well.

The activity of glutathione reductase in haemolysed erythrocytes, measured before and after the addition of flavin-adenine dinucleotide (the FAD effect), is a test for riboflavin deficiency.

Niacin

This term includes nicotinic acid and its amide. Nicotinamide is a component of nicotinamide adenine dinucleotide (NAD) and its phosphate (NADP); these are coenzymes of many dehydrogenases. The body's requirements for nicotinamide are met partly from dietary niacin, but a substantial part normally comes from metabolism of tryptophan via 3-hydroxykynurenine.

Deficiency can be caused by an inadequate dietary intake, especially a diet where maize is the staple food. It may also be caused by conditions in which large amounts of tryptophan are metabolized along abnormal pathways (e.g. carcinoid syndrome, p. 160) and an acute deficiency can be precipitated by isoniazid treatment. Chemical methods for detecting niacin deficiency measure its excretion in urine or the excretion of its metabolites (N'-methylnicotinamide or 2-pyridone).

Pyridoxine (vitamin B₆)

The term vitamin B_6 includes pyridoxine, pyridoxal, pyridoxamine and their 5-phosphate derivatives; the active form of the vitamin, pyridoxal phosphate (PP), is the prosthetic group of many enzymes including the aminotransferases (ALT and AST) and amino acid decarboxylases. Deficiency of vitamin B_6 nearly always occurs as part of a mixed deficiency of the B vitamins.

As a test for suspected pyridoxine deficiency, the activity of ALT or AST in haemolysed erythrocytes can be determined before and after the addition of pyridoxal phosphate (the PP effect). Vitamin B_6 levels can also be measured in plasma, or its main inactive metabolite (4-pyridoxic acid) measured in urine.

Tryptophan load tests provide an alternative way of investigating suspected pyridoxine deficiency. In this test, the 24-hour urinary excretion of xanthurenate or 3-hydroxykynurenine is measured before and after a loading dose of 2 g L-tryptophan. The test stresses pyridoxine-dependent enzymes involved in the further metabolism of kynurenine, normally the main metabolite of tryptophan.

Biotin

This vitamin serves as a coenzyme for carboxylase reactions, including those catalysed by pyruvate carboxylase and acetyl CoA carboxylase.

Deficiency in man has been reported during total parenteral nutrition and very rarely in association with excessive consumption of raw egg whites, which contain the biotin-binding protein avidin. Deficiency symptoms include dermatitis, alopecia, mental depression, nausea and vomiting.

Folic acid

Folic acid functions as a coenzyme in the transport of one-carbon units from one compound to another and is essential for nucleic acid synthesis. Deficiency leads to impaired cell division, especially manifest as a pancytopenia, with defective red cell maturation (megaloblastic anaemia); folate deficiency is one of the commonest vitamin deficiency states in man. Methods of investigation include serum [folate] and erythrocyte [folate]; these tests are usually carried out in haematology departments.

Measurement of formiminoglutamate (FIGLU) in urine, at most a subsidiary investigation in patients with suspected folate deficiency, has sometimes been used in screening patients for suspected intestinal malabsorption. FIGLU is an intermediate in the metabolism of histidine to glutamate; further metabolism of FIGLU requires the presence of tetrahydrofolate. If there is folate deficiency, urinary FIGLU may be increased. However, if a patient with folate deficiency is given 15 g L-histidine by mouth, in a *histidine load test*, this stresses the pathway for conversion of histidine to glutamate and FIGLU excretion may then be greatly increased.

Cyanocobalamin (vitamin B_{12})

Deficiency of vitamin B_{12} is usually diagnosed by haematological examination of blood and bone marrow specimens, and confirmed by measuring serum [vitamin B_{12}] and by investigating vitamin B_{12} absorption from the intestine before and after the administration of intrinsic factor (the Schilling test). These tests are normally all performed by haematology departments.

Examination of gastric secretion for pentagastrin-fast achlorhydria (p. 145), a feature of Addisonian pernicious anaemia, is rarely performed nowadays. Another chemical test of vitamin B_{12} deficiency is measurement of methylmalonic acid (MMA) excretion in urine. Conversion of methylmalonyl-CoA to succinyl-CoA is catalysed by an enzyme that requires vitamin B_{12} as cofactor; urinary excretion of MMA is increased in vitamin B_{12} deficiency.

Ascorbic acid (vitamin C)

Frank scurvy rarely occurs nowadays but its subclinical form is by no means uncommon, especially among elderly people living alone. Ascorbic acid is involved in the hydroxylation of proline and lysine, during the synthesis of collagen.

Plasma [ascorbate] measurements provide a poor index of tissue stores as the concentration falls rapidly when the diet is very deficient in vitamin C. All patients with scurvy have undetectable plasma ascorbate, but not all people with undetectable plasma ascorbate have scurvy. Urinary ascorbate likewise is of no diagnostic value, unless measured as part of a therapeutic trial in an ascorbic acid saturation test.

Buffy layer [ascorbate]. Leucocyte ascorbate measurements provide a reasonable assessment of tissue stores of ascorbate, but difficulties in obtaining leucocytes uncontaminated by other cellular elements mean that the buffy layer, consisting of leucocytes and platelets (and a few erythrocytes), is normally examined instead. Leucocytes and platelets take up ascorbate against a concentration gradient, and may retain most of their ascorbate even when plasma [ascorbate] has fallen to undetectable levels. Buffy layer [ascorbate] falls at about the same time as clinical evidence of scurvy appears, and seems to give a good indication of the body's stores of the vitamin.

Ascorbic acid saturation test. When regular daily loading doses of ascorbic acid (10 mg/kg body weight) are given to patients deficient in vitamin C, the tissues preferentially take up large amounts of the vitamin to replenish their stores and little or none is excreted in the urine for several days or even weeks. In this test, complete collections of urine are made each day until ascorbic acid is detected in the urine. Care must be taken over the preservation of urine specimens as ascorbic acid is unstable. Patients whose vitamin C intake has been adequate begin to excrete large amounts within 1–2 days of starting the test.

Biochemical assessment of nutritional status

Most types of nutritional assessment determine an individual's fat and protein content and depend on comparison with reference ranges derived from extensive population studies. As well as determining the degree of malnutrition or obesity, this type of assessment enables the response to appropriate treatment (e.g. gain in protein and fat content, loss of fat) to be measured. It may also help to define the potential risk of complications of obesity or undernutrition. Nutritional measures include body weight and height, skin-fold thickness as a measure of subcutaneous fat, and mid-arm muscle area (derived from mid-arm muscle circumference and triceps skin-fold thickness). Bioelectrical impedance can be measured to determine total body water content, fat and fat-free mass. Estimates of muscle mass can be based on 24-hour urinary creatinine or 3-methylhistidine excretion; both methods depend on the accuracy of urine collections.

Measurements of serum protein concentrations (particularly albumin, transferrin and pre-albumin) are used to determine nutritional status. However, changes in levels of all these proteins are influenced by factors other than nutritional status such as intercurrent illness, or stress, or changes in fluid volume or distribution.

Nutritional support

Nutritional support is required in the presence of severe undernutrition and malnutrition. In addition, patients who are severely ill with sepsis, multiple trauma or extensive burns may develop marked negative nitrogen balance, demanding nutritional support. Other indications include unconsciousness, clinical cachexia, radiotherapy or chemotherapy, major resection for malignancy, renal failure, the post-operative management of major surgery and complications of surgery, or any circumstances where the GI tract is not available or is unable to support nutrition (e.g. severe inflammatory bowel disease, gut resection, fistula). Nutritional support may range from the presentation of palatable food, through sip or tube feeding, to intravenous feeding.

Intravenous feeding

This is particularly indicated in the short bowel syndrome or in the presence of fistula formation involving the GI tract; it may also be indicated under other circumstances (Table 15.3). Most intravenous feeding is complete, providing all essential nutrients exogenously, and is then known as *total parenteral nutrition* (TPN). Because of the irritant effect on the vascular endothelium of the hypertonic solutions that have to be used , potentially leading to thrombosis, delivery is made into a large central vein to allow rapid dilution of the administered solution. Nutrients can then be given at a pre-defined rate using an appropriate pump and delivery set, usually from a 3 L bag containing all the prescribed ingredients (the '*big bag*') for a 24-hour period.

Table 15.3 Indications for total parenteral nutrition

Category of value	Principal examples
Proven value	Short bowel syndrome, gut atresia, GI tract fistula
Probable value	Pre-operative preparation of malnourished patients After major surgery, especially if complications arise Severe inflammatory bowel disease, severe pancreatitis Severe sepsis Acute renal failure and severe chronic renal failure
Possible value	Malignant disease, as adjunct to radio- or chemotherapy

Composition of the feed

Table 15.4 lists the typical composition of the 'big bag' for a 24-hour period. Such a standard regime would suit the majority of patients on first establishing TPN, though the formulation would be unsuitable for some patients (e.g. in the presence of renal disease). Several principles are important:

1 *Energy content.* The complete intravenous feed must provide adequate calories, typically 2000 kcal/24 h; more may be required in some circumstances (e.g. after severe burns). Calories are normally provided as a mixture of carbohydrate (glucose) and fat. In order to provide 1000 kcal as glucose, it is necessary to use *hypertonic* solutions since about 5 L of 5% dextrose would be needed in order to provide 1000 kcal, whereas the same amount of energy could be provided with 1.25 L of 20% dextrose. Fat, administered as an emulsion, has a higher energy content than glucose, such that 500 mL of a 20% fat emulsion provides about 1000 kcal. The fat emulsion should also provide essential fatty acids.

2 *Nitrogen content.* This is provided in the form of amino acids. The commercially available solutions contain all the essential amino acids. The prescription is

Table 15.4 Total parenteral nutrition: composition of a typical standard 'big bag'*

Organic constituents	Daily amount	Inorganic constituents	Daily amount
Nitrogen, as amino acids	12–14 g	Sodium	70–100 mmol
Fat, 900 kcal	500 mL of 20% emulsion	Potassium	60–100 mmol
Glucose, 1000 kcal	1.25 L of 20% dextrose	Calcium	5–10 mmol
Vitamins, water- and fat-soluble	Each in the amount recommended	Magnesium	5 mmol
		Phosphate	30 mmol
		Trace elements	As for vitamins

The total volume for a 70 kg adult should be 2000–2500 mL.
* *It must be stressed* that the data in this table do no more than provide an example of a suitable *standard regimen*, and that individual patients may have requirements that differ considerably from those listed above.

normally in the range 12–14 g nitrogen/24 h. Some patients require less nitrogen (e.g. renal failure patients or those with severe liver disease), while others require more (e.g. hypercatabolic patients with severe burns, multiple trauma).

3 *Electrolyte content.* The requirements for Na^+ and K^+ over the 24-hour period must be stated on each day's 'big bag' prescription. Typically, the Na^+ requirement will be 70–100 mmol/24 h but more will be needed in the presence of excessive losses of Na^+ (e.g. severe diarrhoea, fistula) and less where there is Na^+ retention (e.g. renal disease, congestive cardiac failure).

Potassium requirements are more variable. Intracellular repletion, or the administration of glucose and insulin, may increase demands for K^+, whereas requirements will be very small in renal failure or where there is extensive tissue breakdown. A stable patient probably requires 60–100 mmol K^+/24 h.

4 *Vitamins and minerals.* The requirements for calcium and phosphate depend on individual patients' needs, but average requirements are about 5–10 mmol/24 h for calcium and 30 mmol/24 h for phosphate. The magnesium requirement is normally about 5 mmol/24 h. Trace metals and both water-soluble and fat-soluble vitamins are also added to the 'big bag'.

5 *Fluid volume.* This is dictated by clinical circumstances, but 2–2.5 L/24 h meets the requirements for most patients. Depending upon the particular energy prescription, a certain minimum volume will be required to deliver the prescribed number of calories.

Chemical monitoring of patients on total parenteral nutrition

The proper monitoring of patients on TPN requires biochemical, haematological and immunological measurements, together with routine anthropometric tests. An important and potentially serious complication of TPN is sepsis introduced via the catheter, and blood and other cultures may be required. Catheter care and the stipulation that, except in extreme emergencies, the catheter must be used *exclusively* for the administration of the feed, are important concepts in feeding patients by the parenteral route. This section considers the biochemical measurements that should be made.

Until the patient is stable, it is advisable to measure the plasma urea, creatinine, Na^+, K^+, total CO_2 and glucose concentrations daily, and to keep accurate records of fluid balance. Where there are potentially large electrolyte losses (e.g. via a fistula after surgery on the GI tract, the diuretic phase of acute renal failure), knowledge of (i) the fluid $[K^+]$ and $[Na^+]$ and (ii) the volume of the fluid lost assists in the interpretation of abnormal plasma electrolyte values and is essential in deciding the amount of K^+ and Na^+ to be added to the 'big bag'.

Plasma calcium, phosphate and magnesium should be measured twice-weekly, in the absence of severe derangements of these analytes. Mild derangements in 'liver function tests' are sometimes observed during TPN, and these tests (p. 107) should also be carried out twice-weekly. Regular measurement of other proteins (i.e. in addition to albumin), used to assay nutritional status, may also be helpful. Measurements of trace metals and vitamins are not often required unless there are specific clinical indications of deficiency.

Twice-weekly 24-hour urine collections should be made so that nitrogen losses can be estimated from the urea excretion; these figures are inevitably underestimates, due to incomplete urine collections and the failure to take account of other routes of nitrogen loss. If proteinuria is significant, these losses must also be determined and taken into account. Despite these drawbacks, the estimated nitrogen losses help to decide if the nitrogen content of the feed is sufficient to maintain positive nitrogen balance.

The nutrition team

It cannot be emphasized too strongly that nutritional support is a multi-disciplinary affair. The clinical biochemist has an important part to play in advising on the selection of tests, recording the results and advising on the metabolic complications which might arise. Ideally, a nutrition team includes representatives from clinical biochemistry, microbiology, pharmacy, dietetics and nursing, in addition to one or more clinicians (often surgeons), all of whom should have special interests in intravenous feeding. Such a team, as well as advising on policy in this costly area, should be able to offer expert advice about the nutritional care of individual patients and be competent to audit nutritional care.

Chapter 16
Disorders of Purine Metabolism

The purine bases, adenine and guanine, and corresponding nucleosides (purine base-ribose, e.g. adenosine) and nucleotides (nucleoside-phosphate, e.g. adenosine 5′-monophosphate, AMP) are present in nucleic acids and in a large number of metabolically important lower mol mass compounds (e.g. ATP). They are obtained partly from the diet and partly from *in vivo* synthesis of adenine or guanine nucleotides. Regulation of *de novo* nucleotide synthesis (Fig. 16.1) probably occurs through the reaction catalysed by 5-phosphoribosyl-1-pyrophosphate amidotransferase (PRPP-amidotransferase); this enzyme is inhibited by 5′-nucleotides, and purine synthesis may thus be controlled by the concentration of AMP and guanosine 5′-phosphate (GMP) within the cell. The nucleotides are incorporated into nucleic acids.

Nucleic acids are broken down by a variety of enzymes, initially to nucleotides; these mix with the intracellular nucleotide pool or are further degraded to nucleosides and then the free bases. Some of the bases so formed (mainly hypoxanthine and guanine) are partly converted to uric acid and excreted as urate. However, a 'salvage pathway' whereby purine bases are partly reused for nucleotide synthesis, by reactions catalysed by hypoxanthine-guanine and adenine phosphoribosyltransferases (HGPRT and APRT, respectively), is also important (Fig. 16.1). These 'salvaged' nucleotides can be used for nucleic acid synthesis.

The body pool of urate, formed by catabolism of dietary and tissue nucleic acids, nucleotides and purines, amounts to about 6 mmol (1 g) in a 70 kg adult. Approximately 50% of the urate pool turns over each day. About 70% of urate excretion normally occurs through the kidney and the rest through the intestine; output via the intestine is increased in renal disease.

Plasma urate

There is a wide variation in plasma [urate], even in health. Much of this can be attributed to physiological factors, which include:

1 *Sex*. Plasma [urate] tends to be higher in males than in females. The *reference range* in adult males is 0.12–0.42 mmol/L and in females 0.12–0.36 mmol/L.

2 *Obesity*. Plasma [urate] tends to be higher in the obese.

3 *Social class*. The more affluent social classes tend to have a higher plasma [urate].

4 *Diet*. Plasma [urate] rises in individuals taking a high protein diet, i.e. a diet also rich in nucleic acids, and in those with a high alcohol consumption.

5 *Genetic factors* are important.

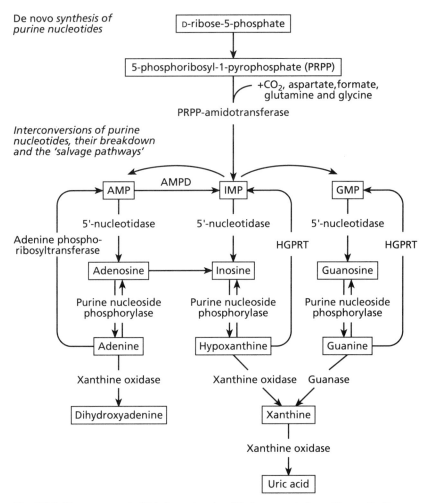

Fig. 16.1 The upper part of this figure is a simplified representation of the synthetic pathway leading to the de novo synthesis of inosinic acid (IMP), a purine nucleotide that can then be converted to adenylic acid (AMP) and guanylic acid (GMP) by complex reactions, indicated by the upper pair of curved arrows.

The lower part of the figure shows the breakdown of AMP, IMP and GMP to their corresponding purines, and their further metabolism to uric acid (the main end-product of purine metabolism) and dihydroxyadenine. It also shows, with another set of curved arrows, the 'salvage pathways' for re-forming AMP, IMP and GMP from their corresponding purine bases, by reactions catalysed by hypoxanthine-guanine phosphoribosyltransferase (HGPRT) and by adenine phosphoribosyltransferase.

The method of analysis can have slight but significant effects on results for urate measurements. Enzymic methods yield lower results (as much as 0.06 mmol/L lower) than less specific colorimetric techniques. Several drugs or their metabolites interfere with colorimetric methods.

Hyperuricaemia

Hyperuricaemia can be defined, on the basis of the reference ranges, as a plasma [urate] greater than 0.42 mmol/L in men and greater than 0.36 mmol/L in women. Its causes are listed in Table 16.1. Solutions of monosodium urate become supersaturated when the concentration exceeds 0.42 mmol/L. However, the relationship between the presence and severity of hyperuricaemia and the development or arthritis or renal calculi is more complex than considerations simply of solubility data might suggest.

Increased plasma [urate] may be attributable to one of several mechanisms, but there must either be overproduction or defective elimination of urate.

Overproduction of urate

Metabolic abnormalities have been defined in a few diseases. The following may occur:

1 Increased activity of the rate-limiting enzyme in *de novo* nucleotide synthesis, PRPP-amidotransferase, or increased concentration of its substrate, PRPP.

2 Increased activity of those pathways of nucleotide metabolism which lead to urate formation, as compared with those which lead to the formation of nucleic acids.

3 Increased rate of nucleic acid breakdown, as occurs whenever there is an increased rate of cell turnover or destruction.

4 Decreased activity of the 'salvage pathway' due to absence or deficiency of HGPRT.

Table 16.1 Examples of causes of hyperuricaemia

Category	Examples
Overproduction of urate	
Increased de novo purine synthesis	
Primary	Idiopathic
	Specific enzymic defects (e.g. PRPP-synthase or PRPP-amidotransferase overactivity)
Secondary	Specific enzymic defects (e.g. complete HGPRT deficiency in the Lesch–Nyhan syndrome, glucose-6-phosphatase deficiency in von Gierke's disease)
Increased turnover of pre-formed purines	
Myeloproliferative disorders	Polycythaemia rubra vera
Lymphoproliferative disorders	Lymphoma, lymphocytic leukaemia, paraproteinaemias (e.g. myeloma)
Miscellaneous	Carcinomatosis, secondary polycythaemia, exfoliative dermatoses
Defective elimination of urate	
Primary	Idiopathic
Secondary:	
Volume depletion	Any cause, if prolonged
Renal disease	Chronic renal failure, lead nephropathy
Drugs	Diuretics, low-dose salicylates
Metabolic acidosis	Lactic acidosis, ketoacidosis

5 Increased activity of xanthine oxidase. When this occurs, it is probably a secondary rather than a primary effect.

Defective elimination of urate

Renal excretion of urate is a complex process. Except for a small fraction bound to plasma proteins, urate is completely filtered at the glomerulus; this is then mostly reabsorbed in the proximal tubule. In the distal tubule, there are *both* active secretion *and* post-secretory reabsorption at a more distal site. These processes can all be affected by disease or drugs:

1 *Glomerular filtration.* When the GFR becomes reduced for any reason, urate retention occurs.

2 *Distal tubular secretion.* Lactic acid, 3-hydroxybutyric acid and some drugs (e.g. thiazide diuretics) compete with urate for this excretory pathway. Any condition giving rise to lactic acidosis or ketosis tends to be associated with hyperuricaemia.

3 *Distal tubular reabsorption.* Most uricosuric drugs (e.g. probenecid) act by decreasing tubular reabsorption of urate.

Salicylates and many other uricosuric agents have paradoxical, dose-dependent, effects on the renal tubular handling of urate. With *low* doses, salicylates mainly reduce distal tubular secretion, tending to cause hyperuricaemia. With *high* doses of salicylates, however, reduction of tubular reabsorption is the dominant effect and there is increased urate excretion.

Hypouricaemia

This is not an important chemical abnormality. It is due to increased urinary urate excretion more often than to decreased production of urate. Treatment with uricosuric drugs (e.g. probenecid) is the commonest cause of increased excretion; renal tubular defects (e.g. Fanconi syndrome) are other, relatively rare, causes. Decreased urate production may occasionally be due to inherited defects of purine metabolism (e.g. xanthine oxidase deficiency) or severe liver disease.

Xanthine oxidase deficiency is a rare cause of very low plasma [urate] and increased urinary xanthine and hypoxanthine excretion. Some patients develop xanthine stones in the urinary tract, but the condition may be asymptomatic.

Primary gout

This condition is characterized by recurrent attacks of arthritis, usually occurring in men. Attacks are often mono-articular, especially in the earlier stages of the disease, and often affect the metatarso-phalangeal joint of the big toe. In patients with hyperuricaemia, it is likely that supersaturation of urate (above 0.42 mmol/L) causes crystals to accumulate in connective tissues, (e.g. joints) over a long period prior to symptoms developing.

The acute symptoms of gout are probably due to crystals of monosodium urate shedding into the joint cavity caused by trauma or local metabolic changes, e.g. increase in plasma [urate]. The crystals are phagocytosed by leucocytes and macrophages and cause damage to membranes within the leucocytes. Lysosomal contents and other mediators of the acute inflammatory response (cytokines, prostaglandins, free radicals, etc.) are then released, causing both the systemic and the local acute manifestation of gout.

Most patients with primary gout have an impaired renal fractional excretion of urate, i.e. an inappropriately low urinary urate output if the raised plasma [urate] is taken into consideration. A minority of patients show clear evidence of *over-production* of urate and markedly *increased* urinary urate output. In a few cases, partial deficiency of HGPRT has been demonstrated.

The risk that a previously asymptomatic individual will develop gout varies with the plasma [urate]. The *annual incidence* in men is very low (about 0.1% per year) when plasma [urate] is below 0.42 mmol/L, but rises progressively with higher concentrations. It is 0.6% per year if plasma [urate] is in the range 0.42–0.54 mmol/L, and 5% per year if the concentration exceeds 0.54 mmol/L.

Patients with primary gout often show deposition of urate as *tophi* in soft tissues. Some also develop *renal stones*, mainly composed of uric acid, but the incidence varies widely, largely depending on the presence of other contributory factors such as dehydration or a low urinary pH.

Diagnosis of primary gout

Diagnosis is often made clinically, on the basis of the distribution of the joint involvement, a past history of similar episodes (especially if responsive to colchicine) and the presence of a raised plasma [urate]. However, not all cases are typical clinically and it should be remembered that:

1 A high plasma [urate] makes the diagnosis of gout probable, but not certain.
2 A small minority of patients with gout have a normal plasma [urate] at the time of an attack.

For the definitive diagnosis of gout, it may be necessary to aspirate joint fluid during an acute attack. This is then examined microscopically and the finding of needle-shaped urate crystals, which show negative birefringence, establishes the diagnosis.

Treatment of primary gout

In an acute attack, anti-inflammatory drugs (e.g. indomethacin) are usually prescribed. Uricosuric drugs and allopurinol should be avoided at this stage.

Long-term treatment aims to reduce plasma [urate]. Factors known to increase plasma [urate], such as a high protein diet, alcohol and certain drugs, should be avoided. Weight reduction, uricosuric drugs (e.g. probenecid) and inhibitors of urate synthesis (e.g. allopurinol) may be required. In patients in whom urate stones seem likely to form, a high fluid intake and alkalinization of the urine reduce the likelihood of stone formation.

Allopurinol (an isomer of hypoxanthine) inhibits xanthine oxidase, thereby causing a fall in plasma [urate] and in urinary urate. It increases urinary excretion of xanthine and hypoxanthine, but usually to a lesser extent than the fall in urinary urate, presumably due to reconversion of hypoxanthine to IMP via the 'salvage pathway' and further conversion of IMP to other purine nucleotides (Fig. 16.1). Allopurinol also reduces the *de novo* synthesis of purines.

HGPRT deficiency

The Lesch–Nyhan syndrome is a very rare, inherited, condition which usually presents in early childhood with choreo-athetosis, mental retardation and self-mutilation. The activity of HGPRT is greatly diminished or undetectable. In the absence of HGPRT, the salvage pathway is inoperative and purines cannot be reconverted to nucleotides (Fig. 16.1); instead, they are converted to urate. Urinary [urate] is greatly increased and uric acid calculi may form in the urinary tract. Plasma [urate] is usually increased.

Partial HGPRT deficiency is another rare, inherited, condition that causes a severe form of primary gout. Patients usually present with this condition in early adult life. Both plasma [urate] and urinary excretion of urate are increased.

Secondary gout

Hyperuricaemia may occur as a complication of several disorders, all of which affect either urate production or excretion, or both. These conditions, although commonly causing hyperuricaemia, are only rarely associated with the joint manifestations of gout. They include:

Myeloproliferative disorders. Almost all of these may be associated with hyperuricaemia, but polycythaemia rubra vera is probably the disease most commonly associated with signs of gout. Hyperuricaemia is due to increased turnover of red cell precursors or leucocytes.

Cytotoxic drug therapy. Patients with malignant disease treated by chemo-therapy, in which the accelerated rate of cell death causes an acute increase in nucleic acid breakdown, are liable to develop acute uric acid nephropathy. In this, there is renal failure due to deposition of urate crystals in the collecting ducts and ureters. Maintenance of a high fluid intake and treatment with allopurinol usually prevent this.

Psoriasis. The hyperuricaemia is thought to be due to an increased rate of cell turnover in the skin.

Hypercatabolic states and starvation. Either one of two mechanisms may be responsible for the hyperuricaemia that develops in these conditions. There may be an increased rate of cell destruction, or there may be an associated lactic acidosis which causes urate retention by diminishing distal tubular secretion of urate.

Chronic renal disease. Plasma [urate] rises in uraemia due to the reduced glomerular filtration rate, but clinical gout is very unusual.

Diuretic therapy. Most effective diuretics (e.g. chlorothiazide, frusemide) cause hyperuricaemia by reducing distal tubular secretion of urate.

Inherited metabolic disorders. Some are associated with lactic acidosis, which causes urate retention. The most striking example is type I glycogen storage disease (von Gierke's disease).

Hypertension and the development of ischaemic heart disease are associated with raised plasma [urate] much more often than would be expected by chance. This may be partly related to the association of both gout and hypertension with obesity, and partly to the urate-retaining effects of some antihypertensive drugs. Hyperuricaemia, by itself, does not appear to be an independent risk factor.

Chapter 17
Abnormalities of Thyroid Function

Thyroxine (T4) and small amounts of tri-iodothyronine (T3) and reverse T3 (rT3) are all synthesized in the thyroid gland (Fig. 17.1). Five stages in the synthesis and release of T4 and T3 from the thyroid can be recognized:

1 *Trapping of iodide* from the plasma by the thyroid gland.
2 *Oxidation of iodide to iodine* by peroxidase.
3 *Incorporation of iodine* into tyrosyl residues of thyroglobulin in the colloid. Mono-iodotyrosine and di-iodotyrosine (MIT and DIT) are formed.
4 *Production of T3 and T4* by coupling iodotyrosyl residues in the thyroglobulin molecule.
5 *Splitting off of T4 and T3* from thyroglobulin following its reabsorption from the colloid and their subsequent release into the circulation.

These stages are shown diagrammatically in Fig. 17.2.

Thyroxine is produced exclusively by the thyroid; it is properly regarded as a pro-hormone. However, it will be mostly referred to here as if it were a hormone, for ease of description. *The biologically active hormone is T3.* About 85% of plasma T3 is formed by extra-thyroidal, outer-ring, mono-deiodination of T4; T3 is produced in most (if not all) tissues, but quantitatively the most important organs

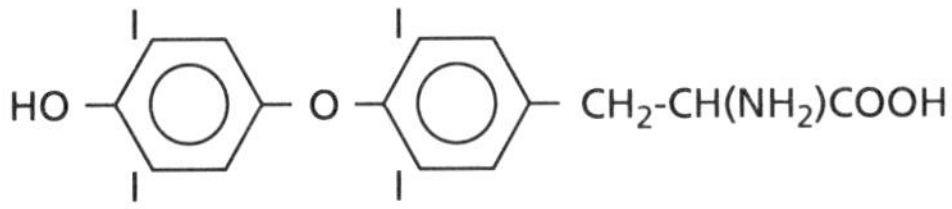

Thyroxine
3:5, 3':5'tetra-iodothyronine (T4)

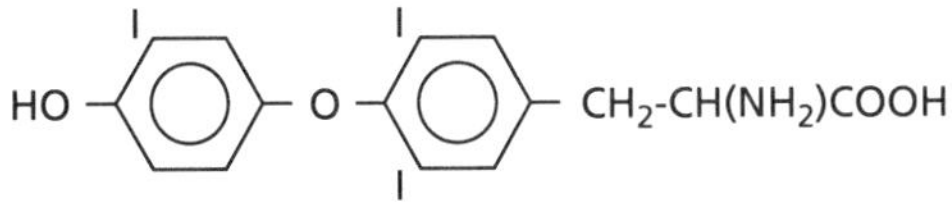

Tri-iodothyronine
3:5, 3'tri-iodothyronine (T3)

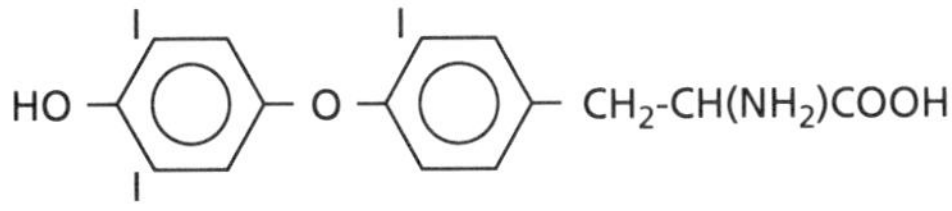

Reverse T3
3, 3':5'tri-iodothyronine (rT3)

Fig. 17.1 The formulae of the thyroid hormones, T4 and T3, and of rT3.

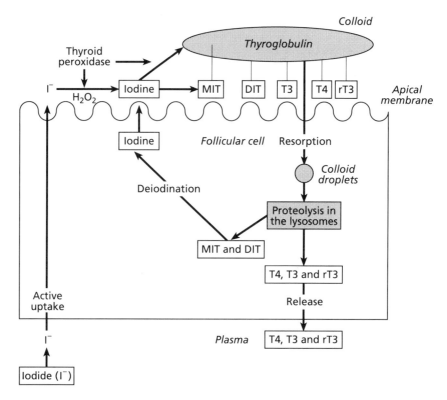

Fig. 17.2 The formation of T4 and T3 in the thyroid gland. The metabolism of T4 is described in Fig. 17.3. Di-iodotyrosine (DIT) and mono-iodotyrosine (MIT) are hormonally inactive; their iodine content is conserved.

for producing the T3 that is present in plasma are the liver, kidneys and muscle (Fig. 17.3). Thyroxine also undergoes inner-ring mono-deiodination in non-thyroidal tissues, with the production of metabolically inactive rT3.

The enzyme systems which perform outer-ring and inner-ring deiodination of T4 may also deiodinate T3 and rT3; the iodine so released is mostly taken up and reused by the thyroid. Various non-thyroidal illnesses (discussed later) and a poor nutritional state lead to diminished outer-ring deiodination which, in turn, results in decreased plasma [T3] and increased plasma [rT3].

Thyroid hormones may also be inactivated by deamination. In addition, about 10% of the T4 and T3 produced each day is excreted in bile, partly conjugated but mainly as the unconjugated hormone. In the intestine, the conjugates are partly hydrolysed; unconjugated T4 and T3 are then reabsorbed and re-enter the pool of circulating thyroid hormones. Small amounts of unmetabolized T4 and T3 are excreted in the urine.

Plasma transport and cellular action

Thyroid hormones are transported in plasma almost entirely bound, reversibly, to plasma proteins. Thyroxine-binding globulin (TBG) is the most important of

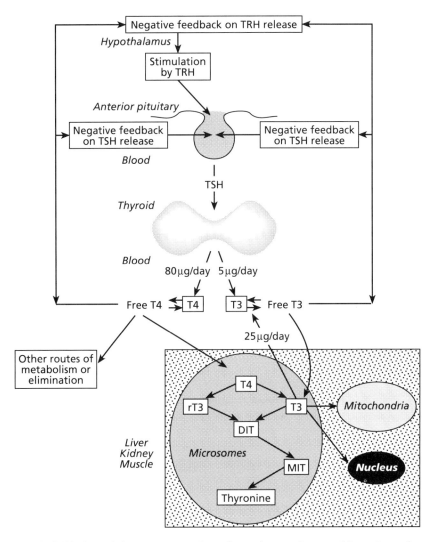

Fig. 17.3 The hypothalamic–pituitary–thyroid axis, showing the sites of formation and release of T4 and T3, and the points of action of the physiological negative feedback control mechanisms. Also shown is the deiodination pathway to thyronine in the microsomes. The other routes of T4 metabolism or elimination (not shown in detail) include conjugation and deamination, and excretion in the bile and urine.

these; it binds about 70% of plasma T4 and 80% of plasma T3. Thyroxine-binding pre-albumin and albumin also bind both T4 and T3.

Approximately 0.05% of plasma T4 and 0.2% of plasma T3 are free (i.e. unbound to protein). It is widely held that only the free fractions can cross the cell membrane and affect intracellular metabolism. This is probably an over-simplification but none the less plasma [free thyroid hormones] correlates better with thyroid status than plasma [total thyroid hormones]. Present evidence suggests that the hormones are actively transported into most cells by an ATP-dependent mechanism. In the cell, T3 can act at various sites (the nucleus, plasma membrane and mitochondria, Fig. 17.3) and influence heat production, amino acid transport and the metabolism of lipids, carbohydrates and proteins.

Regulation of thyroid function (Fig. 17.3)

Thyroid hormone synthesis is regulated by the level of thyroid-stimulating hormone (TSH or thyrotrophin) in the circulation. The release of TSH from the anterior pituitary is stimulated by hypothalamic thyrotrophin-releasing hormone (p. 294). Release of TSH is inhibited by negative feedback of free T3 and free T4 acting directly on the pituitary.

It is thought that the hypothalamus, via TRH, sets the level of thyroid hormone production required physiologically, and that the pituitary acts as a 'thyroidstat' to maintain the level of thyroid hormone production that has been determined by the hypothalamus.

Both free T3 and free T4 may exert some feedback control at the level of the hypothalamus, but this is uncertain. Dopamine, somatostatin and high plasma [cortisol] or [synthetic glucocorticoids] may also all suppress TSH release.

Investigations to determine thyroid status

The tests used to investigate thyroid dysfunction can be grouped into:

1 Tests which establish whether there is thyroid dysfunction, i.e. plasma TSH and thyroid hormone (T4 and T3) measurements.

2 Tests to elucidate the cause of thyroid dysfunction, i.e. thyroid auto-antibody and serum thyroglobulin measurements, thyroid enzyme activities, biopsy of the thyroid, ultrasound and in vivo radioactive iodine tests.

The diagnosis of thyroid dysfunction is often straightforward, using widely available chemical laboratory investigations. These should be performed to determine the patient's thyroid status before invoking the more demanding tests that seek to determine the cause of the thyroid dysfunction.

Plasma thyroid-stimulating hormone (reference range, 0.15–3.5 mU/L)

The use of monoclonal antibodies to measure plasma [TSH] in a basal blood sample by an immunometric assay provides the single most sensitive, specific and reliable test of thyroid status. It is applicable across the entire spectrum of thyroid disease, from overt primary hypothyroidism through mild or subclinical thyroid disturbances to overt hyperthyroidism. In hypothyroidism, increased plasma [TSH] is found whilst in hyperthyroidism plasma [TSH] will be below the detection limits of the immunometric method (i.e. below 0.1 mU/L). There are exceptions to this generalization, and both raised and undetectable plasma [TSH] may be found in some euthyroid patients (Table 17.1).

Radioimmunoassay (RIA) methods for measuring plasma [TSH] are less sensitive and specific and cannot be used to confirm a clinical diagnosis of hyperthyroidism with certainty without having to perform the TRH test (p. 294).

Plasma free thyroid hormones

These measurements indicate the amounts of T4 and T3 that are available to the

Table 17.1 Causes of an abnormal plasma [TSH] in some euthyroid patients

Undetectable plasma [TSH]	Increased plasma [TSH]
Pregnancy, during the first 20 weeks	Subclinical hypothyroidism
Treated hyperthyroid patients within	Amiodarone
6 months of becoming euthyroid	During the recovery stage following
Ophthalmic Graves' disease	various non-thyroidal illnesses*
Various kinds of non-thyroidal illness*	
Non-toxic multinodular goitre	
Treatment with dopaminergic drugs, or	
with high doses of glucocorticoids	

* 'Non-thyroidal illness' is discussed on p. 258.

tissues. Several techniques have been developed, of which equilibrium dialysis is the reference method. However, it is too time-consuming for routine use and is not widely used.

Plasma free thyroxine (reference range, 9–23 pmol/L)

Plasma free [T4] provides a more sensitive and often a more specific index of thyroid status than plasma [total T4]. When interpreting results of free T4 measurements, it must be appreciated that there are two main types of analytical method that are widely used:

1 *Analogue methods.* These depend on the use of labelled hormone analogues. They have been very widely adopted.

2 *Two-step and labelled-antibody methods.* These produce more reliable results than analogue methods. They are becoming more widely available.

These methods produce results that show good agreement in most ambulant patients. However, in patients with various non-thyroidal illnesses (p. 258), results for these methods do not always correlate well with one another.

Free T4 methods are not affected by alterations in plasma [thyroxine-binding proteins] such as occur in pregnancy and in women taking oestrogen-containing oral contraceptives. However, results obtained by most currently available analogue free T4 methods are influenced by reductions in plasma [albumin], and by the presence of certain drugs and endogenous compounds which inhibit the binding of thyroid hormones to albumin.

Euthyroid patients who have a low plasma [albumin], and particularly patients with certain non-thyroidal illnesses (e.g. chronic renal failure), are likely also to have low results for plasma [free T4] when this is measured using an analogue method. When measured by equilibrium dialysis, or by a labelled-antibody or two-step method, normal or raised plasma [free T4] may be found in these patients.

Plasma free thyroxine index (FTI)

This is still measured in a few laboratories. The FTI provides a means of correcting plasma [total T4] results for changes in plasma [thyroxine-binding proteins]. It gives an indirect measure of plasma [free T4]. Calculation of the FTI requires the measurement of both plasma [total T4] and the unsaturated binding capacity of the thyroxine-binding proteins (TBP) in serum.

The FTI correlates well with results determined directly for plasma [free T4] when the tests are performed on patients with *mild* abnormalities of plasma [TBP], as may occur in pregnancy or in women taking oestrogen-containing oral contraceptives. However, the FTI does *not* correct satisfactorily for the presence of TBP abnormalities in elderly patients with non-thyroidal illnesses, nor is it reliable in patients with familial TBG abnormalities or patients with inherited metabolic disorders of thyroid hormone synthesis.

Plasma free tri-iodothyronine (reference range, 3.0–9.0 pmol/L)
Plasma [free T3] is usually measured by an analogue assay; results are, therefore, influenced by changes in plasma [albumin]. Measurements of plasma [free T3] are to be preferred to plasma [total T3] measurements for distinguishing between hyperthyroid and euthyroid states when TBG is abnormal. However, free T3 measurements are of *no value for detecting hypothyroidism* as plasma [free T3] is often normal in these patients. Plasma [free T3] is reduced in many patients with non-thyroidal illnesses.

Plasma total thyroid hormones

Plasma total T4 (reference range, 70–150 nmol/L) and total T3 (reference range, 1.2–2.8 nmol/L)
More than 99% of T4 and T3 circulate in plasma bound to protein. The concentrations of plasma total T4 and total T3 are, therefore, greatly influenced by the plasma concentrations of thyroid hormone-binding proteins, particularly TBG. Both plasma [total T4] and [total T3] change in parallel in euthyroid patients if plasma [TBG] alters, e.g. in women taking oestrogen-containing oral contraceptives or in pregnancy; their concentrations may rise into the hyperthyroid range. However, plasma [free T4] and [free T3] remain normal if pituitary–thyroid homeostasis is maintained.

Plasma [total T4] discriminates well between euthyroid, hyperthyroid and hypothyroid states if there are no abnormalities in plasma [TBG]. Plasma [total T3] also provides a useful test for hyperthyroidism as values are often raised proportionately more than plasma [total T4] in these patients. However, measurement of plasma [total T3] is of *no value* in investigating suspected hypothyroidism as normal results are often obtained in these patients.

Selective use of thyroid function tests

It is not often necessary to carry out more than a limited range of chemical tests in the initial investigation of suspected thyroid disease. The introduction of TSH assays by immunometric methods caused a reappraisal of previous approaches to thyroid investigations since they can be used to detect both overt and subclinical thyroid disorders. However, the results do not give a precise indication of the severity of the disease, this being more a matter of clinical judgment.

Many laboratories now measure basal plasma [TSH] by an immunometric method as the initial chemical test of thyroid function. This test is least likely to produce an abnormal result in non-thyroidal illness and in patients on various

TSH by an immunometric method

	Low	Normal	High
High	Hyperthyroidism	TSH-secreting tumour (this is rare) Also, euthyroidism with T4 auto-antibodies or with variant albumin (both are uncommon), *if* an analogue free T4 assay is used	TSH-secreting tumour (this is rare) Also, hypothyroidism with T4 auto-antibodies (this too is rare), *if* an analogue free T4 assay is used
Normal	Subclinical hyperthyroidism T3-thyrotoxicosis	**Euthyroidism**	Subclinical hypothyroidism
Low	Hypopituitarism (uncommon)	Hypopituitarism (uncommon)	**Hypothyroidism**

(Left vertical axis: Free T4 — High, Normal, Low; right vertical label: Free T4; bottom horizontal axis: Low, Normal, High)

Fig. 17.4 The interpretation of results for plasma [free T4] and [TSH], using a two-step analytical method for measuring [free T4], except where (as stated) results relate to an analogue assay and a sensitive immunometric TSH assay. Low, normal and high indicate that results are below, within or above the reference ranges for the assays.

It is important to note that non-thyroidal illnesses can give rise to almost any combination of results for free T4 and TSH analyses, depending on their severity and the stage of the illness. To avoid confusion, these effects are not shown.

forms of drug treatment. *A normal plasma [TSH] excludes thyroid dysfunction.* If an abnormal result is obtained, plasma [free T4] or [free T3], or plasma [total T4] or [total T3] if preferred, is then measured as a follow-up investigation.

In some laboratories, plasma [total T4] or [free T4] is measured initially, and in others both plasma [TSH] and [total T4] or [free T4] are determined as an initial pair of tests. The latter, combined, strategy is not ideal since quite often the result of one test conflicts with the result for the other (Fig. 17.4). It is essential, therefore, to understand and appreciate the factors which can affect thyroid function and the results of thyroid function tests.

Interpreting results of thyroid function tests

Many factors need to be borne in mind when interpreting the results of thyroid function tests. Some of these can give rise to diagnostic difficulties, if not taken properly into account.

Overt hyperthyroidism

In hyperthyroidism, basal plasma [TSH] is nearly always below 0.1 mU/L, due to feedback inhibition on the pituitary. Very rarely, the cause of the hyperthyroidism is a TSH-secreting tumour. Plasma free and total T4 and T3 concentrations are nearly always increased in patients with overt hyperthyroidism.

In a very small percentage of clinically thyrotoxic patients, plasma [total T4] and [free T4] are both normal whereas both plasma [total T3] and [free T3] are increased. This condition of *T3-thyrotoxicosis* requires plasma free T3 or total T3 measurements for its recognition.

Overt hypothyroidism

Basal plasma [TSH] is invariably increased in *primary hypothyroidism*, as feedback inhibition of the pituitary (Fig. 17.3) is diminished; values often exceed 20 mU/L. It is, however, worth noting that transient and sometimes marked increases in plasma [TSH] may be observed in euthyroid patients while they are recovering from severe non-thyroidal illnesses. Plasma [free T4] and [total T4] are usually low in overt primary hypothyroidism.

Plasma [free T3] and [total T3] measurements are of no value in the investigation of overt or suspected primary hypothyroidism since normal concentrations are often observed. Low values for these tests are also often obtained in elderly patients and in seriously ill patients in the absence of thyroid disease.

In *secondary hypothyroidism*, plasma [TSH] is normal initially but pituitary functional reserve can often be shown to be impaired at this stage by performing a TRH test (p. 294). In fully developed secondary hypothyroidism, basal plasma [TSH] is low in about 50% of these patients and there is little or no TSH response to TRH injection. Plasma [total T4] and [free T4] are usually low in these patients.

Subclinical primary thyroid disease

The clinical diagnosis of mild thyroid disorders is often difficult and the introduction of the sensitive TSH assays has revealed difficulties in categorizing some of these patients as hyperthyroid, euthyroid or hypothyroid. For example, many clinically euthyroid patients with multinodular goitre or with exophthalmic Graves' disease may have a plasma [TSH] below 0.1 mU/L (i.e. undetectable by an immunometric method). They may also show no response in the TRH test, but have plasma [total T4] and [free T4] in the upper part of their respective reference ranges. These patients have a biochemical abnormality, in that their production of TSH has been suppressed despite the fact that their plasma [free T4] is not abnormally high. These patients may remain euthyroid, but in some cases they progress to overt hyperthyroidism. Patients with this combination of chemical findings are said to have 'subclinical hyperthyroidism', but this description is unsatisfactory since it rests solely on the results of chemical investigations.

Some patients who are clinically euthyroid but who are likely to develop overt hypothyroidism (e.g. patients who have been treated by irradiation of the thyroid) may have a raised plasma [TSH] but normal plasma [free T4] and [free T3]. These patients, sometimes described as having 'subclinical hypothyroidism', should be followed up as they frequently progress to clinical hypothyroidism.

Before the diagnosis of subclinical thyroid disease can be made, causes of an abnormal plasma [TSH] other than thyroid disease must be excluded. These include pregnancy, various non-thyroidal illnesses and drug treatment.

Pregnancy

Plasma [TBG] increases during pregnancy and, as a result, plasma [total T4] and [total T3] also increase.

Plasma [free T4] and plasma [free T3] *decrease* as pregnancy progresses and it is important to make use of trimester-related reference ranges (Table 17.2).

In the first trimester and early second trimester, some euthyroid women have low or undetectable plasma [TSH]. This is due to the weak thyrotrophic effect of chorionic gonadotrophin (hCG) which results in slight increases in T4 and T3 production and thus in TSH suppression. Chorionic gonadotrophin concentrations in plasma are highest in the first trimester. After 20 weeks, plasma [TSH] provides a reliable indication of thyroid status in pregnancy.

Transient post-partum thyroid dysfunction may occur in up to 15% of women. In most cases, this is of a subclinical nature.

'Non-thyroidal illnesses' and the 'sick euthyroid syndrome'

The diagnosis of thyroid disease is often straightforward, with both clinical features and biochemical abnormalities being apparent, and in accord with one another. However, this may not be the case in patients attending or admitted to hospital, suffering from any of a wide range of disorders (Table 17.3), since abnormalities in thyroid function tests (if performed) may often be reported even though, when the patients have recovered from these other illnesses, repetition of the thyroid function tests shows that they were in fact euthyroid.

The term 'non-thyroidal illness' is widely used to encompass the range of conditions listed in Table 17.3 (the list is not exhaustive). In addition, drug therapy (see below), major surgery, and the nutritional disturbances that accompany many illnesses may lead to temporary alterations in thyroid function. The effects of these various illnesses and abnormal conditions on thyroid function tests are sometimes described as the 'sick euthyroid syndrome', in which one or more of the following may occur:

1 Alterations in the hypothalamic–pituitary–thyroid axis, e.g. resulting from increased release of dopamine locally or increased plasma [cortisol]; these inhibit TSH release.

2 Changes in the affinity characteristics and in the plasma concentrations of the thyroid hormone-binding proteins. These changes give rise to alterations in the plasma concentrations of both the free and total thyroid hormones.

3 Impaired uptake of thyroid hormones by the tissues.

Table 17.2 Plasma [free thyroid hormones] by analogue methods (trimester-related reference ranges during pregnancy)

Stage of pregnancy	Plasma [free T4] (pmol/L)	Plasma [free T3] (pmol/L)
Non-pregnant state	9–23	3.0–9.0
First trimester	9–23	3.0–9.0
Second trimester	8–20	3.0–7.0
Third trimester	7–17	2.0–6.0

Case 17.1

A 30-year-old housewife attended her general practitioner's surgery. She had been losing weight (6 kg in the previous 6 months), was irritable and had felt very uncomfortable in a recent spell of hot weather. She was taking an oestrogen-containing oral contraceptive and a pregnancy test later confirmed that she was not pregnant. On clinical examination, the doctor noted that her palms were sweaty and that she had a fine tremor of the fingers when her arms were outstretched. There were no thyroid enlargement or bruit, and no abnormal eye signs. The following results were reported in response to the doctor's requests for thyroid function tests:

Analysis	Result	Reference range	Units
[TSH]	< 0.1	0.15–3.5	mU/L
[Free T4]	20	9–23	pmol/L
[Total T4]	160	70–150	nmol/L
[Free T3]	20	3.0–9.0	pmol/L
[Total T3]	6	1.2–2.8	nmol/L

What do you think was the diagnosis in this patient, and on what evidence do you base your diagnosis? This patient is discussed on p. 265.

4   Decreased production of T3 in the peripheral tissues.
5   Changes in the T3 occupancy and function of the T3 receptors.

The results for thyroid function tests reported in patients with non-thyroidal illnesses are liable to vary with the nature and severity of the illness and any associated drug treatment (see below) as well as with the type of analytical method used for measuring thyroid hormones. The subject is very complex, and doctors should not request thyroid function tests on patients with such illnesses unless there are clinical features to suggest that thyroid disease is also present.

The following description indicates the range of adverse effects that non-thyroidal illnesses often have on the results of thyroid function tests in patients with various types of non-thyroidal illness:

Table 17.3 'Non-thyroidal illness' and the sick euthyroid syndrome': examples of illnesses and other conditions that have been reported as leading to abnormal results for thyroid function tests

Acquired immunodeficiency syndrome	Liver diseases (various, acute and chronic)
Adrenocortical dysfunction	Major surgery
Anorexia nervosa	Malnutrition
Burns	Myocardial infarction
Congestive cardiac failure	Neoplastic diseases, various
Crohn's disease (regional ileitis)	Nephrotic syndrome
Diabetes mellitus	Psychiatric disorders, acute
Fasting (prolonged)	Renal failure, acute and chronic
Febrile illnesses (various)	Starvation
Hyperemesis gravidarum	Trauma

1   *Acute phase of the illness.* Plasma [TSH] is usually unaffected, but may be undetectable if the illness is severe or the patient is being treated with glucocorticoids or dopaminergic drugs.

Plasma [total T4] is usually normal or reduced, but it may be increased in patients with non-thyroidal illnesses. Plasma [free T4] may also be normal, increased or decreased with all types of analytical method, and is especially liable to be decreased if analogue-RIA methods are used. Plasma [total T3] and [free T3] are often decreased.

These effects of non-thyroidal illness mean that, for instance, the finding of an undetectable plasma [TSH] and normal plasma [thyroid hormones] is *not* diagnostic of subclinical hyperthyroidism or secondary hypothyroidism. Instead, the tests should be repeated following recovery from the non-thyroidal illness.

2   *Recovery phase.* During recovery from a severe non-thyroidal illness, thyroid hormones gradually return to levels within the reference range, but abnormal levels may still be reported for a considerable time. Plasma [TSH] may rise transiently into the hypothyroid range, as suppression by the stress response is released. It is important to recognize that the combination of low plasma thyroid hormone concentrations and raised plasma [TSH] is not necessarily due to primary hypothyroidism in these patients.

Drug treatment

Several drugs can, by themselves, affect the results of thyroid function tests; examples are given in Table 17.4. The combination of non-thyroidal illness and certain forms of drug treatment can have marked effects on thyroid function test results. In hospitalized patients, abnormal results for these tests are more likely to be due to non-thyroidal illness than to thyroid disease, especially as patients are usually receiving drug treatment for their illness.

Other causes of abnormal results for thyroid function tests

Abnormalities in binding proteins

Alterations in the concentrations or affinities of plasma thyroxine-binding proteins

Table 17.4 Causes of abnormal plasma [thyroid hormones] in euthyroid patients

Increased plasma		Decreased plasma
[total T4]	[total T3]	[total T4] *and* [total T3]
'Non-thyroidal illness'	TBG excess	'Non-thyroidal illness'
T4 auto-antibodies	T3 auto-antibodies	TBG deficiency
Variant albumins		Iodide
TBG excess		Phenytoin
		Lithium
		Salicylates
		Phenylbutazone

Note that all the drugs listed also cause decreased plasma [free T4] and [free T3], when these are measured by analogue assay methods.

can produce the following misleading results for thyroid hormone measurements:

1 *Abnormal plasma TBG concentrations* occur frequently in healthy women and in certain groups of patients (Table 17.5). The affinity and binding capacity of TBG for thyroid hormones may be diminished by the presence of endogenous inhibitors (e.g. free fatty acids) or by drugs (e.g. salicylates). In non-thyroidal illnesses, a modified form of TBG may be produced called 'slow TBG'; this has a low affinity for thyroid hormones. If a patient is euthyroid but has an abnormal plasma [TBG], plasma TSH, free T4 and free T3 concentrations will nevertheless all be normal unless there is co-existing non-thyroidal illness.

2 *Abnormal plasma albumin and pre-albumin concentrations* may influence the results for plasma [total T4] and [total T3], as well as the results for free thyroid hormone measurements, when the free hormones are measured by analogue assay methods.

3 *Genetic variants of both albumin and pre-albumin* have been described in which the affinity of these binding proteins for T4 is increased. These variants give rise to increased plasma [total T4] and, if an analogue assay method is used, plasma [free T4] also appears to be increased due to interference with the assay. Plasma [TSH], [total T3] and [free T3] measurements are usually all normal if the patient is euthyroid, as also is plasma [free T4] if measured by a two-step assay.

Endogenous antibodies

Auto-immune thyroid disease. Endogenous antibodies to T3 or T4, or to both hormones, may occur in patients with auto-immune thyroid disease. These antibodies interfere with many of the T3 and T4 assay methods, and produce apparently grossly elevated results. Plasma [TSH] measurements and [free T4] measured by two-step or labelled-antibody methods provide the most reliable indications of thyroid status in these patients as they are not affected by these auto-antibodies.

Antibodies to mouse immunoglobulins. It is rare for these to be present in patients but, when they are, they are liable to interfere with the measurement of plasma [TSH] by immunometric assay methods and with thyroid hormone assays which use mouse-derived monoclonal antibodies.

Table 17.5 Causes of an abnormal plasma [thyroxine-binding globulin]

Increased plasma [TBG]	Decreased plasma [TBG]
Oral contraceptives	'Non-thyroidal illness'
Pregnancy	Genetic causes
Oestrogen therapy	Protein-losing states
Genetic causes	Corticosteroids
	Androgens

Note that many drugs may bind to thyroxine-binding globulins (TBG) and thereby decrease the affinity and binding capacity of these proteins for thyroid hormones, but without affecting plasma [TBG].

End-organ resistance to thyroid hormones

These are rare causes of abnormal results for thyroid function tests. The resistance may be due to thyroid hormone-receptor defects or to impaired deiodination of T4 to T3 in peripheral tissues.

Monitoring the treatment of thyroid disease

Management of hyperthyroidism

Either plasma [total T4] or [free T4] can be used to provide a satisfactory index of the progress of the untreated disease. These tests also provide the best indications of the adequacy or otherwise of antithyroid drug treatment. The therapeutic objective is to maintain plasma [total T4] or [free T4] in the upper half of the reference range. Plasma [TSH] can also be used to monitor these patients, in which case the aim should be to maintain it within the reference range. However, measurements of plasma [TSH] are not a reliable guide during the first 4–6 months of treatment for hyperthyroidism since TSH levels may still be suppressed even when plasma [total T4] and [free T4] have become abnormally low. Plasma [total T3] or [free T3] must be measured when monitoring the progress of patients with T3-thyrotoxicosis.

After radioactive iodine treatment, the likelihood that patients will eventually develop hypothyroidism is high. Long-term follow-up of these patients with periodic measurements of both plasma [TSH] and either [total T4] or [free T4] is essential. If plasma [TSH] increases above 4 mU/L, this means that the patient is likely to develop hypothyroidism and is a clear indication for more frequent and regular follow-up. However, replacement treatment with thyroxine should not necessarily be instituted on the basis of an increased plasma [TSH] but rather on the basis of clinical assessment coupled with the finding of a low plasma [total T4] or [free T4].

Patients treated by sub-total thyroidectomy are more likely to remain euthyroid than are patients treated with radioactive iodine or with antithyroid drugs. However, they may have temporary disturbances of thyroid function tests in the early post-operative period, and it is advisable to monitor these patients for 6 months before deciding whether thyroid replacement treatment is needed. The decision should then be based on clinical assessment supplemented by measurements of both plasma [TSH] and either [total T4] or [free T4].

Management of hypothyroidism

The objective of replacement therapy in patients with *primary hypothyroidism* is to restore them to the euthyroid state both clinically and, if possible, biochemically. It is desirable to normalize both plasma free T4 (or total T4) and TSH concentrations, but in many patients normal plasma [TSH] can only be achieved in the presence of an elevated plasma [free T4].

Following a change in the prescribed dose of thyroxine, it may be many weeks before the thyroid function tests again stabilize. For instance, when the dose of thyroxine is increased, results do not stabilize for at least 6–8 weeks. If the dose of thyroxine is decreased, it may be many months before normal thyrotroph respon-

---

Case 17.2

A 35-year-old secretary attended for follow-up review of her treatment for Graves' disease. Carbimazole (15 mg three times/day) had been started 1 month before. The results for thyroid function tests were as follows:

Analysis	Result	Reference range	Units
[TSH]	< 0.1	0.15–3.5	mU/L
[Free T4]	<5	9–23	pmol/L
[Free T3]	2.5	3.0–9.0	pmol/L

Would you consider these results acceptable? If not, what would you do? This patient is discussed on p. 265.

---

siveness is restored. Therefore, TSH results must be interpreted with caution during this stabilization period.

Plasma [TSH] should always be measured as part of the follow-up biochemical assessment. This is particularly valuable in the management of hypothyroid patients suspected of not having taken their replacement thyroxine regularly, but who may have taken some shortly before attending the follow-up clinic. Poor compliance is indicated by finding that not only is their plasma [free T4] or [total T4] in the upper half of the reference range, or even abnormally high, but their plasma [TSH] is also abnormally high.

Excessive thyroxine replacement may be recognized from the patient's symptoms and on clinical examination. It may also be suspected or confirmed by finding that plasma [TSH] is less than 0.1 mU/L, or by finding increased plasma [total T3] or [free T3].

Case 17.3

A 65-year-old widow had been being treated for primary hypothyroidism with thyroxine (150 µg/day) for the previous 12 months. She felt well and was clinically euthyroid; her weight was steady. Results for thyroid function tests performed on a blood specimen collected at a routine follow-up clinic visit were:

Analysis	Result	Reference range	Units
[TSH]	0.1	0.15–3.5	mU/L
[Free T4]	28	9–23	pmol/L
[Free T3]	6.0	3.0–9.0	pmol/L

Do you consider that these results indicate that therapeutic control was satisfactory? If not, in what way would you want to adjust the patient's dosage of thyroxine? This patient is discussed on p. 265.

In patients with *secondary hypothyroidism*, the objective of replacement therapy is to maintain plasma [free T4] or [total T4] in the upper half of the reference range.

In patients with papillary and follicular *carcinoma of the thyroid*, the aim of treatment is to give sufficient thyroxine to suppress plasma [TSH] to undetectable levels.

Miscellaneous chemical tests and thyroid disease

Thyroid auto-antibodies

Several types of antibody to thyroid tissue have been detected in serum, usually from patients with thyroid disease. Measuring these antibodies helps to demonstrate the presence of auto-immune disorders.

Complement-fixing antibodies are present in serum in over 80% of patients with Hashimoto's thyroiditis.

Antithyroglobulin antibodies and antimicrosomal antibodies (also known as antithyroid peroxidase) are present in the serum of patients with immunologically-mediated thyroid disease (e.g. Hashimoto's thyroiditis, Graves' disease). They may also be found in a small proportion of healthy individuals, the incidence being higher in relations of patients with hyperthyroidism. The highest titres of these antibodies are found in the serum of patients with Hashimoto's thyroiditis, one or both antibodies being present in 90% of patients. The main indications for measuring antithyroglobulin and antimicrosomal antibodies are to confirm a diagnosis of Hashimoto's thyroiditis and to distinguish ophthalmic Graves' disease from other possible diagnoses.

Thyrotrophin-receptor antibodies are IgG antibodies directed against TSH receptors in the thyroid; they are present in the serum of patients with Graves' disease. Cells to which one group of these antibodies are bound are directly stimulated to produce thyroxine; these antibodies are alternatively called thyroid-stimulating immunoglobulins (TSI). In addition to TSI, there are other immunoglobulins that bind to the thyroid and stimulate its growth but not the production of thyroxine; these are called thyroid-growth immunoglobulins (TGI). Separate measurement of TSI and TGI is a specialized procedure of limited availability. However, serum total thyrotrophin-receptor antibody titres can readily be measured and the results may be of value in predicting which patients with Graves' disease treated with antithyroid drugs are liable to relapse; patients with high antibody titres are likely to relapse when drug treatment is withdrawn.

Thyroid enzymes

Inherited metabolic disorders of thyroid hormone synthesis are all rare. For their specific recognition, measurements of iodinated tyrosines or of the activities of the enzymes involved in thyroxine synthesis may be required.

Thyroglobulin

Some differentiated carcinomas of the thyroid synthesize and secrete thyroglobulin. In these patients, measurement of serum [thyroglobulin] may be of value in monitoring the progress of the disease, and in assessing its response to treatment.

Case 17.4

A 38-year-old factory worker attended her general practitioner because she was always tired and had a feeling of discomfort in her neck. She had been gaining weight. On clinical examination she was found to have a goitre. The following investigations were requested on a blood specimen collected for thyroid function tests:

Analysis	Result	Reference range	Units
[TSH]	45	0.15–3.5	mU/L
[Free T4]	9	9–23	pmol/L
[Free T3]	4.2	3.0–9.0	pmol/L

As follow-up investigations, the laboratory measured the antimicrosomal and antithyroglobulin antibodies in the patient's serum, and found that both were present in very high titre.

What do you think is the diagnosis in this patient? Was it appropriate to request all the thyroid function tests initially requested? This patient is discussed on p. 266.

Tests affected by thyroid dysfunction

Several other chemical tests may be affected by increased or decreased thyroid hormone activity. They require to be briefly mentioned:

Glucose tolerance tests. Hyperthyroid patients may show a diabetic type of response (p. 166).

Plasma calcium. Hyperthyroidism is an occasional cause of increased plasma [calcium] and increased plasma alkaline phosphatase activity. It is one of the rarer causes of metabolic bone disease.

Plasma LDL-cholesterol concentration is often markedly increased in hypothyroidism. It is also sometimes low in hyperthyroidism.

'*Liver function tests*' may be abnormal in hyperthyroidism, especially the results of plasma enzyme activity measurements (e.g. ALT, AST, GGT and alkaline phosphatase).

Medullary carcinoma of the thyroid

This is a tumour of the parafollicular, calcitonin-producing cells (C-cells) of the thyroid gland. The relatively common, non-familial, form accounts for about 10% of cases of carcinoma of the thyroid. Plasma [calcitonin] is often greatly increased in patients with medullary carcinoma of the thyroid, but plasma [calcium] is usually normal.

A few patients have been described with intermittent or persistent hypocalcaemia. In patients with normal plasma [calcitonin], injection of pentagastrin or a drink of whisky (which stimulates the release of gastrin) provokes the release of calcitonin and plasma [calcitonin] rises markedly.

Multiple endocrine neoplasia (MEN) syndromes

Medullary carcinoma of the thyroid occurs rarely as one component of two different forms of MEN II syndromes. The index cases of these familial syndromes usually present in childhood. The two forms of MEN II are:

MEN IIa (MEN 2) or Sipple syndrome. In this form, the thyroid carcinoma occurs in association with phaeochromocytoma and with hyperplasia of the parathyroid glands. In about 20% of patients there is also primary hyperparathyroidism.

MEN IIb (MEN 3). In this form, the thyroid carcinoma occurs in association with phaeochromocytoma but primary hyperparathyroidism is not a feature. MEN IIb is also distinguishable from MEN IIa by the presence of multiple neuromatous lesions, and often a myopathy and Marfanoid features as well.

In MEN II, fasting plasma [calcitonin] should be measured in relatives of the patient; if it is normal, the measurement should be repeated after stimulation by pentagastrin or whisky. As phaeochromocytoma is often present in patients with familial carcinoma of the thyroid, this possibility should be investigated (p. 290) before operation on the thyroid. The diagnosis of primary hyperparathyroidism is discussed elsewhere (p. 203).

Comments on Case 17.1 (p. 258)

The patient had T3 thyrotoxicosis, this diagnosis being based on the increased plasma [free T3] and undetectable [TSH], in the presence of a normal plasma [free T4]. The fact that the patient was taking an oestrogen-containing oral contraceptive would account for the increased plasma [total T4] and [total T3], since the oestrogen content would cause an increase in plasma [TBG].

In patients with thyrotoxicosis but no goitre it is important to perform a thyroid scan to help determine the cause of the hyperthyroidism. This patient's thyroid showed a diffuse and increased uptake of ^{131}I, and TSH-receptor antibodies were detected in her serum.

This patient had Graves' disease but no goitre; this is thought to arise when thyroid-stimulating immunoglobulins are present but thyroid-growth immunoglobulins are absent.

Comments on Case 17.2 (p. 262)

Plasma [TSH] measurements are not a reliable indicator of thyroid status in the early months of treating hyperthyroid patients as the responsiveness of the thyrotrophs lags behind the fall in plasma [free T4] and [free T3] for several weeks. During these early months, plasma [free thyroid hormone] measurements provide the most reliable indication of thyroid status. In this patient, the results for plasma [free T4] and [free T3] clearly indicated the need to reduce the dosage of carbimazole immediately.

Comments on Case 17.3 (p. 262)

The aim of thyroxine replacement treatment for primary hypothyroidism is to maintain the patient clinically euthyroid and to render plasma [TSH] normal (it would have been much increased before thyroxine treatment was started). In about half these patients, it is necessary to give sufficient thyroxine to increase the plasma [free T4] to above the upper reference value in order to normalize plasma [TSH].

In this patient, although clinically euthyroid, the plasma [free T4] was above normal and [TSH] below normal, but not so suppressed as to be undetectable (i.e. it was not < 0.1 mU/L). It was decided not to reduce the thyroxine dosage, and to reassess the patient 3 months later.

Comments on Case 17.4 (p. 264)

The patient has hypothyroidism. However, she still had sufficient functioning thyroid tissue, when stimulated by the very high plasma [TSH], to be able to maintain plasma [free T4] and [free T3] within their reference ranges.

The very high titres of antimicrosomal and antithyroglobulin antibodies in this patient's serum indicate that she had hypothyroidism due to Hashimoto's thyroiditis.

It should be noted that it was not appropriate to have requested the [free T3] measurement, since about 50% of patients with hypothyroidism have a normal plasma [free T3].

Chapter 18
Disorders of the Adrenal Cortex and Medulla

Disorders of the adrenals are uncommon, but they often have to be considered in an individual patient's differential diagnosis. The need for specific and sensitive screening tests is therefore paramount, as well as for other tests to confirm or refute the results of screening tests. In some cases, chemical tests to help determine the specific cause of the adrenal disorder are available.

Regulation of adrenal steroid hormone synthesis and secretion

Three zones can be recognized in the adrenal cortex. The outermost zone (zona glomerulosa) is the site of synthesis of aldosterone, the principal mineralocorticoid. The deeper layers of the cortex, the zona fasciculata and zona reticularis, synthesize glucocorticoids, of which cortisol is the most important in man. Sex steroid production also occurs in the adrenal cortex, mainly in the zona reticularis.

Glucocorticoid secretion

Glucocorticoids have widespread metabolic effects on carbohydrate, fat and protein metabolism. In the liver, cortisol stimulates gluconeogenesis, amino acid uptake and degradation, and ketogenesis. Lipolysis is increased in adipose tissue, and proteolysis and amino acid release promoted in muscle.

Adrenocorticotrophin (ACTH) is the main factor stimulating the release of cortisol. It acts at the cellular level both to elevate intracellular [cyclic AMP] and to stimulate influx of Ca^{2+} into the cell. These intracellular signals lead to an immediate synthesis of cortisol, principally by stimulating cholesterol ester hydrolysis and transport of cholesterol into the inner mitochondrial compartment, to the site of side-chain cleavage where pregnenolone is formed from cholesterol. Little or no hormone is pre-stored and the cellular response depends upon de novo synthesis. In the longer term, ACTH leads to a cyclic AMP-dependent transcriptional activation of certain key steroidogenic enzymes on the glucocorticoid pathway; it also promotes growth of the adrenal cortex in vivo.

Three factors regulate ACTH secretion:

1 *Negative feedback control.* This mechanism is responsible for controlling the release from the hypothalamus of corticotrophin-releasing hormone (CRH). This stimulates the release of ACTH from the anterior pituitary and ACTH, in turn, stimulates the secretion of glucocorticoids. Increased plasma [cortisol] suppresses secretion of CRH, whereas a fall in plasma [cortisol] leads to increased secretion (Fig. 18.1). Synthetic steroids with glucocorticoid activity (e.g. prednisone, prednisolone, dexamethasone) influence the secretion of endogenous glucocorticoids by reducing the secretion of CRH.

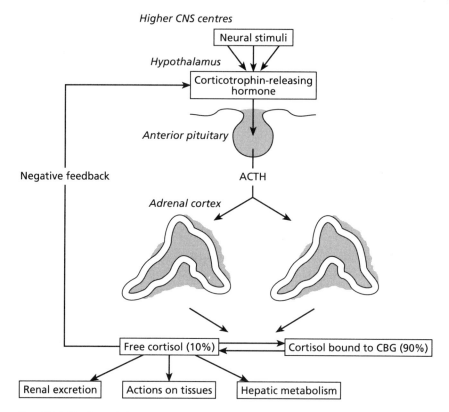

Higher CNS centres

Neural stimuli

Hypothalamus

Corticotrophin-releasing hormone

Anterior pituitary

Negative feedback

ACTH

Adrenal cortex

Free cortisol (10%)   Cortisol bound to CBG (90%)

Renal excretion   Actions on tissues   Hepatic metabolism

Fig. 18.1 The hypothalamic–anterior pituitary–adrenal axis and the fate of cortisol following its release. CBG, cortisol-binding globulin.

2 *The response to stress.* This control mechanism is mediated by CRH and ACTH. It is initiated by centres in the CNS higher than the hypothalamus and results in a sudden large increase in hormone secretion; the negative feedback control mechanism is temporarily overridden. Many stimuli, including surgical operations and emotional stress, can elicit this response. The insulin-hypoglycaemia test provides a standardized stimulus for testing the adrenal's response to stress.

3 *The nychthemeral rhythm of plasma [cortisol].* This control mechanism is related to the rhythm of an individual's sleeping–waking cycle (Fig. 18.2). The pathway for its control also depends on the CRH and ACTH mechanism. It is apparently not due to rhythmic changes in the sensitivity of the adrenals to the effects of ACTH.

In the circulation, the glucocorticoids are mainly bound (about 90%) to proteins; of these, the most important quantitatively is cortisol-binding globulin (CBG), sometimes called transcortin. Changes in plasma [CBG] may occur in the absence of alterations in adrenal function. Plasma [CBG] is increased in pregnancy, in patients receiving oestrogen treatment, and in women taking oestrogen-containing oral contraceptives, whereas in hypoproteinaemic states

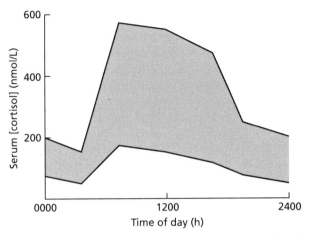

Fig. 18.2 The nychthemeral rhythm of cortisol secretion; the shaded area represents values that lie within the reference range. There is a similar rhythm for the secretion of ACTH by the anterior pituitary.

(e.g. nephrotic syndrome) plasma [CBG] is decreased. Similar changes occur in plasma [cortisol].

The biologically active fraction of cortisol in plasma is the free (unbound) component. This fraction, approximately 10% of circulating cortisol, is in equilibrium with protein-bound cortisol, bound mainly to CBG but also to other plasma proteins. Most clinical biochemistry departments measure the total (i.e. bound plus free) concentration of cortisol in blood specimens.

Aldosterone secretion

The principal physiological function of aldosterone is to conserve Na^+. It does this mainly by facilitating the reabsorption of Na^+ and the excretion of K^+ and H^+ in the distal renal tubule and in other epithelial cells. Although its rate of production is less than 1% of the rate of cortisol production, aldosterone plays a major role in regulating water and electrolyte balance, and blood pressure.

The mechanisms controlling the output of aldosterone are complex. The renin–angiotensin–aldosterone system is the most important of the following three controlling mechanisms, but potassium ions and ACTH also affect aldosterone secretion:

1 *Renin* is a proteolytic enzyme produced by the juxtaglomerular apparatus of the kidney. Its release into the circulation is stimulated by a fall in circulating blood volume or renal perfusion pressure, and by loss of Na^+. Its action on renin substrate is described on p. 39.

2 *Potassium.* Changes in plasma $[K^+]$ can have marked effects on aldosterone output. In response to increases in plasma $[K^+]$, aldosterone is released and exerts its effects on the distal renal tubule, causing an increased output of K^+ in the urine.

3 *ACTH.* This control mechanism is relatively unimportant, except possibly in stress conditions and in congenital adrenal hyperplasia due to 21-hydroxylase deficiency.

No specific aldosterone-binding protein comparable to cortisol-binding globulin has been demonstrated. A higher percentage of aldosterone circulates in plasma in the unbound form than in the case of cortisol.

Cortisol and ACTH measurements

Chemical tests of glucocorticoid metabolism are used firstly to support a clinical diagnosis of adrenal hypofunction or adrenal hyperfunction, by helping to classify the level of activity as normal, reduced or increased. Further chemical tests may provide information about the nature of the underlying disease process.

Serum (or plasma) cortisol

Most clinical biochemistry laboratories use radioimmunoassay (RIA) techniques because of their high degree of specificity and relative freedom from interference. When a specific antiserum is used, significant interference is only likely to be encountered in patients being treated with prednisone or prednisolone. In general, serum measurements provide more reliable results than plasma assays, and we shall refer solely to serum [cortisol] from now on.

Specimen collection

Specimens for measurement of serum [cortisol] must be collected at standard times because of the nychthemeral rhythm (Fig. 18.2). The times widely adopted are between 0800 h and 0900 h, and between 2200 h and 2400 h since the most reliable reference ranges have been defined for these times, i.e. 160–565 nmol/L and less than 205 nmol/L, respectively. Several important points need to be observed when collecting blood specimens for measuring serum [cortisol]:

1 *Anxiety.* Temporary, often large, increases in serum [cortisol] may be observed as a response to emotional stress. An indwelling venous catheter can help in this respect, especially when repeated blood sampling is necessary. Because of the anxiety associated with hospital admisssion, it is necessary to admit the patients 48 hours before assessing the nychthemeral rhythmn.

2 *Venous stasis* must be avoided or misleadingly high results will be obtained because cortisol is mainly bound to proteins in plasma.

3 *Storage.* The need to store specimens prior to analysis arises frequently, especially for samples collected at 2200 h. After collection, blood specimens are best kept at 4°C; they must *not* be frozen. If the analysis is to be delayed more than 12 hours, serum (or plasma) should be separated and then frozen.

Plasma ACTH

This can only be measured reliably in a few specialized laboratories. Since ACTH is unstable, the detailed instructions that these laboratories issue for collecting, preserving and transporting specimens must be followed.

There is a nychthemeral rhythm in the secretion of ACTH, and specimens for plasma ACTH measurements must be collected at the specified times for which reference ranges have been established, e.g. between 0800 h and 0900 h, and between 2200 h and 2400 h. Stress must be avoided when collecting specimens. Plasma [ACTH] is normally below 20 mU/L at 0800 h.

Urinary cortisol excretion
Cortisol is removed from plasma by the liver and mostly converted to a number of metabolically inactive compounds. These are excreted in the urine mainly as conjugated metabolites (e.g. glucosiduronates, often called glucuronides). These metabolites mostly retain the side-chain (at position 17 on the steroid nucleus) and the hydroxyl group at the 17 position.

A small amount of cortisol is excreted unchanged in the urine; this can be measured by specific RIA methods. Urinary cortisol excretion is related to the output of cortisol by the adrenal cortex during the period of urine collection, and to the plasma [free cortisol], i.e. the level of active hormone to which tissues have been exposed. In normal individuals, the excretion of cortisol in urine is less than 300 nmol/24 h and the cortisol : creatinine ratio in an early morning specimen of urine is less than 50 µmol cortisol : mol creatinine.

Investigation of suspected adrenocortical hyperfunction
Adrenocortical hyperfunction leads to the group of symptoms and signs known as Cushing's syndrome; its causes are listed in Table 18.1. With the exception of glucocorticoid therapy (iatrogenic Cushing's syndrome), these all result from adrenocortical hyperfunction. Most ACTH-dependent forms of Cushing's syndrome lead to diffuse adrenocortical hyperplasia, but a stimulated gland may become autonomously overactive, leading to micronodular or macronodular hyperplasia.

Some of the tests used in the investigation of suspected adrenocortical hyperfunction are time-consuming and a logical scheme is essential to prevent unnecessary tests. The following order of investigations provides one such scheme:

1 *Screening tests (out-patient).* To assess whether a clinical diagnosis of adrenocortical hyperfunction is likely to be correct.

2 *Confirmatory tests (in-patient).* To confirm or exclude the provisional diagnosis of adrenocortical hyperfunction. At this stage the diagnosis is based on both clinical findings and the results of screening tests.

3 *Tests to determine the cause.* Having already confirmed that there is adrenocortical hyperfunction, these further tests are performed in order to help answer the following questions:

(a) *What is the site* of the pathological lesion? Is it in the adrenal cortex, the pituitary or elsewhere?

(b) *What is the nature* of the pathological lesion?

Table 18.1 Causes of adrenocortical hyperfunction

ACTH-dependent causes	ACTH-independent causes
Cushing's disease	Adrenal adenoma
Ectopic production of ACTH	Adrenal carcinoma
Iatrogenic: ACTH therapy	Adrenal micronodular hyperplasia*
Ectopic production of CRH or related peptides	Iatrogenic: glucocorticoid therapy

* This condition is partially ACTH-dependent.

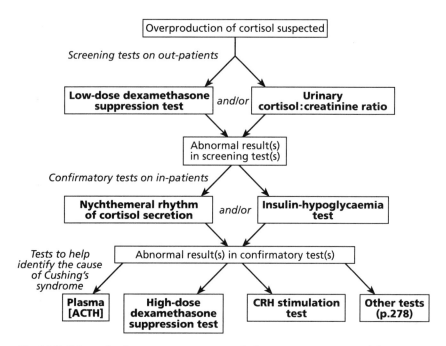

Fig. 18.3 Scheme for the stepwise investigation, by hormone measurements, of patients in whom adrenal hyperfunction (Cushing's syndrome) is thought to be the diagnosis.

A suggested plan of investigation is shown in Fig. 18.3. The details of the tests to be performed depend on the tests available to the clinician from the laboratory. Table 18.2 gives a summary of the commonly observed (but not invariable) findings in these hormonal tests.

Screening tests

The clinical suspicion that adrenocortical disease may be present arises quite commonly in hospital practice, whereas the incidence is very low if drug-induced (i.e. iatrogenic, usually due to steroid treatment) causes are discounted. Effective screening tests are therefore required. These need to be sensitive (i.e. they should detect all patients with adrenocortical disease) but do not have to be specific, since further tests will need to be performed in order to confirm the provisional diagnosis of adrenocortical disease.

Screening tests that can be performed on an out-patient basis are to be preferred. More detailed investigations can, thereafter, be carried out on an in-patient basis on the small minority of patients in whom the results of screening tests are abnormal. The initial screening investigations for adrenocortical hyperfunction should consist *either* of a low-dose dexamethasone (or betamethasone) suppression test *or* measurement of urinary free cortisol. If both tests are performed, this needs to be on *separate* occasions. Both of these screening tests can be satisfactorily performed on out-patients.

Table 18.2 Results of hormonal tests in patients with adrenal hyperfunction

Test	Cushing's disease	Adrenal tumour	Ectopic ACTH-secreting tumour
Tests to confirm the diagnosis			
Serum [cortisol]	Increased	Increased	Increased
Dexamethasone, low-dose test	Not suppressed	Not suppressed	Not suppressed
Urinary cortisol*	Increased	Increased	Increased
Nychthemeral rhythm	Lost	Lost	Lost
Insulin-induced hypoglycaemia	No response	No response	No response
Tests to differentiate the cause			
Plasma [ACTH]	Normal or increased	Not detectable	Increased or much increased
Dexamethasone, high-dose test	Suppressed	Not suppressed	Not suppressed
CRH test (p. 296)	Increased response	No response	No response

* This test may be performed on a 24-hour collection of urine or on an early morning specimen when the results are expressed as the urinary cortisol : creatinine ratio.

Low-dose dexamethasone suppression test

Dexamethasone normally suppresses the output of CRH temporarily via the negative feedback control mechanism (Fig. 18.1), even when given in small dosage, and hence suppresses the secretion of ACTH and cortisol. Several versions of this test are available.

In the *overnight suppression test*, the patient takes dexamethasone at 2200 h the night before attending the out-patient clinic; the dose used varies, being either 1 mg or 2 mg. Serum [cortisol] is measured on a blood specimen collected at the clinic the following morning, about 0900 h. Ingestion of 1–2 mg dexamethasone normally results in suppression of serum [cortisol]. The higher dose (2 mg) gives an unacceptably high rate of false negatives; this is less of a problem with the 1 mg dose but, with it, a greater number of false positives occur and these require further investigation to exclude Cushing's syndrome.

The *48-hour suppression test* (Table 18.3) can also be carried out on an out-patient basis but may also be performed in hospital, as a preliminary to a high-dose dexamethasone test (p. 277). In it, dexamethasone (0.5 mg) is taken every 6 hours, beginning at 0900 h on the first day, and serum [cortisol] is measured 48 hours later. The true-positive rate is reported to be better than 97%, with a false-negative rate of less than 1%. For these reasons, the 48-hour low-dose dexamethasone suppression test is to be preferred to the overnight suppression test.

Drugs which induce hepatic microsomal enzymes (e.g. phenytoin, phenobarbitone) may cause an increased rate of metabolism of dexamethasone to such an extent that its blood level may be lowered prematurely below that normally required to achieve suppression of CRH secretion. Patients taking these drugs may, therefore, show no suppression of serum [cortisol] in these tests.

Table 18.3 A protocol for a low-dose dexamethasone test followed by a high-dose dexamethasone test

Day of test	Dexamethasone (oral dose)*	Serum [cortisol] at 0800–0900 h (specimen description)
1	Nil	Basal
2	Nil	Basal
3	0.5 mg 6-hourly	Basal
4	0.5 mg 6-hourly	'Low-dose'
5	2 mg 6-hourly	'Low-dose'
6	2 mg 6-hourly	'High-dose'
7	Nil	'High-dose'

*The dosage of dexamethasone for the ensuing 24-hour period is started at the time that the blood specimen is collected for measuring serum [cortisol].

Urinary free cortisol

This is a good screening test, but it suffers from the disadvantage that an incomplete collection of urine may lead to a false-negative result. It is better to determine the *urinary cortisol : creatinine ratio* on an early morning specimen, collected at the out-patient clinic. The ratio is normally less than 50 μmol cortisol : mol creatinine.

Interpretation of screening tests

The screening tests usually serve to distinguish simple, non-endocrine, obesity from obesity due to Cushing's syndrome. Abnormal results for these screening tests may, however, be obtained in depressed or extremely anxious patients, or in alcoholism.

If the results of screening tests are normal, there is usually no need to proceed to further investigation of cortisol production, unless there is strong clinical suspicion that the patient has adrenocortical hyperfunction. However, if the result of a screening test is abnormal, the patient needs to undergo further investigation to confirm the clinical diagnosis of adrenocortical hyperfunction.

Confirmation that there is cortisol overproduction

The investigations described here require the patient to be in hospital, to enable the tests to be performed under properly controlled conditions. Alcoholism may mimic Cushing's syndrome, and patients may show abnormal results in the screening tests, but the biochemical abnormalities revert to normal when alcohol intake ceases following hospital admission.

Loss of nychthemeral rhythm

The characteristic finding at an *early* stage of Cushing's syndrome, whatever the cause, is an increase in serum [cortisol] in a blood specimen collected at 2200 h, accompanied by loss of the nychthemeral rhythm. In some patients, even at this early stage, there is also an increase in serum [cortisol] in the 0800 h specimen.

At a later stage, abnormally high serum [cortisol] can be detected throughout the 24 hours.

Insulin-hypoglycaemia test

In the absence of adrenal disease, the common causes of abnormal results in all the tests for investigating suspected adrenocortical hyperfunction so far described are depressive illness (exogenous or endogenous) and any cause of stress to the patient. The insulin-hypoglycaemia test distinguishes these causes of increased cortisol production from Cushing's syndrome.

Insulin provides a convenient and reproducible means of inducing stress, and the insulin-hypoglycaemia test is the most widely used stress test of hypothalamic-pituitary-adrenal (HPA) axis integrity. The adrenal response to a rapid reduction in plasma [glucose], induced by an intravenous injection of insulin, is assessed by measuring serum [cortisol]. The test is contraindicated in patients with epilepsy or heart disease.

Preparation for the test. The patient fasts overnight, and has nothing to eat or drink (apart from water) on the morning of the test. An indwelling intravenous needle should be inserted at least 30 minutes before the test, and the patient warned that the test may induce sweating or a feeling of drowsiness.

The dose of insulin, to be given as a single intravenous injection, must be related to the weight of the patient and to the tentative clinical diagnosis; the standard dose of soluble insulin is 0.15 units/kg. The patient must not be left unattended at any time during the test; a syringe and 50% glucose solution must be immediately available so that the test can be terminated rapidly if signs of marked hypoglycaemia appear (e.g. severe and prolonged sweating, loss of consciousness or fits).

Performing the test. At least 30 minutes after inserting the indwelling needle, specimens of blood are collected for measurement of basal serum [cortisol] and plasma [glucose]. Insulin is then given via the indwelling needle and further blood specimens collected 30, 45, 60 and 90 minutes later for cortisol and glucose measurements. The test is ended by giving the patient a glucose-containing drink and a meal.

It is essential to produce an adequate degree of hypoglycaemia for the test to be valid. This is usually defined as a rapid fall in plasma [glucose] to less than 2.2 mmol/L. In patients with Cushing's syndrome, if adequate hypoglycaemia is not induced with the standard dose of insulin, the test can be repeated with increasing doses of insulin, incremented in steps of 0.05 units/kg; up to 0.30 units/kg may be required.

Interpretation of results. The cortisol response to the stimulus of hypoglycaemia depends on the integrity of the whole HPA axis. Serum [cortisol] normally reaches its maximum at 60 or 90 minutes, the level reached being at least 425 nmol/L with an increment above the basal (pre-insulin) level of at least 145 nmol/L.

A high basal serum [cortisol] may be due to anxiety, or to insufficient time having been allowed between inserting the indwelling needle and starting the test. However, these patients show a normal response to insulin-induced hypoglycaemia. The response is usually normal also in patients with simple obesity, and in patients with depression.

Patients with Cushing's syndrome, whatever the cause, do not respond normally to insulin-induced hypoglycaemia. There is a high basal serum [cortisol] and usually little or no increase in serum [cortisol] despite the production of an adequate degree of hypoglycaemia. The test is very valuable, therefore, in confirming a clinical diagnosis of Cushing's syndrome.

Determining the cause of Cushing's syndrome

Once the diagnosis of Cushing's syndrome has been established, the results of other investigations may help to determine the cause of the adrenocortical hyperfunction (Table 18.2). Although the diagnosis of Cushing's syndrome is relatively straightforward, the differentiation of its cause, particularly between ectopic ACTH production and Cushing's disease, may be difficult by means of chemical tests. The results need to be considered together with the findings from other methods of investigation, particularly radiological (e.g. CT scanning).

Plasma [ACTH]

The first investigation in differential diagnosis is the measurement of plasma [ACTH], carried out on blood specimens collected both in the morning and the evening (e.g. at 0800 h and 2200 h).

If ACTH is undetectable, this is diagnostic of an adrenal tumour as the cause of the Cushing's syndrome, and should be confirmed by an abdominal CT scan to detect an adrenal mass.

If the patient has Cushing's disease, ACTH will be present in plasma in normal or increased amount (5–50 mU/L), particularly in the evening specimen due to loss of the nychthemeral rhythm. Results for plasma [ACTH] overlap considerably for patients with Cushing's disease and ectopic ACTH secretion. However, a very high plasma [ACTH] points to an ectopic ('non-endocrine') origin.

Differentiation between ectopic and pituitary hypersecretion of ACTH can sometimes be made by measuring 'big ACTH', a high mol mass form of normal ACTH that is usually present in plasma when ACTH production is ectopic. 'Big ACTH' is not present in patients with Cushing's disease unless the pituitary tumour is large and invasive.

High-dose dexamethasone suppression test

This test is carried out in an identical fashion to the 48-hour low-dose suppression test (p. 273), except that 2 mg dexamethasone is given 6-hourly for 48 hours. A protocol for the high-dose dexamethasone test is given in Table 18.3. If the response is determined by measuring serum [cortisol], suppression is defined as a fall to less than 50% of basal values, usually to less than 125 nmol/L. If the response is being determined on the basis of urinary cortisol measurements, the 24-hour outputs on days 4 and 5 are compared with the basal output; suppression is again defined as a fall in output to less than 50% of the basal level.

Suppression of cortisol production in the high-dose dexamethasone suppression test *suggests* that the patient has Cushing's disease. However, about 10% of patients with Cushing's disease do not show suppression of cortisol output and may even show a paradoxical increase in serum [cortisol].

Most patients (90%) with ectopic ACTH production or with adrenal tumours do not show suppression. Since measurements of plasma [ACTH] and CT scanning readily establish the diagnosis of adrenal tumour, the high-dose dexamethasone test is helpful in distinguishing ectopic from pituitary-dependent origins for ACTH-dependent Cushing's syndrome because, having excluded an adrenal tumour as the cause, failure of suppression on the high-dose dexamethasone test strongly suggests that the patient has an ectopic ACTH-secreting tumour.

CRH stimulation test

This test (p. 296) may also help to distinguish Cushing's disease from ectopic ACTH production. Most patients with Cushing's disease show normal or exaggerated ACTH and cortisol responses to synthetic CRH, whereas patients with ectopic ACTH-secreting or adrenocortical tumours show no response. However, about 10% of patients with Cushing's disease fail to respond. False-positive responses in patients with ectopic ACTH production are unusual. By performing both the high-dose dexamethasone suppression test and the CRH test, the combined results provide almost 100% specificity and sensitivity in the diagnosis of Cushing's disease.

Other chemical tests

Potassium. Hypokalaemic alkalosis is a prominent feature of ectopic ACTH production. The finding of a low plasma [K^+] before any drug treatment is started in a patient with Cushing's syndrome, therefore, helps to distinguish ectopic ACTH production from a pituitary tumour since hypokalaemia is rarely found in untreated Cushing's disease. However, patients with Cushing's syndrome (whatever the cause) are often treated with diuretics (for hypertension and oedema) and this treatment may itself lower the plasma [K^+]. Hypokalaemia may also occur with adrenal tumours.

The mechanism whereby hypokalaemia is produced by ectopic ACTH-secreting tumours, and sometimes by adrenal neoplasms, is poorly understood but there may be increased output of mineralocorticoids. High levels of cortisol may also have a mineralocorticoid effect. These steroids cause renal retention of Na^+ and water, and loss of K^+ and H^+ in the urine.

Tumour markers. In ectopic ACTH production, increased plasma concentrations of markers (e.g. CEA, gastrin, somatostatin and calcitonin) may be found. As many as 70% of patients with ectopic ACTH secretion also secrete one or more marker peptides; such increases are rarely observed in patients with Cushing's disease or adrenal neoplasm.

Selective venous sampling. Blood specimens may be collected from selected sites for measurement of plasma [ACTH], to help identify the region of the body from which excess ACTH is being released. For instance, if plasma [ACTH] is highest in specimens collected from the internal jugular vein, this tends to confirm that the patient has Cushing's disease. If a specimen obtained from a vein draining

---

Case 18.1

A 34-year-old housewife was admitted to hospital with a provisional diagnosis of Cushing's syndrome. As an out-patient, her serum [cortisol] had not been suppressed when an overnight dexamethasone suppression test (2 mg dexamethasone) had been performed. She was obese (weight, 74 kg; height, 1.7 m), hypertensive (blood pressure, 165/105 mmHg) and had wasting of the proximal limb muscles. The following results were obtained for adrenal function tests:

Test	Time	Result	Reference range
Nychthemeral rhythm	0800 h	400 nmol/L	160–565 nmol/L
of serum [cortisol]	2200 h	380 nmol/L	Up to 205 nmol/L

Insulin-hypoglycaemia test		Basal value	Maximum response
Plasma [glucose]		4.5 mmol/L	1.5 mmol/L after 30 min
Serum [cortisol]		435 nmol/L	480 nmol/L after 60 min

Dexamethasone	Basal value	After 48 h on	After 48 h on
suppression tests		0.5 mg q.i.d.	2 mg q.i.d
Serum [cortisol]	420 nmol/L	410 nmol/L	500 nmol/L

Plasma [ACTH] at 0800 h: less than 2 mU/L (reference range, 2–20 mU/L)

How would you interpret these results? This patient is discussed on p. 292.

---

an intrathoracic site contains the highest plasma [ACTH], a tumour responsible for ectopic ACTH production is likely to be the cause and to be located in the related tissues.

Pituitary function tests (Chapter 19) may be abnormal in Cushing's syndrome due to the suppressive effect of cortisol on the hypothalamus and pituitary. The responses to LH-RH and to TRH are both impaired, the increases in plasma [LH] and [TSH] being less than normal. The increase in plasma [growth hormone] in response to hypoglycaemia is also impaired.

Glucose tolerance test. Patients with adrenocortical hyperfunction may develop steroid-induced diabetes and have a diabetic type of response to an oral glucose tolerance test (p. 166).

Metyrapone test. This test is based on the fact that, in Cushing's disease, inhibition of 11β-hydroxylase in the adrenal cortex by metyrapone suppresses cortisol production leading to a rise in plasma [ACTH] and increased formation of the steroid proximal to the block, 11-deoxycortisol. This does not occur in adrenocortical tumours. However, the test is very poor at distinguishing Cushing's disease from ectopic ACTH production and is now regarded as *obsolete*.

Investigation of suspected adrenocortical hypofunction

The causes of Addison's disease are listed in Table 18.4. In recent years it has become evident that adrenal lesions can also occur in *HIV-infected patients*. Whilst clinical features of adrenocortical insufficiency may be a late event in these

Table 18.4 Causes of adrenocortical hypofunction

Primary adrenocortical insufficiency (Addison's disease)	Adrenocortical insufficiency secondary to pituitary disease
Auto-immune adrenalitis	Congenital deficiency*
Secondary tumour deposits	Post-partum haemorrhage
Congenital adrenal hypoplasia	Trauma
Infections (e.g. tuberculosis, histoplasmosis, cytomegalovirus, meningococcal)	Iatrogenic (e.g. surgery, radiotherapy)
	Infections (e.g. tuberculosis, syphilis)
Congenital adrenal hyperplasia	Secondary tumour deposits
Drugs (e.g. etomidate)	Secondary to hypothalamic disease

* The deficiency may be isolated or accompanied by growth hormone deficiency.

patients, glucocorticoid (i.e. cortisol) responses may be impaired at an earlier stage. The adrenocortical pathology has been attributed to opportunistic infection by cytomegalovirus (CMV) or mycobacterial species, or to auto-immune adrenalitis, or to the effects of drug therapy. Mineralocorticoid deficiency has also been reported in AIDS.

In suspected adrenocortical crisis, blood should be collected for basal measurements of plasma urea, electrolytes and glucose, and serum cortisol concentrations *before* the patient is given cortisol. Definitive tests for the diagnosis of this condition should be carried out later, after the crisis is over.

Some of the tests used in the investigation of suspected adrenocortical hypofunction are time-consuming and a logical scheme is essential to prevent unnecessary tests. Tests that stimulate the gland directly (with ACTH or tetracosactrin) should *always* be performed before tests that stimulate the gland indirectly (e.g. insulin-hypoglycaemia test). A suggested plan of investigation is shown in Fig. 18.4, and the tests will be considered in the following order:

1 *Screening tests*, to assess whether adrenal hypofunction is likely.
2 *Confirmatory tests*, to confirm or exclude the presence of adrenocortical hypofunction.
3 *Tests to help determine the cause* of the adrenocortical hypofunction.

Table 18.5 summarizes the commonly (but not invariably) observed pattern of results for the principal investigations that should be performed, stepwise, on patients with adrenocortical hypofunction.

Screening tests

Measurements of basal serum [cortisol] and 24-hour urinary excretion of cortisol in patients with suspected Addison's disease may be of little value, by themselves, since their results may be normal in patients with even quite marked degrees of adrenocortical hypofunction. In particular, a normal serum [cortisol] at 0800 h does *not* exclude Addison's disease; patients may be able to maintain a normal basal output but be unable to secrete adequate amounts of cortisol in response to stress. Nevertheless, a serum [cortisol] that is below 50 nmol/L at 0800 h is strong presumptive evidence for Addison's disease, whilst a value (at 0800 h) of 550 nmol/L or more (in the absence of steroid therapy) makes the diagnosis

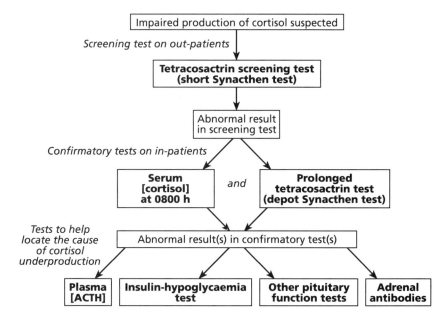

Fig. 18.4 Scheme for the stepwise investigation, by means of hormone measurements, of patients in whom adrenal hypofunction (Addison's disease) is thought to be the diagnosis.

extremely unlikely. For the many patients who have intermediate values, it is necessary to investigate the response of the adrenal cortex to stimulation, in order to assess its reserve capacity.

Tetracosactrin screening test (short Synacthen test)

ACTH is a single polypeptide chain composed of 39 amino acids, with the biological activity lying in the N-terminal sequence of 24 amino acids. Tetracosactrin (most often used in the form of Synacthen) is a synthetic polypeptide with a structure identical to the N-terminal 24 amino acids of ACTH. Tetracosactrin has a short duration of action. Its use as a stimulus to the adrenal cortex provides a

Table 18.5 Results of hormonal tests in patients with adrenal hypofunction

Test	Primary hypoadrenalism	Secondary hypoadrenalism	Congenital adrenal hyperplasia
Serum [cortisol]	Decreased or normal	Decreased or normal	Decreased or normal
Tetracosactrin tests			
(a) Screening test	No response	No response	Not indicated
(b) Prolonged test	No response	Response*	Not indicated
Plasma [ACTH]	Increased	Decreased or normal	Increased

* Tetracosactrin (depot) injections may need to be given for 6 days, instead of the 4 days that are normally adopted in this test, in order to elicit a response.

convenient and rapid screening test in the investigation of suspected adrenocortical hypofunction. The test can be performed with the patient on a normal diet, and as an out-patient, as follows:

1 A blood specimen is collected for measuring basal serum [cortisol].

2 Tetracosactrin, 0.25 mg, is given by intramuscular injection.

3 Further blood specimens for serum cortisol measurements are collected exactly 30 and 45 minutes after the injection.

A normal response is defined as a rise in serum [cortisol] to at least 425 nmol/L and an increase of at least 145 nmol/L over the basal concentration. It is advisable to collect at least two pre-test samples, at 15-minute intervals, to establish the true baseline concentration of serum [cortisol].

A normal response excludes primary adrenocortical insufficiency. Adrenocortical hypofunction secondary to hypothalamic or pituitary disease is also extremely unlikely if the response is normal since, in the prolonged absence of ACTH, the cells of the adrenal cortex would have atrophied. However, an impaired or absent response requires further investigation by a prolonged tetracosactrin test.

Emotional stress can increase serum [cortisol], so any anxiety that the patient may feel must be allayed as much as possible beforehand. Other reasons that may invalidate the test include treatment with glucocorticoids within 12 hours prior to the tetracosactrin injection, and the taking of oestrogen-containing oral contraceptives. Where a patient with suspected Addison's disease is receiving steroid therapy, it is important to prescribe a steroid which does not cross-react in the cortisol assay; dexamethasone is normally suitable (p. 283).

Confirmation of cortisol underproduction

If the response to the tetracosactrin screening test is impaired or absent, the patient should be admitted to hospital for further investigation. The serum [cortisol] at 0800 h should be measured and a prolonged (depot) tetracosactrin test is then performed. There are several ways of performing these tests, one of which is described here.

Prolonged tetracosactrin test (depot Synacthen test)

Tetracosactrin adsorbed on to a zinc phosphate complex (Synacthen depot) is used in this test; it has a longer duration of action than tetracosactrin. The principal diagnostic value of this test lies in the assessment of adrenocortical function when prolonged stimulation is needed. The patient can remain ambulant and on a normal diet throughout the test. The procedure is as follows:

Day 1 A tetracosactrin screening test is performed, as described above. As soon as the 45-minute blood specimen has been collected, 1 mg tetracosactrin zinc phosphate complex is injected intramuscularly.

Day 2 A further injection of 1 mg tetracosactrin zinc phosphate complex is given.

Day 3 As for day 2.

Day 4 A second tetracosactrin screening test is performed.

If the response on day 1 is seriously subnormal, dexamethasone (1 mg daily) can be given as steroid replacement treatment during the rest of the 4-day tetracosactrin test without affecting its interpretation.

The response is assessed by comparing the results of the first tetracosactrin screening test, performed on day 1, with the results of the second test, performed on day 4. A normal response is defined in the same way as for the tetracosactrin screening test. There should be a rise in serum [cortisol] to at least 425 nmol/L *and* an increase of at least 145 nmol/L over the basal concentration.

Subnormal or absent responses on both day 1 and day 4 indicate the presence of primary adrenocortical insufficiency. A definite but slight increase on day 4, as compared with day 1, with maximum serum [cortisol] greater than 550 nmol/L, indicates that the patient has secondary adrenocortical insufficiency. Occasionally, patients with secondary hypofunction fail to produce an adequate response to tetracosactrin after 3 days of injections, but do so if the test is continued for another 2 days.

Poor responses to prolonged tetracosactrin tests may occur in patients with hypothyroidism, whether primary due to thyroid disease or secondary to pituitary insufficiency. *In patients with hypothyroidism, adrenal function cannot be satisfactorily assessed until the thyroid deficiency has been corrected.*

Determining the cause of adrenocortical hypofunction

Plasma ACTH

Measurement of plasma [ACTH] is valuable in confirming the presence of minor degrees of primary hypofunction of the adrenal cortex. Results may be very high in these patients, and disproportionately high when related to the corresponding results for serum [cortisol]. In patients with secondary adrenocortical hypofunction, plasma [ACTH] is almost invariably low. The measurement of plasma [ACTH] thus provides the definitive way of distinguishing between primary and secondary adrenocortical hypofunction by chemical tests.

Hypothalamic–pituitary–adrenal (HPA) axis function tests

Stress in various forms normally induces an increased secretion of ACTH and corticosteroids. Patients shown to have adrenal hypofunction by the results of tests of basal secretion, but in whom the adrenal cortex responded to direct stimulation in a prolonged tetracosactrin test, can have the functional integrity of the HPA axis tested by means of an insulin-hypoglycaemia (stress) test.

Insulin-hypoglycaemia test. In patients with adrenocortical hypofunction, the initial dose of soluble insulin should be 0.10 units/kg. Indeed, this dose of insulin should be used initially whenever it seems likely that a patient might be unduly sensitive to insulin, as in patients with hypothalamic or pituitary hypofunction, or in patients who are severely undernourished (e.g. anorexia nervosa). The test is strongly contraindicated if there is unequivocal panhypopituitarism.

Apart from using a reduced dose of insulin, the test is performed as described on p. 275. For the test to be valid, it is essential to produce an adequate degree of hypoglycaemia. However, in patients with adrenocortical hypofunction, the baseline plasma [glucose] may be low and it may therefore be inappropriate to attempt to produce a rapid fall of plasma [glucose] to hypoglycaemic levels (less than 2.2 mmol/L). Instead, careful observation of the patient for symptoms of hypoglycaemia may be a safer and more satisfactory criterion for assessing the stress that has been produced by insulin injection.

An absent or impaired rise in serum [cortisol], despite the production of an adequate degree of hypoglycaemia, may be due to hypothalamic, pituitary or adrenal hypofunction. Responses are also absent or impaired in patients with anorexia nervosa, or severe malnutrition due to some other cause.

Failure to respond to the insulin-hypoglycaemia test, combined with an adequate response to a prolonged tetracosactrin test, confirms that there is secondary hypofunction of the adrenal cortex, but fails to distinguish between the pituitary or the hypothalamus, or 'higher centres', as the site of the disease.

In patients with established hypothalamic-pituitary disease or post-hypophysectomy patients, the short Synacthen test alone is adequate in predicting the requirement for glucocorticoid therapy. The insulin-hypoglycaemia test is, however, important in assessing adrenocortical function after withdrawal of long-term steroid therapy.

Other pituitary function tests

Chemical tests of pituitary, thyroid and gonadal function may help to locate the cause of adrenocortical hypofunction as, by the time hypopituitarism is severe enough to cause secondary adrenocortical hypofunction and reduced serum [cortisol], other pituitary functions will almost certainly be abnormal. It is usual in these patients, therefore, to measure basal concentrations of free T4 and TSH, LH and FSH in plasma or serum and to investigate the growth hormone response to insulin-induced hypoglycaemia (p. 297) in addition to the cortisol response.

Other tests

Adrenal antibodies. One of the causes of primary hypofunction of the adrenal cortex is auto-immune disease. A diagnosis of auto-immune Addison's disease can be made in patients who have idiopathic Addison's disease, if they have adrenal antibodies in their serum.

Electrolytes. In patients with adrenocortical hypofunction, there are important effects on electrolyte metabolism. However, changes in plasma electrolyte concentrations tend only to appear at a relatively late stage in the development both of Addison's disease and of secondary adrenocortical hypofunction.

There is loss of Na^+ in urine, the volume of ECF tends to fall, and there may be hyponatraemia; this can become severe in untreated patients, especially in Addisonian crisis. There is retention of K^+, with diminished urinary excretion and a tendency to hyperkalaemia. Acid–base disturbances are not usually observed unless complications develop (e.g. due to vomiting).

Investigations in patients being treated with steroids

There are sometimes circumstances in which it is necessary to investigate adrenocortical function while the patient is still receiving steroids. If the patient is being treated with cortisol or cortisone, the drug should be replaced by one of the more powerful synthetic steroids (e.g. dexamethasone, betamethasone), since these do not interfere with RIA measurements of serum [cortisol] or urinary [cortisol]. However, prednisone and prednisolone are not suitable, as they interfere with the cortisol assay.

Having satisfactorily stabilized the patient on the low dosage of steroid, baseline values for serum [cortisol] or 24-hour urinary cortisol excretion are determined. A prolonged tetracosactrin test is then performed. The majority of patients who are receiving long-term treatment with steroids, or who have received such treatment in the past, usually respond quickly to stimulation by tetracosactrin zinc phosphate complex injections. However, in these patients it is advisable to continue the injections (1 mg daily) for 6 days, since the adrenal response may be delayed due to suppression caused by long-term steroid therapy.

Hyperaldosteronism

Primary hyperaldosteronism, Conn's syndrome or low-renin hyperaldosteronism, is due to an adrenal adenoma in the majority of cases (65%) with bilateral nodular hyperplasia (idiopathic hyperaldosteronism) responsible for most of the rest. Adrenal carcinoma is a very rare cause of primary hyperaldosteronism.

Conn's syndrome is a rare cause of hypertension. One of the suggestive but by no means constant features is the finding of a reduced plasma $[K^+]$, which occurs in about 80–90% of patients. The depletion of K^+, consequent upon renal loss, has several effects, principally muscle weakness and renal tubular defects; more severe hypokalaemia can lead to life-threatening cardiac arrhythmias. There are, however, other causes of hypertension occurring in association with a reduced plasma $[K^+]$ (e.g. diuretic therapy), and these need to be considered in the differential diagnosis.

Secondary hyperaldosteronism occurs much more commonly than primary but, unlike primary hyperaldosteronism, it is only sometimes associated with hypertension. It is due to conditions which stimulate the secretion of renin, possibly caused by an abnormality of Na^+ metabolism.

Secondary hyperaldosteronism occurs in association with a wide range of disorders that do not directly involve the adrenal cortex. These include Na^+ deprivation, K^+ excess, haemorrhage, congestive cardiac failure, the nephrotic syndrome, cirrhosis with ascites, and renal artery stenosis. In many of these conditions the diagnosis is clear, and there is no need to consider investigating the renin–angiotensin–aldosterone system. Probably the commonest cause of secondary hyperaldosteronism is diuretic therapy.

Investigation of primary hyperaldosteronism

The definitive identification of primary hyperaldosteronism depends on investigations which are expensive and of limited availability. It is important, therefore, to undertake preliminary studies designed to show whether primary hyperaldosteronism is likely to be present. These screening studies depend on the fact that aldosterone causes retention of Na^+ by the kidney, associated with loss of K^+ and H^+ in the urine. The changes in plasma $[K^+]$ are potentially of greatest diagnostic value.

Plasma potassium

This is the principal investigation used for initial screening. Essential precautions include finding out whether the patient is being treated with diuretics, which may lower plasma $[K^+]$, and ensuring that no form of liquorice or carbenoxolone preparation is being taken since these stimulate mineralocorticoid receptors directly, thereby producing a syndrome similar to primary hyperaldosteronism. Ideally, plasma $[K^+]$ should be measured either before the patient starts treatment with hypotensive drugs or diuretics, or after the patient has been taken off such treatment (and off liquorice, etc.) for at least 1 month. Care must also be taken to prevent spuriously high plasma $[K^+]$, by avoiding venous stasis and forearm exercise when collecting blood specimens; it is important to measure *plasma* $[K^+]$, not serum $[K^+]$, in these patients.

The finding of a reduced plasma $[K^+]$ in an untreated hypertensive patient is an important first step in the diagnostic process. It may be lower than 3.0 mmol/L, but values of 3.3 mmol/L and below should be regarded as suspicious. There may also be a slight increase in plasma $[Na^+]$, a mild metabolic alkalosis, and urinary K^+ excretion that is inappropriately high in the presence of hypokalaemia.

Primary aldosteronism is occasionally associated with an intermittently reduced plasma $[K^+]$. If the first result is normal but the diagnosis is still considered probable on clinical grounds, plasma $[K^+]$ should be measured again at intervals of a few weeks. Alternatively, or additionally, patients can be placed on a high Na^+ intake (150–200 mmol/day) for 2 weeks, after which plasma $[K^+]$ is measured again. Patients who develop hypokalaemia should be further investigated.

Special investigations

Patients requiring further investigation will be hypertensive and will have had certain other causes of hypertension excluded (e.g. phaeochromocytoma, coarctation of the aorta). Also, they will have been found to have hypokalaemia, or to be liable to develop hypokalaemia in the presence of an Na^+ load. Other causes of hypokalaemia (e.g. diuretics, laxatives, liquorice) should have been excluded.

Plasma renin activity (PRA). Primary hyperaldosteronism can be distinguished from secondary hyperaldosteronism by measuring either PRA or angiotensin II. We prefer to base the initial distinction on PRA measurements. The reasons for preferring PRA measurements are:

1   The rate-limiting factor in the formation of angiotensin II is PRA, except in patients with severe liver disease in whom synthesis of renin substrate may be so reduced as to make plasma [renin substrate] the rate-limiting factor.

2   Renin has a half-life in plasma of 20 minutes, whereas the half-life of angiotensin II is only 1 minute.

3   Plasma renin activity assays are more widely available than angiotensin II.

It is common practice for PRA and aldosterone measurements to be requested at the same time, whenever the index of suspicion of primary hyperaldosteronism is high. Differentiation between primary and secondary hyperaldosteronism can then be made on the basis of the PRA results:

1   *If PRA is low*, the patient may have primary hyperaldosteronism. Further

investigation of these patients requires measurement of plasma [aldosterone] or 24-hour urinary excretion of aldosterone, or both. If results for these tests are high, this confirms the diagnosis.

2 *If PRA is high*, the patient has secondary hyperaldosteronism and steps should be taken to identify its cause, if not already apparent.

Distinction between adenoma and hyperplasia

It is important to distinguish between an aldosterone-producing adenoma, the commonest cause of Conn's syndrome, and idiopathic adrenal hyperplasia. Adenomas are curable by surgery whereas surgery only occasionally cures patients with adrenal hyperplasia.

Adrenal vein sampling with measurement of the aldosterone : cortisol ratio can be used to localize an adenoma. If the patient has an adenoma, the ratio is higher in the adrenal vein draining this gland than in the inferior vena cava whereas the contralateral gland shows suppression, with the aldosterone : cortisol ratio being lower in its adrenal vein than in the inferior vena cava. In contrast, the aldosterone : cortisol ratio is higher in both adrenal veins than in the inferior vena cava in patients with idiopathic adrenal hyperplasia.

An alternative method is to measure the plasma [aldosterone] at 0800 h, before the patient gets up, and again at 1130 h after being up and about. For this test, it is important that the patient should be 'volume expanded'; this is achieved by the prior administration of a high Na^+ diet plus a mineralocorticoid (e.g. fludrocortisone). In patients with idiopathic adrenal hyperplasia the plasma [aldosterone] is higher at 1130 h, whereas plasma [aldosterone] is lower at 1130 h in patients who have an adenoma. This difference between the two causes of Conn's syndrome may depend upon the fact that, whereas the hyperplastic gland is still under some degree of renin–angiotensin control, the adenoma is predominantly under ACTH control. Since ACTH levels are falling over the period 0800 h to 1130 h, plasma [aldosterone] also falls; any residual renin–angiotensin regulation of the adenoma can be minimized by the prior volume expansion.

Congenital adrenal hyperplasia

Striking anatomical changes take place in the adrenal cortex immediately after birth; these are associated with marked alterations in the pattern of steroid output. There is a period of transition during the first 6 months of an infant's life, during which the pattern of fetal steroid metabolism changes to the normal childhood pattern, which closely resembles the adult pattern. Soon after delivery, cortisol begins to be synthesized by the infant's adrenal cortex at a rate similar to that found in adults, if corrected for the surface area of the body, and the infant adrenal becomes fully able to respond normally to stress.

Several inherited enzymic defects affecting the synthesis of cortisol have been identified in congenital adrenal hyperplasia (CAH). These mostly relate to the hydroxylation reactions in the final stages of steroid biosynthesis. However, other defects have been described that affect earlier stages in the synthetic pathway (i.e. 20,22-desmolase and 3β-hydroxysteroid dehydrogenase defects). In a patient with CAH, the defect is usually a deficiency of a single enzyme. All the conditions that comprise CAH are rare, and the non-virilizing group is extremely rare. Only the commoner conditions will be considered here.

21-hydroxylase defect (Fig. 18.5)

Classical CAH results from a defect in 21-hydroxylase (OH-21) activity and is an autosomal recessive disorder with an incidence of about one in 10 000 live births in Caucasians. This enzyme is a microsomal cytochrome P450. Defective activity may lead to cortisol deficiency with resulting increased compensatory secretion of ACTH and overproduction of the precursors to the block, 17α-hydroxy-progesterone (17α-OHP) and 17α-hydroxypregnenolone; 17,20-lyase activity leads to excessive conversion of these precursors to androstenedione and dehydroepiandrosterone, respectively.

Androstenedione is a moderately strong androgen which can be converted in peripheral tissues to testosterone. Hence, in more severe defects of 21-hydroxylase, the effects of androgen excess may lead to virilization of the female

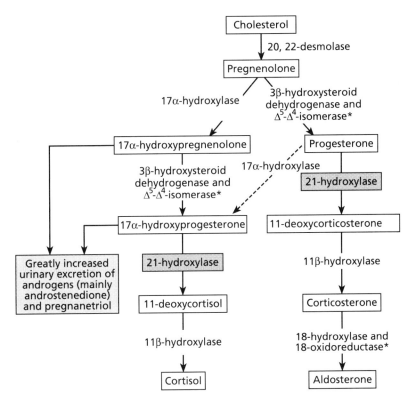

Fig. 18.5 The pathways in the synthesis of cortisol and aldosterone from cholesterol, showing the sites of the enzymic block in congenital adrenal hyperplasia that are due to the 21-hydroxylase defect, and the principal steroids that are excreted in abnormal amounts in this disease. The enzymes that are marked with asterisks are single enzymes that possess both the catalytic activities that the names describe.

fetus and to precocious sexual development in the male. About 50–75% of the severe defects also have an associated defect in aldosterone biosynthesis, with salt wasting and potential adrenal crisis. The increased ACTH secretion leads to hyperplasia of the adrenal glands.

The clinical presentation is variable and several clinical forms have been recognized; these are the classical salt-losing form, the simple virilizing form, and a late-onset form. In the simple, virilizing variant, sufficient aldosterone is produced to prevent salt depletion. Genetic analysis has established that the OH-21 gene is closely linked to the HLA major histocompatibility complex on the short arm of chromosome 6. Two OH-21 genes are recognized, OH-21A and OH-21B, adjacent to genes coding for the fourth component of complement. The product of OH-21B is the active OH-21 enzyme, whereas the OH-21A gene-product does not appear to be active in steroidogenesis; it is a pseudogene. A number of mutants have been recognized, including deletion of the active OH-21B gene and conversion of the active OH-21B to the inactive OH-21A gene, in addition to point-mutations leading to an inactive gene-product. The relationship of these different genetic disorders to the different clinical presentations is not yet clearly defined.

Diagnosis

This is usually confirmed by measuring plasma [17α-OHP]. However, it is important not to collect the blood specimen until at least 48 hours after birth since plasma [17α-OHP] is usually increased till then because of the continuing presence of 17α-OHP of maternal origin. Plasma [17α-OHP] is normally less than 15 nmol/L; in patients with 21-hydroxylase deficiency, it is usually over 100 nmol/ L, and may exceed 1000 nmol/L. Urinary excretion of pregnanetriol is usually greatly increased. Plasma [17α-OHP] may also be considerably raised in premature and in sick infants in the absence of CAH.

Prenatal diagnosis is possible by measurement of amniotic fluid [17α-OHP] and HLA-typing of amniotic cells. However, both methods require amniocentesis at about 16 weeks' gestation, by which time female virilization will have occurred. Although amenable to treatment after birth, it would clearly be preferable to prevent the intra-uterine development of ambiguous genitalia in affected females (with the potential need for corrective surgery). There is some evidence that administration of dexamethasone to the mother of an affected female child from 10 weeks' gestation can, by suppressing ACTH production, prevent excessive androgen secretion. Such an approach would depend upon chorionic villus sampling before the end of 10 weeks' gestation combined with HLA-linkage analysis or direct probing of the OH-21 gene.

Neonatal screening for 21-hydroxylase deficiency is possible, using a micro-scale filter-paper assay of blood [17α-OHP]. This extension of the Guthrie test (p. 329) has not been widely adopted, but it may be justified in areas of high incidence (e.g. Alaska).

Treatment

Since the overproduction of cortisol precursors and their metabolites is due to failure of the negative feedback control mechanism, treatment with glucocorticoids (e.g. cortisol) suppresses the excessive output of ACTH. In turn, this limits the excessive androgen production, though adequate androgen suppression may only be possible at the expense of iatrogenic Cushing's syndrome. Where salt loss is marked, it may also be necessary to administer a mineralocorticoid. The biochemical effectiveness of treatment can be assessed by measuring plasma [17α-OHP] or [androstenedione] or urinary pregnanetriol excretion; these rapidly revert to normal if cortisol dosage is adequate.

11β-hydroxylase defect (Fig. 18.6)

This accounts for most of the remaining 10% of cases of congenital adrenal hyperplasia. The block in synthesis of cortisol, at 11-deoxycortisol, leads to increased excretion of metabolites of 11-deoxycortisol and, to a lesser extent, metabolites of its precursor, 17α-OHP. Plasma 11-deoxycortisol measurements provide the diagnostic test.

The 11β-hydroxylase (OH-11) defect is usually only partial, and the nature of the clinical presentation is influenced by the severity of the defect. Adequate

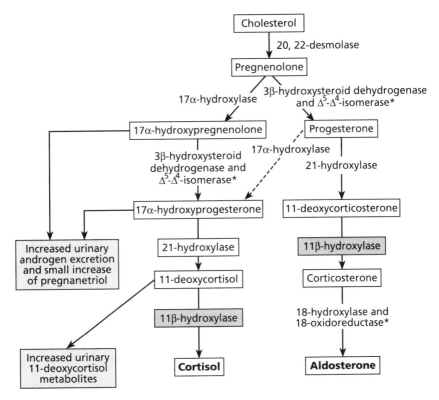

Fig. 18.6. The pathways in the synthesis of cortisol and aldosterone from cholesterol, showing the sites of the enzymic block in congenital adrenal hyperplasia due to the 11β-hydroxylase defect, and the principal steroids that are excreted in abnormal amounts in this disease. The enzymes marked with asterisks are single enzymes that possess both the catalytic activities that the names describe.

amounts of cortisol are usually synthesized in response to the increased output of ACTH by the pituitary. The block on the pathway to aldosterone synthesis leads to a build-up of 11-deoxycorticosterone and this is responsible for the hypertension which may be a feature of 11β-hydroxylase deficiency.

As with 21-hydroxylase deficiency, pre-natal diagnosis is possible by measurement of amniotic fluid [17α-OHP]. The genetics of OH-11 deficiency are less well understood than for 21-hydroxylase deficiency; it is known that the gene is located on chromosome 8 and is, therefore, not HLA-linked. Restriction fragment length polymorphisms (p. 355) have been used to follow segregation of the defect within affected families.

Phaeochromocytoma

These tumours arise from chromaffin cells. In 90% of cases they are in the adrenal medulla; the remaining extra-adrenal tumours can occur anywhere from the base of the brain to the testes. About 5% of tumours are bilateral. They secrete excessive amounts of either noradrenaline or adrenaline, but usually both these catecholamines, and there is excessive excretion of catecholamines and their metabolites in the urine. The tumours may produce marked pharmacological effects.

Phaeochromocytoma is a rare cause of hypertension. Characteristically, this is episodic. Even when the hypertension is present all the time, episodic attacks of symptoms (e.g. headache, pallor, palpitations, sweating) tend to occur. These features are important, when selecting the time for collecting specimens for laboratory investigation.

Phaeochromocytoma sometimes occurs as a familial condition, in association with medullary carcinoma of the thyroid, and quite often also with hyperparathyroidism in the MEN IIa syndrome (p. 265).

Urinary catecholamines and metabolites

Chemical tests usually involve measurement of 24-hour urinary excretion of catecholamine metabolites, mostly excreted as their 3-O-methyl derivatives (metadrenaline and normetadrenaline) and as 4-hydroxy, 3-methoxy mandelic acid (HMMA), the metabolite normally excreted in the largest amount. 'Total metadrenalines' in urine are usually about 10–20% of HMMA output. Only small amounts of catecholamines are excreted unchanged or conjugated. Most laboratories routinely perform one (occasionally more) of the following investigations:

1 *Metadrenaline and normetadrenaline*, and their conjugated derivatives. Many laboratories measure 'total metadrenalines' ('total metanephrines'), which include metadrenaline and normetadrenaline and their conjugates. A few laboratories determine these metabolites separately. Methods can be adapted for use as screening tests, with a false-negative rate of only 1–2%.

2 *HMMA*, sometimes still wrongly called vanillyl mandelic acid (VMA), is a widely available investigation. Formed from both noradrenaline and adrenaline, HMMA measurements cannot be used to estimate the separate output of the individual catecholamines.

3 *Noradrenaline and adrenaline*, and their conjugated derivatives. A few laboratories measure total urinary catecholamines, after hydrolysing the conjugates; very few measure noradrenaline and adrenaline separately. These measurements are technically difficult.

Most patients in whom there is a phaeochromocytoma can be diagnosed on the basis of an increased 24-hour urinary excretion of 'total metadrenalines' or HMMA. However, it can be difficult to decide the significance of slightly increased outputs, since these may also occur in patients with essential hypertension and in otherwise healthy individuals subjected to stress.

Performance of urine excretion tests

Several points concerning the collection and timing of urine specimens for catecholamine investigations should be noted:

1 *Drugs.* Many drugs increase the release of catecholamines (e.g. vasodilators, diuretics); others decrease the amounts released (e.g. reserpine) or affect their metabolism (e.g. monoamine oxidase inhibitors). Some drugs (e.g. methyldopa, labetalol) interfere with some analytical methods. Patients should preferably be investigated for phaeochromocytoma *before* drug treatment is started.

2 *Diet.* Some analytical methods are liable to interference from certain dietary constituents. The laboratory's requirements for any dietary restriction must be observed.

3 *Timing of urine collections* is important, in order to minimize the number of false-negative results. *Where the clinical index of suspicion is high*:

(a) *Patients who have 'attacks'.* If the patient is normotensive between attacks, a single baseline set of measurements should be made, and the patient instructed to start a second 24-hour urine collection when the next 'attack' occurs.

(b) *Patients with persistent hypertension.* Determination of 24-hour urinary excretion of catecholamines or metabolites need only be performed once.

Where the clinical index of suspicion is low (e.g. a middle-aged or elderly patient presenting with hypertension, but without paroxysmal symptoms), there is little or no justification for requesting these investigations. Hypertension is common and phaeochromocytoma is rare. In general, *only with young patients who are hypertensive is screening of urine specimens worthwhile* for abnormal excretion of catecholamines or their metabolites.

Plasma catecholamines

This measurement is becoming more widely available. In some studies, it has been found to be a more sensitive test for phaeochromocytoma than the urinary metabolite determinations just described, but this has not been universal experience. Plasma and urinary measurements provide different information.

Urinary excretion of catecholamines and their metabolites relate to total catecholamine production during the collection period. Plasma measurements only reflect catecholamine output in the previous few minutes; plasma free noradrenaline has a half-life of about 2 minutes in plasma. Thus, if a tumour is secreting catecholamines intermittently, plasma measurements may fail to detect any abnormality whereas results for urinary measurements may be abnormally high.

Plasma catecholamine measurements can be used to help localize an extra-adrenal phaeochromocytoma, by determining concentrations in blood specimens obtained from veins draining possible tumour sites. However, this is rarely needed as CT scanning and imaging techniques are usually more satisfactory for this purpose. If plasma catecholamines are to be requested, strict attention to the sampling procedures (as detailed by the laboratory) is essential.

Comments on Case 18.1 (p. 278)

These results are consistent with a diagnosis of Cushing's syndrome due to an adrenal adenoma or nodular adrenal hyperplasia. These tumours account for 5–10% of all cases of Cushing's syndrome.

Ultrasound examination, CT and ^{75}Se-cholesterol scans confirmed the presence of an adrenal tumour in the right adrenal, and the patient was treated successfully by right adrenalectomy.

Chapter 19
Hypothalamic and Pituitary Hormones

The hormones and factors secreted by the hypothalamus, and the corresponding hormones secreted by the pituitary, will be considered in this chapter. As far as the anterior pituitary hormones are concerned, much valuable information can be obtained from measurements of hormones secreted by their target glands (e.g. T4 and T3, cortisol, gonadal steroids), and this information considered collectively may provide chemical evidence pointing to disease in the hypothalamic-pituitary region. Investigation of the functions of these target glands is considered in other chapters, where the value of measurements of TSH, ACTH, FSH and LH are also discussed. The insulin-hypoglycaemia test for assessing the hypothalamic–pituitary–adrenal axis is also described elsewhere (p. 275, 282).

Hypothalamic and anterior pituitary hormones

The hypothalamus secretes several hormones or factors. These control the release of hormones from the anterior pituitary, in some cases by stimulating hormonal release and in others by inhibiting it (Table 19.1). The hormones produced by the target glands controlled by the anterior pituitary may exert negative feedback effects on the secretion of the corresponding hypothalamic hormone (e.g. plasma

Table 19.1 Hypothalamic and anterior pituitary hormones and factors

Hypothalamic stimulating hormone or factor	Anterior pituitary hormones(s) released	Feedback control hormone or compound
Corticotrophin-releasing hormone (CRH) and factors	ACTH β-Lipotrophin (LPH)	Cortisol Cortisol
Growth hormone-releasing factor (GH-RF)	Growth hormone (GH)	GH release-inhibiting hormone
Gonadotrophin-releasing hormone (Gn-RH)	Follicle-stimulating hormone (FSH) Luteinizing hormone (LH)	Gonadal steroids and inhibin Gonadal steroids
No stimulating factor identified	Prolactin	Prolactin release-inhibiting hormone, dopamine
Thyrotrophin-releasing hormone (TRH)	Thyroid-stimulating hormone (TSH) (and prolactin)	Free T4, free T3

[free cortisol] influences the output of CRH). Release of hypothalamic hormones is also influenced by stimuli from higher CNS centres.

Thyrotrophin-releasing hormone (TRH) and TSH

TRH is a tripeptide, pyroglutamyl-histidyl-prolinamide; it controls the secretion of thyrotrophin or thyroid-stimulating hormone (TSH) by the anterior pituitary. Release of TRH is influenced by plasma [free T4], but free T4 exerts its main feedback effects directly on TSH secretion (Fig. 17.3, p. 251).

TSH is a glycoprotein (M_r, 28 kDa) composed of an α-subunit that is common to LH, FSH and hCG, and a β-subunit specific to TSH. The place of TSH measurements in the investigation of thyroid function has been discussed in Chapter 17.

TRH test

The TRH test can be used to confirm or exclude a provisional diagnosis of hyperthyroidism. However, it has been largely replaced for this purpose by sensitive and specific immunometric assay methods for measuring plasma [TSH] (p. 252). The main indication for the TRH test is for the investigation of pituitary function in patients thought to have secondary hypothyroidism.

To perform the test, 200 μg TRH is injected intravenously. Blood is taken for measuring plasma or serum [TSH] before the injection (basal level) and 20 and 60 minutes after the injection. In normal subjects, serum [TSH] increases by more than 2 mU/L above the basal level at 20 minutes with maximal values falling between 4 and 30 mU/L. At 60 minutes the serum [TSH] has normally returned to below the 20-minute value and lies in the range 3–24 mU/L.

In the absence of hyperthyroidism, a TSH response of less than 2 mU/L is an indication of pituitary disease, but a normal response is found in about 50% of patients with pituitary disease.

Thyrotroph adenoma

These are very rare pituitary tumours, characterized by increased plasma [thyroid hormones] in the presence of increased plasma [TSH], or at least a plasma [TSH] that is inappropriately high in the presence of increased plasma [free T4] and [free T3]. These findings may also be reported in patients who have abnormal nuclear T3 receptors.

Serum [α-subunits] of TSH are increased, often markedly, in patients with thyrotroph adenomas whereas normal concentrations are present in patients with abnormal T3 receptors. Serum [α-subunits] may also be slightly increased in healthy post-menopausal women.

Gonadotrophin-releasing hormone (Gn-RH), FSH and LH

Gn-RH is a decapeptide released from the hypothalamus in pulses into the hypothalamic-hypophyseal portal circulation. The release of Gn-RH is modified by oestrogens, progesterone and androgens. A Gn-RH test similar to the TRH test can be used to investigate gonadotrophin reserve.

Follicle-stimulating hormone (FSH) and luteinizing hormone (LH) are glycoproteins, each containing a common α-subunit (shared with TSH and hCG) and a specific β-subunit responsible for hormone action. Secretion of both FSH and LH is controlled by Gn-RH, and in males inhibin exerts an additional control on FSH release. LH is released in pulses at 5–20-minute intervals; the release of FSH is less pulsatile.

FSH and LH measurements are important in the investigation of gonadal failure; they help to differentiate primary failure of the gonads from failure secondary to pituitary dysfunction (pp. 305, 308). In organic pituitary disease, the ability to secrete FSH and LH are among the earliest functions to be lost.

After the menopause, plasma [FSH] and [LH] both increase, but in the child-bearing period increased plasma [FSH] and [LH] indicate gonadal failure.

Gn-RH test

This test is often normal even in the presence of clinical hypogonadism. It may, however, be of value in the investigation of delayed puberty. There is no point in performing the test when there are raised basal gonadotrophin levels.

In the Gn-RH test, a basal blood sample is obtained before giving the patient an intravenous injection of 50 µg Gn-RH; further blood samples are collected at 20 and 60 minutes. Peak levels of plasma [LH] are 10–40 IU/L in both sexes; peak levels of plasma [FSH] are 5–25 IU/L in females and 2–14 IU/L in males. The FSH : LH response ratio is usually greater than one when delayed puberty results from hypopituitarism, but less than one in constitutional delayed puberty. Subnormal responses may be seen in Cushing's syndrome as well as in hypopituitarism.

Gonadotroph adenoma

These tumours may arise as a result of long-standing gonadal failure (e.g. Klinefelter syndrome). There is an increased plasma [FSH] but low concentrations of gonadal steroids in plasma. Plasma [LH] is normal or low. There is usually enlargement of the pituitary fossa.

Corticotrophin-releasing hormone (CRH) and ACTH

CRH is composed of 41 amino acids. It is the main component among a number of corticotrophin-releasing factors (CRF) involved in the control of the pituitary–adrenal axis. Its release is subject to negative feedback control by plasma [free cortisol] (Fig. 18.1, p. 268). A CRH (or CRF) test has been described (see below) that helps sometimes to differentiate Cushing's disease from adrenal tumours and from ectopic ACTH-secreting tumours (p. 277).

ACTH is a polypeptide of 39 amino acids (M_r, 5600 Da); its biological activity is contained in the 24 amino acids at the N-terminal end (p. 280). Secretion of ACTH is controlled by CRH. ACTH and β-lipotrophin (β-LPH, 93 amino acids) exist next to each other at the C-terminal end of a much larger precursor molecule, pro-opiomelanocortin. Separating β-LPH from the pro-ACTH component, and similarly separating the ACTH component from pro-γ-MSH (melanocyte-stimulating hormone), are residues of two basic amino acids, lysine and arginine. Proteolysis appears to occur simultaneously at these sites, releasing ACTH and β-LPH into the circulation. In ectopic ACTH production, it seems that there is abnormal processing of pro-opiomelanocortin resulting in the release of 'big ACTH'.

There is a nychthemeral rhythm of ACTH output by the pituitary. This, in turn, is responsible for the rhythm in the secretion of cortisol (Fig. 18.2, p. 269). Specimens for measuring plasma [ACTH] must be collected under specified conditions (p. 270). These measurements are of value in the investigation of adrenocortical hyperfunction (p. 275) and in differentiating between primary and secondary adrenocortical hypofunction (p. 282).

CRH stimulation test

Corticotrophin-releasing hormone (CRH) can be used to test the response, measured as changes in plasma [ACTH] and serum [cortisol], following an intravenous injection of CRH. In this test, a basal blood sample is obtained before the patient is given a rapid injection of 100 µg synthetic CRH. In normal individuals, the peak serum [cortisol] occurs 60 minutes after the injection and does not exceed 820 nmol/L.

Patients with Cushing's disease have been reported as showing an exaggerated response to CRH; serum [cortisol] either exceeds 820 nmol/L after CRH, or rises more than 25% above the basal level in patients in whom the basal serum [cortisol] is greater than 820 nmol/L. Little or no response to CRH has been reported as occurring in patients with Cushing's syndrome due to ectopic ACTH production or to adrenal tumour. As with the other chemical tests described, however, there is overlap between these groups of patients and the value of the CRH stimulation test is still not fully established.

Growth hormone

Growth hormone (GH) is a polypeptide (M_r, 21 kDa). It is structurally similar to prolactin and human placental lactogen. Its functions are to stimulate protein synthesis and growth; it also has metabolic effects that oppose the action of insulin (Table 11.2, p. 163).

Release of GH is stimulated by GH-RF and inhibited by somatostatin. Hypothalamic GH-RF has not been characterized but two factors which cause acromegaly have been isolated from pancreatic tumours. Somatostatin inhibits the release of several pituitary hormones, including GH and TSH. GH release can also be suppressed by high doses of glucose and this response is used in the investigation of suspected acromegaly and giantism.

Measurement of basal plasma [GH] is of little value as it cannot be detected in more than 50% of normal individuals by present assay methods. Increases in plasma [GH] can be caused by stress or exercise and this forms the basis of the insulin-hypoglycaemia stress-response test.

Insulin-hypoglycaemia test

This is the best of the stress tests of anterior pituitary function, as the stress can be standardized. It is used for the investigation of suspected hypopituitarism in adults and of short stature in children. The test is performed as described on p. 275 but the initial dose of insulin is reduced to 0.10 units/kg. The response, when used as a pituitary function test, can be assessed by measuring serum [cortisol] or plasma [ACTH], or both, as well as plasma [GH]. Normally, hypoglycaemia causes a marked increase in plasma [GH] to more than 20 mU/L, but this increase is not observed in severe pituitary dysfunction. A limited response, with plasma [GH] rising to less than 20 mU/L, may be observed in patients with partial pituitary failure. It is more convenient to measure serum [cortisol] than plasma [ACTH]; maximal cortisol levels should normally exceed 425 nmol/L, with an increment above basal of greater than 145 nmol/L.

Acromegaly and giantism

These disorders are caused by adenomas of the anterior pituitary. Giantism results if the disorder occurs before closure of the epiphyses of the long bones, acromegaly if it occurs after their closure.

Basal plasma [GH] is often very high in these patients, but the concentrations are too variable for accurate diagnosis. In all these patients, the diagnosis should be confirmed by measuring the response of plasma [GH] to an oral glucose tolerance test (p. 166). Normally, plasma [GH] falls to less than 2 mU/L at some time during this test. However, in patients with acromegaly or giantism, plasma [GH] does not fall in response to the stimulus of hyperglycaemia, and may even increase.

Prolactin

This hormone is distinct from growth hormone, but the two have some common structural features. Prolactin is a single polypeptide (M_r, 22.5 kDa), secreted by the lactotrophs. It is responsible for lactation, and has a role in the complex processes controlling gonadal function.

Prolactin secretion is pulsatile and is normally under tonic inhibitory control (unlike the other pituitary hormones) by one or more prolactin release-inhibiting hormones (PRIH), the most important of which is dopamine. Prolactin secretion increases in response to oestrogens and to suckling.

There is a nychthemeral rhythm of prolactin secretion, with highest levels during sleep and lowest between 0900 h and 1200 h. Superimposed on these gradual changes, there are occasional sharp (pulsatile) increases in plasma [prolactin]. Increases also occur in response to stress. It can, therefore, be difficult to interpret the results of single measurements. Plasma [prolactin] is much higher in women of child-bearing age, especially during pregnancy, than it is in girls before puberty, in post-menopausal women or in males.

There are many causes of hyperprolactinaemia other than pituitary disease (Table 19.2). Before collecting blood for measuring plasma [prolactin], it is particularly important to enquire about the intake of drugs.

Prolactin measurements should be performed in the investigation of amenorrhoea, oligomenorrhoea and subfertility, whether or not there is galactorrhoea (p. 308). Plasma [prolactin] should also be measured in any patient with spontaneous inappropriate lactation. A significant proportion of subfertile female patients have hyperprolactinaemia; these may respond to bromocriptine (a dopamine agonist) therapy.

Pituitary tumours

Plasma [prolactin] greater than 700 mU/L (reference range, 60–390 mU/L) may indicate the presence of a pituitary tumour. However, before this interpretation is made, the measurement must be repeated as a high result may represent a response to stress, and other non-pathological causes of a raised level should also be eliminated (Table 19.2).

Pituitary tumours may secrete prolactin directly (prolactinoma) or, alternatively, a non-prolactin-secreting tumour may give rise to hyperprolactinaemia because the tumour exerts pressure on the pituitary stalk and prevents dopamine from reaching the pituitary from the hypothalamus.

Prolactinomas only secrete prolactin; in many of these patients no other evidence of pituitary dysfunction can be detected. Approximately one-third of prolactinomas are associated with moderate increases in plasma [prolactin], in the range 700–1000 mU/L, but basal levels of plasma [prolactin] greater than 1000 mU/L strongly suggest that a tumour is present. If, in addition, radiological abnormalities are visible in the pituitary fossa, this supports the diagnosis of prolactinoma rather than functional hyperprolactinaemia in these patients.

Increased plasma [prolactin] occurs in some patients with acromegaly, when there is a tumour that secretes both GH and prolactin. Also, some ectopic hormone-secreting tumours produce prolactin.

Melanocyte-stimulating hormone (MSH)

Pro-opiomelanocortin contains within its molecule three components with MSH activity: α-MSH in the ACTH component, β-MSH in the LPH component, and a

Table 19.2 Causes of hyperprolactinaemia

Category of cause	Examples
Physiological	Pregnancy
	Suckling
	Stress
Drugs	
(a) Dopamine receptor-blocking agents	Phenothiazines
	Butyrophenones
	Tricyclic antidepressants
	Metoclopramide
(b) Dopamine-depleting drugs	Methyldopa
	Reserpine
(c) Histamine receptor agonists	Cimetidine
(d) Monoamine oxidase inhibitors	Phenelzine
	Isocarboxazid
Pathological	Prolactinoma
	Other pituitary tumours
	Idiopathic
	Chronic renal failure
	Primary hypothyroidism

Case 19.1

A 31-year-old nurse was admitted to hospital with severe renal colic, which was treated satisfactorily. During her admission, however, it was noted that she had a Cushingoid appearance and excessive bruising on her forearms; she was also hypertensive. Her urinary cortisol : creatinine ratio was measured and was found to be 120 µmol/mol (reference range, < 50 µmol/mol). Her discharge from hospital was delayed by an acute psychiatric episode. She was later readmitted for further investigation of the provisional diagnosis of Cushing's syndrome, when the following results were obtained:

Test	Time	Result	Reference range
Nychthemeral rhythm	0800 h	470 nmol/L	160–565 nmol/L
of serum [cortisol]	2200 h	485 nmol/L	Up to 205 nmol/L

Insulin-hypoglycaemia test		Basal value	Maximum response
Plasma [glucose]		3.7 mmol/L	1.2 mmol/L after 30 min
Serum [cortisol]		470 nmol/L	510 nmol/L after 60 min

Dexamethasone	Basal value	After 48 h on	After 48 h on
suppression tests		0.5 mg q.i.d.	2 mg q.i.d.
Serum [cortisol]	565 nmol/L	370 nmol/L	65 nmol/L

Plasma [ACTH] at 0800 h: 15 mU/L (reference range, 2–20 mU/L)

How would you interpret these results? Are there other hormone investigations that you would consider appropriate in this patient? This patient is discussed on p. 301.

third component with melanocyte-stimulating activity, γ-MSH. The importance of these various peptides with MSH activity is unknown. Whether or not they are at least partly the cause of the excessive pigmentation that occurs (e.g. in the mouth, limb flexures) in Addison's disease, for instance, is uncertain; ACTH also possesses melanocyte-stimulating activity.

Some patients with pituitary dysfunction (e.g. Cushing's disease, Nelson's syndrome) show excessive pigmentation as do some patients with ectopic ACTH-secreting tumours. In most of these patients, changes in plasma [ACTH] and plasma [MSH] occur in parallel.

Anterior pituitary disease and its investigation

A wide range of diseases can affect the anterior pituitary and result in localized or diffuse lesions. Pituitary dysfunction can be manifest by either excessive hormone production or hormone deficiency; in both cases, one or more of the pituitary hormones may be affected. In some patients, pituitary failure may be secondary to hypothalamic disease.

Hypopituitarism

The most common causes of hypopituitarism are pituitary tumour, particularly prolactin-secreting tumours, and therapeutic action such as the removal of a pituitary tumour or irradiation. Failure may be total (panhypopituitarism) or partial, in which case secretion of one or more pituitary hormones is retained. Specific congenital deficiencies in the production of anterior pituitary hormones do occur and deficiencies of GH, LH, FSH, ACTH and TSH have all been described; these are all rare.

Initially, impairment of function will usually only be revealed by the use of stimulation tests. Later, basal concentrations of the pituitary hormones in blood will be affected. In general, the secretion of GH, LH and FSH are affected relatively early in disease involving the anterior pituitary, whereas ACTH, TSH and prolactin are not affected until much later.

Some basal measurements may provide diagnostic information prior to performing dynamic tests. Plasma [free T4] may be decreased and plasma [TSH] normal or decreased in secondary hypothyroidism, and plasma LH, FSH and sex steroid concentrations may all be diminished in secondary hypogonadism. The presence of a prolactin concentration of over 700 mU/L may indicate the presence of a pituitary tumour and suggests the need for further investigation.

Combined pituitary function test

When hypopituitarism is thought to be very probable, a combined test of pituitary function may be performed to assess the anterior pituitary reserve for ACTH, GH, FSH and LH production. In this test, a blood sample is collected for measurement of basal serum FSH, LH, oestradiol-17β or testosterone, cortisol, TSH, free T4, GH and prolactin concentrations. Insulin (0.10 units/kg), TRH (200 µg) and Gn-RH (50 µg) are then injected and further blood specimens are collected at 20, 30, 60, 90 and 120 minutes. Responses in this combined function test are interpreted in the same way as when the tests are performed separately.

Hyperfunction

This is almost always restricted to the overproduction of one hormone, by a pituitary adenoma. In all patients where the presence of an adenoma has been established, the functional reserve of the anterior pituitary for the production of its other hormones should be assessed.

Posterior pituitary hormones

The posterior pituitary is an integral part of the neurohypophysis. Its secretion is directly subject to nervous control. It produces at least two hormones, arginine vasopressin (AVP), often called the antidiuretic hormone (ADH), and oxytocin. Investigation of posterior pituitary function is mainly based on tests affected by the output of AVP.

Arginine vasopressin (AVP)

Synthesized in the hypothalamus and combined with neurophysin II, the AVP-containing neurosecretory granules migrate to the posterior pituitary. AVP, a nonapeptide (M_r, about 1000 Da), is normally released in response either to a rise in plasma osmolality or to a fall in ECF volume. It increases the permeability of the distal tubules and collecting ducts of the kidney to water.

The syndrome of inappropriate secretion of ADH (SIADH) is defined as the excessive secretion of AVP (or ADH) in the absence of either of the normal major stimuli for AVP secretion. This syndrome gives rise to water retention, dilutional hyponatraemia and reduced osmolality of the ECF and ICF (p. 42). The finding of plasma [Na$^+$] less than 125 mmol/L, accompanied by a urine osmolality that is inappropriately high, supports the diagnosis. Determination of plasma [AVP] confirms the diagnosis, but can only be performed by a few laboratories.

Overproduction of AVP may occur in association with head injury, cerebral tumour, cerebral abscess, pneumonia, pulmonary tuberculosis, acute porphyria, ectopic hormone-secreting tumours, hypothyroidism, hypoadrenalism, the Guillain–Barré syndrome, etc. In some of these conditions, AVP appears to be of pituitary origin; in others, the diseased tissue produces AVP or a peptide with similar pharmacological actions.

Deficiency of AVP gives rise to diabetes insipidus. Its causes include primary (idiopathic, familial) and several secondary causes which are all related to disease or injury in or close to the pituitary. Deficiency of AVP may be the sole hormonal abnormality, or there may be disturbances of anterior pituitary hormone production as well in patients with secondary AVP deficiency. Recognition of hyposecretion of AVP depends on urine concentration tests, i.e. the fluid deprivation test and the DDAVP test (p. 129). Measurements of plasma [AVP] are not usually required.

Comments on Case 19.1 (p. 299)

The diagnosis of Cushing's syndrome was confirmed by the loss of the nychthemeral rhythm of serum [cortisol], and the failure to show a significant response in the insulin-hypoglycaemia test despite adequate hypoglycaemia. In the presence of an abnormal serum [cortisol], the patient's plasma [ACTH] was inappropriately high (it should normally be suppressed), and this suggested that she had pituitary-dependent Cushing's disease; the dexamethasone test result supported this diagnosis.

This patient was further investigated with a combined pituitary function test that gave the following results in response to Gn-RH, insulin-hypoglycaemia and TRH:

Time (minutes)	0	20	60	Units
Plasma [glucose]	4.3	2	2.2	mmol/L
Serum [cortisol]	510	490	500	nmol/L
Plasma [growth hormone]	< 0.7	1.8	1.1	mU/L
Plasma [prolactin]	300	–	–	mU/L
Plasma [FSH]	3.9	8.2	8.8	IU/L
Plasma [LH]	3.1	16.9	15.3	IU/L
Plasma [TSH]	0.9	5.1	3.1	mU/L

Normally hypoglycaemia causes an increase in plasma [GH] to over 20 mU/L, and Gn-RH causes increases in plasma [FSH] to at least twice the basal level (peak 5–25 IU/L) and plasma [LH] to at least four times the basal level (peak 10–40 IU/L). TRH normally causes plasma [TSH] to rise at least 2 mU/L above the basal level in the 20-minute specimen.

Abnormal results in pituitary function tests are often found in Cushing's syndrome, whatever its aetiology, these being caused by the sustained high plasma [cortisol]. Abnormal results in these other tests, therefore, do not necessarily indicate pituitary-dependent Cushing's disease.

After radiological investigations, the patient had a pituitary adenoma removed. It is worth noting that determining the urinary cortisol : creatinine ratio, during her first admission, was inappropriate as she was clearly under considerable stress at that time.

Chapter 20
Gonadal Function and Pregnancy

Male gonadal function

Spermatogenesis takes place in the seminiferous tubules. Formation and maturation of sperm require both the Leydig and the Sertoli cells to be functioning normally. Each type of cell has distinct biochemical functions.

Leydig cells are under the control of luteinizing hormone (LH), via specific membrane receptors. Receptor activation by LH leads to increased production of testosterone, the principal androgen; dehydroepiandrosterone (DHA) and androstenedione are also formed in the testes. Testosterone acts locally, or is released into the plasma to exert its actions on other tissues.

Sertoli cells provide other testicular cells with nutrients; they possess follicle-stimulating hormone (FSH) receptors. Stimulation of Sertoli cells by FSH results in the production of several regulatory proteins, of which inhibin and androgen-binding protein (ABP) are the best characterized. Inhibin is important in controlling secretion of FSH, and ABP is thought to be important in maintaining high intratesticular [testosterone].

Spermatogenesis and its control

Spermatogenesis requires the entire hypothalamic–pituitary–testicular axis (Fig. 20.1) to be functioning normally. Gonadotrophin-releasing hormone (Gn-RH) from the hypothalamus stimulates release of LH and FSH; its effects on LH release are more marked than on FSH release. The secretion of Gn-RH, and thus of LH, occurs in pulses; the secretion of FSH is less markedly pulsatile. The amplitude and frequency of the pulses of LH release from the pituitary may be important for LH in exerting its normal effects on testosterone production.

The secretion of LH is under negative feedback control from plasma [free testosterone]. Release of FSH is inhibited by inhibin.

Spermatogenesis requires FSH for its initiation and high testicular [testosterone] for its maintenance. High testicular [testosterone] is ensured by the anatomical proximity of Leydig, Sertoli and spermatogenic cells, and by the local release of androgen-binding protein.

Transport and metabolism of testosterone

In the circulation, about 65% testosterone is bound to sex hormone-binding globulin (SHBG) and 30% to albumin. It is the free (unbound) fraction, about 2% of the testosterone in plasma, that gains access to tissues and exerts its biological activity. Target tissues for androgens have high-affinity cytosolic receptors that

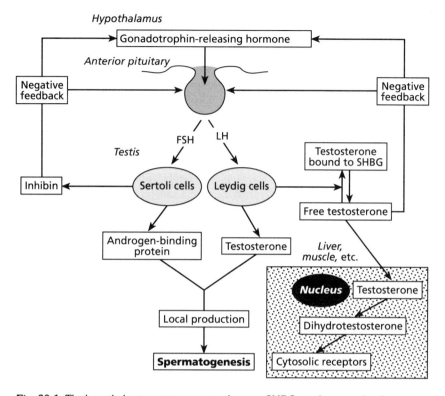

Fig. 20.1 The hypothalamic–pituitary–testicular axis. SHBG, sex hormone-binding globulin.

transport androgens into the cell nucleus; these receptors can bind other androgens besides testosterone.

Many tissues contain steroid 5α-reductase. This converts testosterone to 5α-dihydrotestosterone (5α-DHT), which binds more strongly to the cytosolic receptors than does testosterone. It has been suggested that testosterone is a pro-hormone and that 5α-DHT is the principal male hormone.

Investigation of male hypogonadism and infertility

A sperm count should be determined first, before requesting chemical investigations; if it is normal on two occasions, tests of endocrine function are not required. If the count is low, the principal investigations are measurements of plasma LH, FSH and testosterone concentrations (Fig. 20.2). Reference ranges for these hormones in men are as follows:

FSH   1.5–9.0 IU/L   Testosterone   10–30 nmol/L
LH   1.5–9.0 IU/L   Free testosterone   250–750 pmol/L

Plasma [prolactin] should also be determined (p. 298), as hyperprolactinaemia can lead to hypogonadism and impotence (reference range, 60–390 mU/L).

Specimens for LH and FSH measurements should be collected at standard

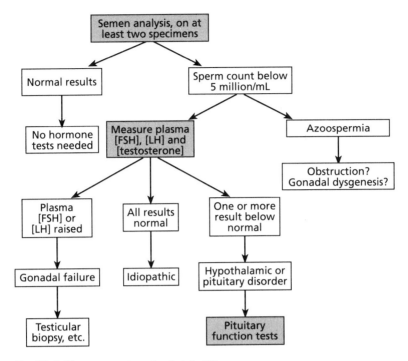

Fig. 20.2 The investigation of male infertility.

times (e.g. in the 0800 h–1000 h region), to minimize the effects of diurnal variation. More than one specimen needs to be collected, on different days, to allow for the possibility that misleadingly high values might be observed in a single specimen, because of the pulsatile release of Gn-RH.

Plasma [total testosterone] can be measured by a specific radioimmunoassay method. The results are affected by changes in plasma [SHBG] and, to a lesser extent, by changes in plasma [albumin]. Plasma [free testosterone] can be estimated indirectly by measuring salivary [testosterone], or by determining both plasma [total testosterone] and [SHBG] and calculating plasma [free testosterone] from these results.

Hypergonadotrophic and hypogonadotrophic hypogonadism

It is convenient to distinguish two forms of hypogonadism, depending on whether the primary defect is, respectively, in the testes or in the hypothalamic–pituitary region. Both forms lead to infertility. However, the majority of infertile men do not fit into either of these categories. Instead, they are eugonadotrophic with normal plasma [FSH], [LH] and [testosterone]; they have oligospermia due to failure of the seminiferous tubules. Their plasma hormone concentrations are often at the lower end of the reference ranges.

Hypergonadotrophic hypogonadism. This group of conditions includes Klinefelter syndrome (usually 47XXY). The primary abnormality is in the testes, and plasma [testosterone] is reduced. There may be increased plasma [LH], indicating failure of function of the Leydig cells, whereas increased plasma [FSH] indicates failure of function of the Sertoli cells. This summary description is an over-simplification.

Hypogonadotrophic hypogonadism. The primary abnormality is in the hypothalamus or the pituitary. There may be selective deficiency of production of both LH and FSH, or only of LH. Alternatively, the deficiency may be part of a generalized failure of pituitary hormone production. Plasma [LH] and [testosterone] are both reduced; usually, there is low plasma [FSH] as well.

Human chorionic gonadotrophin (hCG), injected daily for several days, can be used to help differentiate between hypergonadotrophic (primary) and hypogonadotrophic (secondary) hypogonadism; plasma [testosterone] or 24-hour urinary testosterone output is measured to assess the effect of the hCG injection.

Disorders of male sex differentiation

Many conditions have been described, all rare. In some, the gonads degenerate; in others, there is an enzyme defect affecting steroid synthesis. In a third group there is androgen resistance at the end organ, and a fourth group consists of the true hermaphrodites.

The testicular feminization syndrome is probably due to a receptor defect or end-organ resistance to androgens; plasma [testosterone] is abnormally high. In many of the other conditions, plasma [testosterone] is low, both in childhood and in adult life.

Gynaecomastia in males

Breast development occurring in males other than during puberty usually has a pathological cause. The principal causes are conditions which lead to an imbalance of oestrogen and androgens. These include decreased androgen activity in hypogonadism and increased oestrogen production resulting from a variety of endocrine tumours; these tumours may synthesize oestrogens or secrete hCG, which then acts as a stimulus of oestrogen production. Various drugs with anti-androgen activity or oestrogenic activity may also cause gynaecomastia.

These patients require to be investigated, by measuring plasma or urinary androgens (e.g. testosterone, androstenedione) and oestrogens (e.g. oestradiol-17β, total oestrogens).

Female gonadal function

Menstrual disorders and infertility

The changes that occur in normal menstrual cycles depend on cyclical variations in the output of FSH and LH, influenced by the output of Gn-RH. The effects of Gn-RH on LH and FSH release, in terms of the amounts secreted at different stages of the menstrual cycle, are strongly influenced by negative feedback control effects exerted by oestradiol-17β and progesterone.

The developing Graafian follicles in the ovaries respond to the cyclical stimulus of gonadotrophins by secreting two oestrogens, oestradiol-17β and oestrone; these are metabolized to a third oestrogen, oestriol. After ovulation, the corpus luteum secretes progesterone as well as oestrogens. The changes in the uterus are determined by the ovarian steroid output at each stage. These changes are modified if pregnancy occurs.

Changes in plasma concentrations of FSH, LH and the principal gonadal steroids in the normal menstrual cycle (i.e. a cycle unmodified by oral contraceptives) are shown diagrammatically in Fig. 20.3. Reference ranges for these hormones are given in Table 20.1.

Oestrogens act on several target tissues, including the uterus, vagina and breast; progesterone mainly acts on the uterus. Both oestrogens and progesterone are important in the control of the hypothalamic–pituitary–ovarian axis. Oestradiol-17β may stimulate or inhibit the secretion of gonadotrophins, depending on its concentration in plasma; the stimulating effect of oestradiol-17β can be prevented by high plasma [progesterone].

Ovarian dysfunction and its investigation

The relationships between the hypothalamus, pituitary and ovary in the control of gonadal function mean that abnormality in any of these organs may cause abnormal menstruation and infertility. Other endocrine diseases (e.g. Cushing's syndrome, thyroid disease) can also have these effects, as may excessive production of androgens of adrenal or ovarian origin.

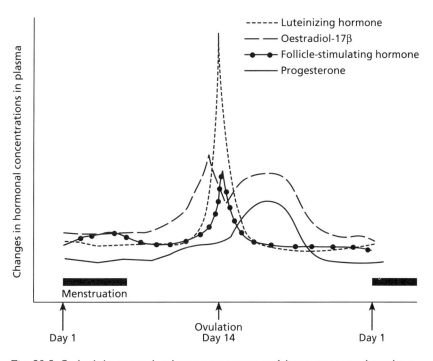

Fig. 20.3 Cyclical changes in the plasma concentrations of the pituitary gonadotrophins and the principal ovarian steroid sex hormones in a normal 28-day menstrual cycle.

Table 20.1 Reference ranges in women for the plasma concentrations of the pituitary gonadotrophins and of the principal female sex hormones, and serum testosterone (data kindly provided by Dr J. Seth)

Hormone	Menstruating female			Post-menopausal
	Early follicular	Mid-cycle	Luteal	
Follicle-stimulating hormone (IU/L)	3.0–15.0	< 20	3.0–15.0	30–115
Luteinizing hormone (IU/L)	2.5–9.0	< 30	2.5–9.0	30–115
Oestradiol-17β (pmol/L)	110–180	550–1650	370–700	< 100
Progesterone (nmol/L)	< 2.0		> 15	< 2.0

Serum [total testosterone], 0.8–2.8 nmol/L; serum [free testosterone], 10–50 pmol/L

Case 20.1

A 17-year-old boy was investigated for the delayed onset of puberty. There was nothing of note in his medical history, and he had not been on any drugs; his 14-year-old brother was already more advanced developmentally. The patient was on the 25th centile for height and had poorly developed secondary sexual characteristics. There were no other signs of endocrine disturbances. However, it was noted that the patient had a poor sense of smell. Hormone investigations on blood specimens gave the following results (reference ranges are for adult males):

Hormone analysis	Result	Reference range	Units
[LH]	1.2	1.5–9.0	IU/L
[FSH]	ND*	1.5–9.0	IU/L
[TSH]	1.3	0.15–3.5	mU/L
[Free T4]	21	9–23	pmol/L
[Prolactin]	200	60–390	mU/L
[Testosterone]	2	10–30	nmol/L
[Cortisol] at 0800 h	500	160–565	nmol/L

* ND = not detected (i.e. below the limits of sensitivity of the assay).

How would you interpet these results in the light of the patient's history and the findings on clinical examination? This patient is discussed on p. 319.

Amenorrhoea

In this discussion, we shall assume that physiological causes of amenorrhoea (pregnancy, lactation) and anatomical abnormalities have all been excluded as the possible cause. Amenorrhoea may be primary, i.e. the patient has never menstru-

Table 20.2 Endocrine causes of amenorrhoea and infertility

Site of lesion	Examples
Hypothalamus	Anorexia nervosa Severe weight loss Stress (psychological and/or physical) Gn-RH deficiency (Kallman's syndrome) Tumours (e.g. craniopharyngioma, acromegaly)
Anterior pituitary	Hyperprolactinaemia Hypopituitarism Functional tumours (e.g. Cushing's disease) Isolated deficiency of FSH or of LH
Ovaries	Polycystic ovary syndrome Ovarian failure* Ovarian tumours
Receptor defect	Testicular feminization syndrome
Other endocrine diseases	Diabetes mellitus Thyrotoxicosis Adrenal dysfunction (e.g. late-onset CAH)

* Ovarian failure may be auto-immune, chromosomal, iatrogenic (e.g. surgery) or idiopathic.

ated, in which case abnormal development is the likely cause, or secondary to various causes (Table 20.2).

For the investigation of amenorrhoea, measurements of plasma concentrations of prolactin, FSH, LH, oestradiol-17β, TSH and free T4 may all be required. In addition, plasma testosterone, androstenedione and dehydroepiandrosterone sulphate (DHAS) concentrations may need to be measured if there is hirsutism or virilization. Figure 20.4 summarizes the investigations commonly performed in patients with menstrual abnormalities. Plasma [prolactin] is measured first and further investigations depend on whether the results are high or normal.

Plasma [prolactin] high. This finding needs to be confirmed by repeating the investigation. Even then, it must be interpreted with caution (p. 297). About 20% of women with secondary amenorrhoea and ovulatory failure have *hyperprolactinaemia*; some of these patients have galactorrhoea. These patients may respond to bromocriptine.

Plasma [prolactin] normal. As indicated in Fig. 20.4, the next stage of investigation involves measurement of plasma concentrations of FSH, LH and oestradiol-17β or other oestrogens:

1 *Plasma [FSH] and [LH] high, [oestradiol-17β] low.* There is primary ovarian failure, due to a chromosomal abnormality, chemotherapy or auto-immune disease, or it may be idiopathic due to a premature menopause.

2 *Plasma [LH] high, [FSH] and [oestradiol-17β] low* or at the lower limit of their reference ranges. The patient may have the polycystic ovary syndrome (pp. 310, 312).

3 *Plasma [FSH], [LH] and [oestradiol-17β] all low,* or at the lower limits of

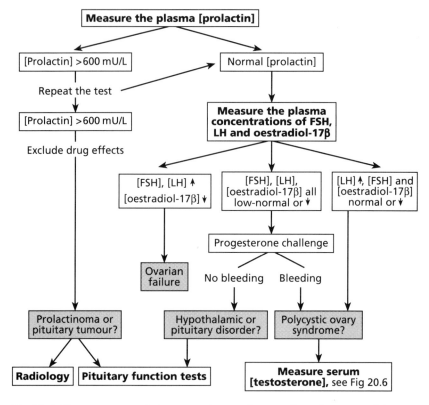

Fig. 20.4 The investigation of oligomenorrhoea and amenorrhoea. It is assumed that other endocrine causes of these conditions (e.g. thyroid disease) have been excluded.

their reference ranges. The patient may have hypothalamic, pituitary or other endocrine disease but, before this possibility is investigated, a progesterone challenge test should be performed. In this test, the patient takes 5 mg medroxy-progesterone daily for 5 days. Menstrual bleeding in the week following progesterone withdrawal indicates that there has been adequate priming of the endometrium by oestrogens; in these patients, polycystic ovary syndrome may be the diagnosis.

Infertility

Table 20.2 summarizes the endocrine causes of infertility that may have to be considered, especially if there are menstrual abnormalities also. Having established that the patient is not taking oral contraceptives, and that other endocrine diseases (e.g. diabetes mellitus, hypothyroidism) are not the cause of the infertility, investigation should proceed according to the schemes outlined in Figs. 20.4 and 20.5, depending on whether or not the patient has normal menstruation.

In patients who menstruate normally (Fig. 20.5), it is important to establish whether the cycles are ovulatory or anovulatory. Serum [progesterone] should be measured daily between days 19 and 23 of the cycle on three separate occasions.

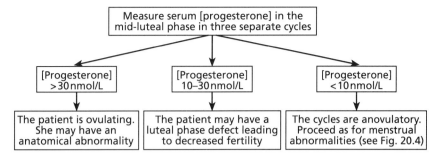

Fig. 20.5 The investigation of female infertility in patients with normal menstrual cycles. In the luteal phase of the menstrual cycle, serum [progesterone] is normally > 15 nmol/L.

If the serum [progesterone] is greater than 30 nmol/L, this indicates an ovulatory cycle whereas levels less than 10 nmol/L strongly suggest anovulatory cycles. In patients who have a serum [progesterone] between 10 and 30 nmol/L, it is thought that the cycles are ovulatory but that there may be a defect in the luteal phase leading to decreased fertility.

In patients who have a low luteal-phase serum [progesterone] or anovulatory cycles, clomiphene may be used for treatment. It acts by blocking oestrogen receptor sites in the hypothalamus and pituitary, thereby inhibiting the normal negative feedback control by plasma oestrogens. Normally, therefore, clomiphene stimulates release of gonadotrophins and these stimulate steroid output from the ovaries.

Hirsutism and virilism

Hirsutism is a fairly common complaint among women. Most hirsute women have normal menstruation and no evidence of virilism. By itself, hirsutism rarely signifies an important disease but it still requires investigation because patients with ovarian or adrenal tumours have been described with normal menstrual cycles. Patients who have menstrual disorders in addition to hirsutism are more likely to have endocrine dysfunction.

Figure 20.6 outlines a scheme for the investigation of female hirsutism. Serum [testosterone] and [DHAS] should be measured; in females, DHAS is a specific adrenal product. Most hirsute women have *idiopathic hirsutism* with normal levels of these steroids. Detailed investigation, however, may reveal evidence of androgen excess due, for instance, to low plasma [SHBG] accompanied by increased serum [free androgens], or to increased conversion of testosterone to 5α-DHT in the skin.

A second group of hirsute women (Fig. 20.6) have moderately increased serum [testosterone], 2.8–7.0 nmol/L, secondary to increased production by the ovaries or the adrenals, and often associated with menstrual irregularity. If the underlying cause is *late-onset congenital adrenal hyperplasia* (CAH), due to partial deficiency of 21-hydroxylase (p. 287), this can be confirmed by injecting tetracosactrin (250 mg intramuscularly) and measuring serum [17α-hydroxyprogesterone] 1 hour later. In a patient with CAH, there will be an

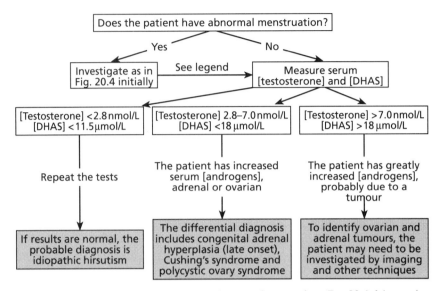

Fig. 20.6 The investigation of hirsutism in females. Continue from Fig. 20.4 if the results there indicate the need to measure serum [testosterone]. Reference ranges for testosterone and for dehydroepiandrosterone sulphate (DHAS) in females are, respectively, 0.8–2.8 nmol/L and 1.5–11.5 μmol/L.

increase in serum [17α-OHP] to more than twice the upper reference value. About 5% of hirsute women have late-onset CAH. *Polycystic ovary syndrome (Stein–Leventhal syndrome)* is another cause of hirsutism, irregular menses and moderately increased serum [testosterone]. It may be associated with moderately increased serum [DHAS] and increased plasma [LH].

A third group of hirsute women (Fig. 20.6) have considerably increased serum [testosterone] and [DHAS], and may show signs of virilism. Late-onset CAH should be excluded before investigating these patients for rarer causes of these abnormalities, e.g. ovarian or adrenal tumours.

Metabolic effects of steroid contraceptives

Steroid contraceptives, principally those containing oestrogens, may cause diverse metabolic effects unrelated to their contraceptive action. Contraceptives that only contain progestogens are largely free from these effects.

Carbohydrate metabolism. About 75% of women develop a minor, usually temporary, impairment of glucose tolerance when they start to take oestrogen-containing oral contraceptives. This can be detected in an oral glucose tolerance test (p. 166), but fasting plasma [glucose] usually remains normal.

Lipid metabolism. Low-oestrogen oral contraceptives tend to cause small increases in plasma [triglycerides] and [HDL-cholesterol], and a fall in plasma [LDL-cholesterol]; progestogens have the opposite effects.

Plasma proteins. The concentrations of a large number of carrier proteins (apolipoproteins, hormone-binding proteins, transferrin, etc.) and coagulation factors (fibrinogen, factors VII and X) may be increased, sometimes markedly. As

---

Case 20.2

A 17-year-old girl consulted her doctor because she was embarrassed by the amount of dark hair that was growing on her face. She told the doctor that her menstrual periods had never been regular (menarche, age 13) and that she had not had a period for over 4 months. She was not pregnant.

On examination, the doctor found that the patient was slightly over-weight, and that she had an extensive growth of dark hair on her lower abdomen (an escutcheon) as well as much dark hair on her upper lip, arms and legs. The patient was referred to an endocrinologist. After confirming that a pregnancy test gave a negative result, the following hormones were measured in blood (reference ranges are for the early follicular phase, where relevant):

Hormone analysis	Result	Reference range	Units
[Prolactin]	450	60–390	mU/L
[LH]	23	2.5–9.0	IU/L
[FSH]	5	3–15	IU/L
[Oestradiol-17β]	250	110–180	pmol/L
[Testosterone]	3.5	0.8–2.8	nmol/L
[DHAS]	12	1.5–3.5	µmol/L
[TSH]	0.2	0.15–3.5	mU/L
[Free T4]	18	9–23	pmol/L

What do you think is the most likely diagnosis in this patient? What is your differential diagnosis? This patient is discussed on p. 319.

---

a result, plasma [cortisol], [total T4] and [total T3] may all be increased by as much as 50%, but the free hormone fractions remain normal.

Pregnancy and the fetoplacental unit

The placenta produces several proteins including (human) chorionic gonadotrophin (hCG) and (human) placental lactogen (hPL). It also produces large amounts of steroid hormones and is the main source of progesterone during pregnancy.

Proteins of trophoblastic origin

There are several pregnancy-specific proteins, all of which normally originate in the trophoblast. The two most commonly measured are hCG and hPL.

Human chorionic gonadotrophin

Following synthesis, hCG is secreted into the maternal circulation. There is a surge in maternal [hCG] in early pregnancy, peak blood levels being reached at 12 weeks; thereafter, production of hCG rapidly declines, except for a small and unimportant rise about the 34th week. It is metabolized rapidly by the liver and kidneys, only a small fraction being excreted unchanged in the maternal urine. Measurement of urinary hCG is an early test for pregnancy, and commercial test kits are widely available to the public.

Although described as a 'pregnancy-specific protein', hCG is produced in other conditions besides pregnancy, by *tumours of the trophoblast*. These tumours can occur in males and females; they include hydatidiform mole and choriocarcinoma, both of which may secrete hCG in very large amounts. A female who is found to be excreting hCG, and who is not pregnant, most frequently has a tumour of the trophoblast; in males, testicular teratoma is the commonest source. In addition, hCG is a non-specific marker for a number of carcinomas, and hCG or hCG-like proteins are secreted by a minority of non-trophoblastic, non-gonadal neoplasms, especially those of GI origin.

Human placental lactogen

This is produced from an early stage of pregnancy, the output being proportional to placental mass; it can be detected in plasma by about 6 weeks' gestation. The output rises progressively thereafter until the last few weeks of pregnancy; the high output is then normally sustained until term. In the last few weeks of pregnancy, the placenta may produce about 12 g hPL/day, and the peak plasma [hPL] is about 8 mg/L. Measurements of plasma [hPL] have been largely replaced by ultrasound monitoring of the later stages of pregnancy.

Steroids in pregnancy

Oestrogens and progesterone are secreted by the corpus luteum during the first 6 weeks of pregnancy, but after this the placenta is the most important source of these steroids. Oestriol is the oestrogen produced in greatest amount, but oestradiol-17β and oestrone are also produced in large amounts. The placenta cannot synthesize oestriol *de novo*, but it can produce oestriol from C-19 adrenal steroids which are supplied by the fetal adrenal in the form of DHAS. The oestriol produced in this way is secreted into the maternal and fetal circulation. Oestriol production thus requires the involvement of both the placenta and the fetus and recognition of this interdependence led to the concept of the fetoplacental unit.

Measurements of plasma [oestriol] have been used in the past to monitor fetoplacental function. Low levels give an indication of a failing fetoplacental unit. These tests have now largely been replaced by ultrasound monitoring.

Other chemical changes in pregnancy

Hormones: Plasma [prolactin], [total T4] and [total T3] are all increased whereas the concentrations of growth hormone and the pituitary gonadotrophins are decreased. In the first trimester, plasma [TSH] is low due to the thyrotrophic effect of hCG. Plasma [free T4] and [free T3] fall in the later months of pregnancy, but this is usually without pathological significance.

Hyperthyroidism is particularly common in women in the 25–40 age-group, and the need to consider the diagnosis occurs quite often in pregnant women. It is important in these patients to measure plasma [TSH] and plasma [free T4] or [free T3], rather than plasma [total T4] or [total T3], and to make use of appropriate sets of trimester-related reference ranges (Table 17.2, p. 257) if potentially misleading conclusions are to be avoided.

There are large increases in serum [cortisol] due to increased plasma [CBG], but the nychthemeral rhythm is retained. There is also an increase in serum [free cortisol] and in the 24-hour urinary excretion of cortisol, probably due to the production of an ACTH-like substance by the placenta. This may help to explain why pregnant women often show intolerance of glucose, and occasionally develop Cushingoid features.

Plasma [1 : 25-DHCC] is increased and there is enhanced absorption of calcium. Plasma [PTH] may be slightly raised near term.

Plasma volume. During pregnancy, the plasma volume increases, sometimes by as much as 50%. This is accompanied by decreases in, for example, plasma [Na^+], [urea] and [albumin]. However, some plasma constituents increase in concentration during pregnancy, e.g. plasma [triglycerides].

Alkaline phosphatase. In pregnancy there is an additional (heat-stable) isoenzyme of alkaline phosphatase detectable in plasma, originating from the placenta. Plasma total alkaline phosphatase activity is sometimes as much as three times the activity normally present in non-pregnant women.

Iron and ferritin. During pregnancy there is a greater demand for iron. This arises from increased maternal red cell synthesis and from transfer of iron to the developing fetus. Although greater absorption of iron may enable part of this increased requirement for iron to be met, plasma [iron] usually falls unless dietary supplements are given. Plasma [ferritin] also falls; after 20 weeks' pregnancy, it is often less than 20 μg/L in women who are not receiving iron supplements.

There is an increase in plasma [transferrin] during pregnancy, so plasma TIBC increases although the percentage saturation of the iron-binding capacity falls unless iron supplements are given.

Maternal complications in pregnancy

Diabetes mellitus

When women attend the antenatal clinic, most doctors consider that urine specimens should be routinely tested for glucose (p. 14), and plasma [glucose] is usually measured at the first clinic attendance. Detection of glucosuria does not necessarily indicate the presence of diabetes mellitus; the renal threshold for glucose is often lowered in pregnancy, and the glucosuria usually disappears after delivery. Interpretation of these simple 'side-room' tests, therefore, is not altogether straightforward in pregnancy and a glucose tolerance test may be needed if gestational diabetes mellitus is suspected (p. 169). Up to 10% of pregnant women with glucosuria have diabetes, as defined by the WHO criteria (p. 165).

There are special problems associated with the diagnosis of diabetes mellitus in pregnancy. Fasting plasma [glucose] is usually slightly increased and glucose tolerance slightly impaired, possibly as a result of the presence of hPL and the increase in plasma [cortisol], both of which tend to produce resistance to insulin.

Case 20.3

A 23-year-old housewife was 4 months pregnant when she told her general practitioner that she had been feeling very uncomfortable during a recent spell of hot weather. She was concerned because, 20 years before, her mother had had similar symptoms and had been found to have Graves' disease. The patient had no signs of thyroid disease. However, the doctor decided to request the following thyroid function tests:

Analysis	Result	Reference range	Units
[TSH]	< 0.1	0.15–3.5	mU/L
[Free T4]	19	8–20	pmol/L
[Total T4]	190	70–150	nmol/L
[Free T3]	3.5	3.0–7.0	pmol/L
[Total T3]	3.0	1.2–2.8	nmol/L

How would you interpret these results? Would you request any further thyroid-related investigations? This patient is discussed on p. 319.

Pre-eclampsia

At the antenatal clinic, urine specimens should be routinely tested for protein. Proteinuria, if detected, may be the first evidence of pre-eclampsia and, as the condition worsens, proteinuria in excess of 1 g/24 h may occur. Patients with pre-eclampsia may develop impaired renal function with increasing plasma [creatinine] and [urea] as the renal impairment worsens, or as a result of vomiting and dehydration. In pregnancy, a plasma [urea] of 7.0 mmol/L should be regarded as definitely abnormal, since plasma [urea] is normally reduced in pregnancy due to the increase in plasma volume.

Plasma [urate] may be measured to assess the severity of pre-eclampsia, and to provide an index of prognosis. The upper reference value in non-pregnant women is 0.36 mmol/L. A plasma [urate] greater than 0.35 mmol/L before 32 weeks' gestation, or greater than 0.40 mmol/L after 32 weeks, is significantly raised; impaired renal function causes reduced tubular clearance of urate.

Jaundice in pregnancy

Intrahepatic cholestasis is an uncommon feature of pregnancy. It is associated with the occasional development of idiosyncratic jaundice in women when taking oral contraceptives. There is retention of bilirubin (mainly conjugated) and bile acids, and bilirubinuria. The increase in plasma alkaline phosphatase activity in these patients is partly hepatic in origin, and partly placental.

Prenatal diagnosis of fetal abnormalities

Neural tube defects

The fetal liver begins to produce α_1-fetoprotein (AFP) from the sixth week of gestation onwards, and the highest concentration of AFP in fetal serum occurs at about 13 weeks, after which it falls progressively until term. If the fetus has an open neural tube defect, abnormal amounts of AFP are present in amniotic fluid in about 95% of cases at 16 weeks' gestation, and in maternal serum in about 80% of cases at that time.

In many countries, maternal serum [AFP] (MSAFP) is measured as a screening test for neural tube defects, carried out with a view to identifying those women who should be further investigated by ultrasound and then, in appropriate cases, by amniocentesis. If the diagnosis of open neural tube defect is confirmed before the 20th week, termination of pregnancy can be offered.

It is essential to know the gestational date for the interpretation of results, since MSAFP concentrations vary considerably with the length of gestation. The best discrimination between normality and abnormality is obtained at 16–18 weeks' gestation. There is, even then, considerable overlap between [MSAFP] in normal pregnancies and in women carrying affected fetuses. If an upper reference value at the 95% percentile for the normal population (a value which is about 2.5 times the median value for this population) is selected as the level above which further investigations should be performed, less than 10% of women with 'abnormal' [MSAFP] defined in this way will, in fact, be carrying affected fetuses. In other words, the MSAFP test is a screening test used to identify a 'high risk' group of women.

Other causes of high [MSAFP] include multiple pregnancy and some rare, non-neurological, fetal abnormalities (e.g. oesophageal or duodenal atresia, exomphalos).

Amniocentesis before 20 weeks' gestation

If an abnormal result for [MSAFP] is reported, it is usual to repeat the serum measurement and, if the result is again abnormal, to proceed to ultrasound examination. This detects multiple pregnancy and will also often detect neural tube defects. Ultrasound examination helps with placental localization for subsequent amniocentesis, if this is to be performed. Amniocentesis would not be indicated, for instance, if the ultrasound examination revealed twins or an anencephalic fetus.

Amniocentesis carries a risk to the fetus estimated to be between 0.5% and 2% loss. To justify its performance, there must be a high index of suspicion that a fetal abnormality is present. An appropriate course of action must be available in the event that an abnormality is diagnosed as a result of amniocentesis. The risks of chorion villus sampling, important in the prenatal diagnosis of inherited metabolic disease (p. 327), are correspondingly low, but are likewise not negligible. Two chemical tests are normally carried out if amniocentesis is performed for confirming a diagnosis of neural tube defect:

1 *Amniotic fluid [AFP]*. This is abnormal in over 95% of cases where there is a neural tube defect. However, false-positive results may be obtained when the fluid is blood-stained, or when certain other defects (e.g. exomphalos) are present.

2 *Amniotic fluid acetyl cholinesterase activity*. This is increased when the fetus has a neural tube defect, presumably due to leakage of the enzyme (which is

relatively specific for the nervous system) through the defect. The test (electrophoresis) distinguishes acetyl cholinesterase from the relatively non-specific cholinesterase (p. 81) normally present in plasma and in amniotic fluid, and is more sensitive and specific than amniotic fluid [AFP] measurements. It is not affected by contamination of the fluid with maternal blood. However, amniotic fluid acetyl cholinesterase activity may be increased if there is fetal exomphalos.

If the results for maternal serum [AFP], measured on two occasions, and for amniotic fluid [AFP] and amniotic fluid acetyl cholinesterase are all abnormal, the diagnosis of neural tube defect can be made with a fairly high degree of confidence. However, certain other uncommon congenital abnormalities (e.g. exomphalos) may yield a similar pattern.

Screening for Down syndrome

Down syndrome (trisomy of chromosome 21) is the commonest congenital cause of mental retardation. The overall incidence is $1:1000$ births and affected pregnancies can be identified by chromosome analysis of cells obtained at amniocentesis in the mid trimester. The incidence of Down syndrome varies greatly with maternal age, and women over 35 years of age have a risk of at least $1:250$ of carrying an affected fetus whereas in women aged less than 20 years the risk is $1:2000$. However, since women aged over 35 years old represent only 5–7% of total pregnancies, only 30% of Down syndrome pregnancies can be detected by performing amniocentesis in this older group.

Abnormalities in a number of maternal serum analytes are associated with Down syndrome pregnancies. These include decreased [MSAFP], increased serum total [hCG], increased [free β-subunit of hCG], increased [unconjugated oestriol] and decreased [pregnancy-associated plasma protein A]. Each of these measurements shows overlap between Down syndrome pregnancies and the normal population but, if the distributions of the concentrations of these analytes for Down syndrome pregnancies and normal pregnancies are known, a 'likelihood ratio' or the risk of the fetus having Down syndrome can be calculated for an individual woman. Calculation of the risk is most conveniently done by entering the test results, gestational age and maternal age into a computer program which holds the distribution profiles of the analytes. The risk of Down syndrome based on maternal and gestational age is then calculated. Patients with a high risk of carrying an affected child may then be offered amniocentesis. Individual maternity units can determine at what level of risk amniocentesis should be offered to ensure an acceptable workload.

Amniocentesis late in pregnancy

This is occasionally performed to investigate fetal well-being and to detect potentially serious but treatable conditions. Preparations can then be made for treatment to start immediately after birth, or sometimes even before birth. Chemical examinations on the amniotic fluid may include:

1   *Lecithin.* Fluid in fetal lung tissues normally contributes to the formation of amniotic fluid. Before its discharge, this fluid is in contact with alveolar epithelial cells; these produce a surface-active material containing a large amount of phospholipid. Amniotic fluid [lecithin] can be used as an index of fetal lung

maturity, and to assess the likelihood that an infant will develop the respiratory distress syndrome.

2 *Bilirubin*. Small amounts are normally detectable in amniotic fluid. However, if a fetus is affected by Rhesus haemolytic disease the concentration rises, often in direct relation to the severity of the haemolytic process. False predictions of the risk to the fetus, based on measurements of amniotic fluid [bilirubin], have been reported in an appreciable percentage of patients.

Monitoring the fetus during labour

If monitoring of the fetal heart rate suggests the onset of fetal distress, fetal scalp blood sampling and measurement of blood $[H^+]$ may be performed. As an indicator of fetal acidosis, the finding of blood $[H^+]$ over 63 nmol/L (pH below 7.20) is a serious finding; it is usually a sign of fetal hypoxia. Once the cervix is dilated, fetal oxygenation can be continuously monitored transcutaneously by measuring blood Po_2.

The increasing availability in labour wards of equipment for measuring blood $[H^+]$, Po_2 and other indices of fetal well-being places growing emphasis on the reliable performance by ward staff of measurements hitherto regarded as the province of trained laboratory workers. The developing subject of ward-based chemical equipment is considered on p. 17.

Comments on Case 20.1 (p. 308)

The findings suggest that the patient had hypogonadotrophic hypogonadism as the sole endocrine abnormality, but a combined test of pituitary functional reserve (p. 300) would be worth considering; it would provide information about growth hormone.

The lack of a sense of smell is typical of Kallman's syndrome, in which there is an isolated deficiency of Gn-RH. Stimulation with exogenous Gn-RH can be used both diagnostically and as treatment, but usually puberty is induced in these patients with sex steroids.

Comments on Case 20.2 (p. 313)

This girl had the clinical and biochemical features of polycystic ovary syndrome (PCOS). The slight increase in plasma [prolactin] is not of pathological significance; it may, for instance, be due to stress. The gonadotrophin pattern excludes hypogonadotrophic hypogonadism and ovarian failure as the cause of amenorrhoea (pregnancy had already been excluded), and the testosterone and DHAS concentrations were such as to make it most unlikely that the patient had an androgen-secreting tumour. Late-onset CAH can present with all the features of PCOS, and should be excluded by measuring the 17α-OHP response to tetracosactrin stimulation (p. 311).

Comments on Case 20.3 (p. 316)

Plasma [TSH] was below the limits of sensitivity of a very sensitive immunometric assay. Undetectable TSH could be due to hyperthyroidism, but it could also be due to the mild thyrotrophic action of the high plasma [hCG] that is found until about the 15th week of pregnancy.

Plasma [TBG] increases in pregnancy. This causes increases in plasma [total T4] and [total T3], without at the same time causing the levels of the free thyroid hormones to become abnormal. When interpreting results for plasma [free T4] and [free T3] in pregnant women, it is important to use the appropriate trimester-related reference ranges. In this patient, the results for these analyses were both normal, so elevated free thyroid hormone values as a cause of the low plasma [TSH] could be eliminated.

As a follow-up investigation, a blood specimen was examined for TSH-receptor antibodies. As these could not be detected, this supported the conclusion that TSH was undetectable due to the effects of hCG; it did not indicate that the patient had Graves' disease.

Chapter 21
Clinical Biochemistry in Paediatrics and Geriatrics

Clinical Biochemistry in Paediatrics will be considered first. Chemical investigations can be very helpful in the diagnosis and management of diseases affecting infants and children provided that satisfactory specimens are collected for analysis. Also the laboratory must have available the appropriate range of investigations and be able to perform them reliably and quickly on very small volumes of blood or other specimens.

Improvements in specimen-collection techniques and the development of microanalytical procedures together mean that as wide a range of commonly performed analyses can be offered for the investigation of neonates, infants and children as for adults. However, much greater emphasis has to be placed on selecting the investigations most appropriate for individual patients because of the limited amounts of blood available, especially in premature babies. In addition to the uses of analyses discussed elsewhere in this book, many diagnostic problems are particularly relevant to Paediatrics, e.g. the identification of suspected inherited metabolic disorders. These special problems can also be investigated by a growing range of sophisticated analytical techniques that require very small samples.

Specimen collection from neonates and children

The collection of blood specimens is often the responsibility of a team of specimen-collecting staff, who obtain at one time all the specimens required for haematology and clinical biochemistry investigations. This minimizes the upset to patients, by reducing the frequency of disturbance. It requires coordination of requests for investigations, and indications of test priority to ensure that the clinically most important specimens are obtained first. Capillary blood should be collected whenever possible in Paediatrics, to avoid not only the occasional hazards of venepuncture but also the mental stress that preparations for performing a venepuncture tend to produce.

Blood specimens from babies are best obtained by heel prick, from the fleshy (lateral) parts of the heel. It is important not to use the central part of the heel as the calcaneus is very close to the surface and injury to it, by the blood-collecting lancet, can cause necrotizing osteochondritis.

In older children, the sides of the fingers provide the best sites, especially where repeated sample collection may be needed (e.g. diabetics), *not* the dorsum of the finger below the nail. The sides of the fingers, over the terminal phalanges, have relatively few nerve endings and the procedure is much less painful and less likely to cause damage than collecting blood from the nail-bed area. The ear lobes are also sometimes used, but blood-collecting from this site can be very painful.

The site chosen for specimen collection must be warm to ensure a free flow of blood, and cleanliness of operation is essential. Glass capillary collection tubes, heparinized, should be used as these maximize the yield of plasma; they are filled by gently touching each droplet of blood with the edge of the lip of the tube as drops form on the skin.

Reference ranges in Paediatrics

For interpreting the results of analyses, it is essential to make use of reference ranges appropriate for the age-group of the patient (Table 21.1), and comprehensive lists of age-related reference ranges should be available from all specialist paediatric biochemistry laboratories. Data such as those in Table 21.1 represent an over-simplification as, for example:

1 In the first few hours after birth, plasma [bilirubin] and [total T4] normally show wide variations in concentration.

2 In the first few months, the nature of the diet significantly influences the reference ranges for plasma [calcium], [phosphate], [amino acids], etc.

3 Some plasma constituents normally vary in their activity or concentration with different levels of osteoblastic activity or in relation to different stages of genital development (e.g. alkaline phosphatase activity, gonadotrophin and gonadal steroid concentrations).

4 Much of the work of a paediatric biochemistry laboratory is concerned with the investigation and management of low-birthweight or premature (often very premature) infants, for whom there may be no satisfactory reference ranges. Even in the absence of complicating disease, the results of chemical investigations on these patients depend both on gestational age at the time of birth and on post-natal age.

Table 21.1 Examples of plasma reference ranges that are age-dependent (data for children kindly provided by Dr A. Westwood)

Constituent	Neonates	Infants	Childhood	Adults
Albumin (g/L)	30–42	34–46	36–47	36–47
Alkaline phosphatase (IU/L)*	70–550	70–550	125–400	40–125
Bilirubin, total (μmol/L)	< 200		< 26	2–17
Calcium (mmol/L)	1.60–3.00	2.10–2.80	2.12–2.62	2.12–2.62
Creatinine (μmol/L)	40–80	30–60	30–80	55–120
Gamma-glutamyl transferase (IU/L)	< 200	< 120	< 35	10–55 (M) 5–35 (F)
Phosphate, fasting (mmol/L)	1.3–3.0	1.0–2.1	1.0–1.9	0.8–1.4
Potassium (mmol/L)	4.0–6.6	4.1–5.6	3.3–4.7	3.3–4.7
Protein, total (g/L)	51–68	55–78	60–80	60–80
Thyroid-stimulating hormone (mU/L)	< 25		0.15–3.5	0.15–3.5
Thyroxine, free (pmol/L)	10–50		9–23	9–23
Thyroxine, total (nmol/L)	140–440	90–195	70–180	70–150

* Activities measured by a different technique from the one used for adults but the results for the paediatric method have been divided by two so as to make them accord with the adult reference range for alkaline phosphatase activity (p. 79).

Inherited metabolic disorders

Many inherited metabolic diseases are due to an inborn error. The spectrum of disorders subdivides into two main groups:

1 Disorders due to the addition or deletion of chromosomes or parts of chromosomes. This group has an incidence of about six per 1000 live births, and leads to clinically significant abnormalities (e.g. Down syndrome, Turner syndrome) in about three per 1000 live births. Clinical biochemistry investigations at present play little part in the diagnosis and management of chromosomal abnormalities.

2 The Mendelian disorders, in which the primary defect is probably in the structure of the gene. This group includes a wide variety of conditions, mostly very uncommon. Chemical investigations (often detailed in nature) are needed for the proper characterization of these genetic disorders.

The primary defect in each of the Mendelian disorders is probably a change in the base sequence of a gene. This change affects the synthesis of a protein, which may be a structural protein, or a transport protein, or an enzyme etc. The consequences depend on the functions of the protein affected by the primary alteration in the gene, and can be illustrated by discussing a defect that gives rise to a marked reduction (rarely a complete absence) of activity of an enzyme (E) involved in the metabolism of a compound, A, at one stage in the following reaction sequence:

$$A \xrightarrow{E_1} B \xrightarrow{E_2} C \xrightarrow{E_3} D \xrightarrow{E_4-E_n} R$$

We shall later on make the important assumption that the defect resulting from the Mendelian disorder renders the reaction catalysed by the affected enzyme the rate-limiting step in the pathway.

Diagnosis in the neonatal period

An increasing number of inherited metabolic disorders can be detected in the neonatal period, some by screening programmes (see below) and others on clinical examination or by means of widely available investigations (e.g. amino acid chromatography). The incidence of individual disorders is low but *collectively* they are not at all uncommon; examples of these conditions are given in Table 21.2. Some

Table 21.2 Incidence in the UK of some metabolic diseases detectable in neonates (approximate frequency in terms of numbers of cases per 100 000 live births)

Disorder	Incidence	Disorder	Incidence
Cystic fibrosis	50	Histidinaemia	5–10
α_1-Protease inhibitor deficiency	50	Mucopolysaccharidoses	5–10
Hypothyroidism	20–30	Urea cycle defects	2–5
Duchenne muscular dystrophy	20–30	Galactosaemia	1–2
Phenylketonuria	10–20	Homocystinuria	1
21-Hydroxylase deficiency	10	11β-Hydroxylase deficiency	1
Cystinuria	5–10	Maple syrup urine disease	1
Hartnup disease	5–10	Non-ketotic hyperglycinaemia	1

Table 21.3 Examples of inherited metabolic disorders that may produce acute illness, especially in the neonatal period (after Haan & Danks, 1981)

Metabolic group and examples	Site of enzymic block
Amino acid disorders	
Hereditary tyrosinaemia	Fumarylacetoacetate hydrolase
Maple syrup urine disease	Decarboxylation of branched-chain ketoacids
Non-ketotic hyperglycinaemia	Glycine decarboxylase system
Carbohydrate disorders	
Galactosaemia (commonest form)	Galactose-1-phosphate uridylyltransferase
Glycogen storage disease type I (von Gierke's disease)	Glucose-6-phosphatase
Glycogen storage disease type IIa (Pompe's disease)	α-D-Glucosidase
Hereditary fructose intolerance	Fructose-1-phosphate aldolase
Organic acid disorders	
Dicarboxylic aciduria	Fatty acid β-oxidation
Isovaleric acidaemia	Isovaleryl-CoA dehydrogenase
Propionic acidaemia	Propionyl-CoA carboxylase
Urea cycle defects	
Argininosuccinic aciduria	Argininosuccinate lyase
Citrullinaemia	Argininosuccinate synthetase
Hyperammonaemia type I	Ornithine carbamoyltransferase
Steroid synthesis defects	
Congenital adrenal hyperplasia	21-Hydroxylase, 11β-hydroxylase, desmolase, etc.

inherited metabolic disorders may present acutely in the first few days or weeks of life, and Table 21.3 illustrates the diversity of these conditions. They form one group of causes among the many that might account for an infant failing to thrive or being seriously ill.

Most of the inherited metabolic disorders that present in the neonatal period give rise to non-specific symptoms such as feeding difficulties (e.g. vomiting when protein or carbohydrate feeding is started) or failure to thrive. There may be respiratory difficulties, fits, jaundice, or hepatomegaly but rarely are there unusual signs such as the smell of maple syrup urine disease. In the salt-losing forms of congenital adrenal hyperplasia, the patient may present in adrenal crisis. In families where there has been no index case, the recognition that there is a metabolic disease present, and thereafter the precise identification of its nature, can present complex diagnostic problems. About 10% of deaths in infancy in Britain are due to genetic disorders.

The index case

It is worth testing the infant's urine in the 'side room' for reducing substances and for protein (p. 14), as long as this is not at the expense of providing the laboratory with an adequate specimen for its investigations. Tests for glycosuria may detect fructose or galactose, in addition to glucose. Laboratory confirmation of a provisional diagnosis of the commonest form of galactosaemia or hereditary fructose intolerance should follow quickly, but meanwhile appropriate dietary treatment can be started without detriment to the patient. Identification of the two much rarer enzymic defects in galactosaemia can take much longer (p. 179).

Depending on the infant's clinical condition, blood-gas studies and measurements of plasma concentrations of bilirubin, calcium, creatinine or urea, glucose, potassium and sodium may all be required. If an inherited metabolic disorder is suspected, the aim must be to make a specific diagnosis, but the wideranging nature of the conditions can make it difficult to achieve this aim quickly. The following investigations help to narrow the differential diagnosis considerably:

1 *Chromatography.* Serum or plasma and urine studies can help to identify fairly precisely most of the conditions listed in the various groups included in Table 21.3. Separate chromatographic examinations are performed for amino acids, monosaccharides, organic acids and steroid metabolites, but not all are necessarily required in every case.

2 *Blood [NH$_3$].* This is probably the best initial investigation if a urea cycle defect is suspected.

It should be noted that clinical management of a very sick infant, such as dextrose–saline infusions or exchange transfusion, can interfere seriously with the investigation of suspected metabolic disorders. It is important, therefore, to collect appropriate specimens early.

Confirmation of the diagnosis

The specific recognition of an inherited metabolic disorder cannot usually be made solely on the basis of blood and urine examinations, although identification of a precursor that has accumulated in plasma, or detection of abnormal amounts of the precursor or one of its metabolites in urine, may strongly indicate the site of the primary defect. Tissue preparations are usually needed (e.g. leucocyte concentrates, erythrocyte haemolysates) or biopsy specimens (e.g. liver, skin, thyroid or brain) for precise diagnosis.

In the index case, intracellular enzyme studies may be essential if the diagnosis is to be established. These assume particular significance for the future if the infant's condition deteriorates. The downward progression of some inherited metabolic diseases can be very rapid in the neonatal period and the possible need for intracellular enzyme studies may not be appreciated until the infant is already very seriously ill. Under these circumstances, if death seems imminent, arrangements should be made for the collection and preservation of those specimens that a laboratory specializing in the identification of metabolic disorders will require, for later detailed studies.

Permission should be obtained for a needle biopsy of the liver to be performed while the patient is still alive. Other specimens to be obtained include serum and urine (i.e. in addition to the residues of specimens previously collected and examined), blood for lymphocyte and erythrocyte studies, CSF and a specimen of skin for fibroblast culture. Specimens collected later, after death, are rarely as satisfactory for these metabolic studies, although if possible a post-mortem examination should be carried out also.

It is important to make a diagnosis in the index case since the specific recognition of the inherited metabolic disorder forms the basis for any search for affected relatives. It is also relevant to planning the management and investigation of any subsequent pregnancy since knowledge of the metabolic defect in the index case is essential if either enzyme studies or DNA analyses are to be performed for pre-natal diagnosis of the disorder in later pregnancies. Genetic counselling may be required for parents who have had a child affected by one of the inherited metabolic disorders. Such counselling is more acceptable if it is soundly based on the results of scientific investigation, and is not long delayed in being given.

Several other inherited metabolic disorders may present less acutely than the conditions listed in Table 21.3, but may nevertheless carry a very poor prognosis and (unless treatable) progress inexorably to death in infancy or childhood; examples are given in Table 21.4. It is again very important to make the diagnosis precisely, so as to be able to advise parents about possible future pregnancies. The approach to the diagnosis of the specific metabolic defect in the index case with these patients is similar to the approach described above. However, with conditions such as those listed in Table 21.4, there is usually more time in which to reach the diagnosis.

Table 21.4 Inherited metabolic diseases that may present less acutely than the examples listed in Table 21.3, but which have a very poor prognosis in the index case and for which termination of pregnancy may be advised in later pregnancies

Category and examples	Enzyme defect
Glycogen storage diseases	
Anderson's disease (type IV)	1,4-α-glucan branching enzyme
Hug's disease (type VIII)	Phosphorylase (liver)
Lipid storage diseases	
Fabry's disease*,†	α-D-Galactosidase
Niemann–Pick disease*	Sphingomyelin phosphodiesterase
Gaucher's disease*	Glucosylceramidase
Tay–Sachs disease	β-N-acetyl-D-hexosaminidase (hexosaminidase A)
Mucopolysaccharidoses (MPS)	
Hurler disease (MPS 1H)*	α-L-Iduronidase
Sanfilippo A disease	Sulphoglucosamine sulphamidase
(MPS IIIA)	(heparan-N-sulphatase)
Purine metabolism	
Lesch–Nyhan syndrome†	Hypoxanthine-guanine phosphoribosyltransferase

* A few patients have been successfully treated by bone marrow transplantation.
† These conditions have sex-linked recessive inheritance. The other conditions listed in this table all have autosomal recessive inheritance.

Screening for heterozygotes

This is at present mainly confined to screening the relatives of patients found to have an inherited metabolic disorder. The programme is normally restricted to the specific abnormality identified in the index case.

The effect of the metabolic defect can sometimes be assessed directly and quantitatively. Usually, however, the effect of the mutant gene can only be detected by investigating the metabolic reaction directly as an enzymic assay, or indirectly by measuring the effects of the block or partial block when subjected to a loading test. For instance, a phenylalanine loading test can be used to screen for PKU heterozygotes. Heterozygote detection depends increasingly on DNA analysis, using the same techniques as are being developed for pre-natal diagnosis.

Early diagnosis of inherited metabolic disease

The aim of identifying disorders that will prove severely handicapping, untreatable and eventually fatal is to be able to offer the mother the opportunity of a therapeutic abortion if the fetus is found to be affected in the same way as a previous child. Table 21.4 includes examples of conditions that can be detected *in utero* by chorion villus biopsy or amniotic fluid studies.

Pre-natal diagnosis: chorion villus biopsy

This technique enables pre-natal diagnosis of inherited metabolic disorders to be made at a much earlier stage of pregnancy than amniocentesis, i.e. about the ninth week of pregnancy. The biopsy can be used for karyotyping and for gene probe diagnosis. The whole process of gene probe analysis, using DNA from chorion villus tissue, takes about 10 days. The technique has been applied particularly to the diagnosis of haemoglobinopathies, but also to several other conditions including cystic fibrosis and Duchenne muscular dystrophy (p. 360).

Pre-natal diagnosis: amniotic fluid studies

Amniocentesis can be carried out about the 15th week of pregnancy for cyto-genetic reasons (e.g. to detect Down syndrome), or for the detection of the appropriate *one* of a wide range of rare untreatable metabolic disorders in families where there has already been an index case and where the nature of the defect to be sought in the current pregnancy has previously been identified. Diagnosis is usually made on the basis of enzyme studies carried out on fibroblasts cultured from the amniotic fluid. Although culture and the subsequent specialized investigations take time, they should be able to be completed by 20 weeks' gestation.

For pre-natal diagnosis of metabolic disorders to be carried out reliably, it is essential that the specimen of amniotic fluid be cultured and examined by one of the few laboratories that possess the requisite skills. The laboratory must be informed about the *precise nature* of the metabolic disorder for which the cultured cells are to be examined. This diagnosis will, in most instances, have been established on the basis of enzyme studies previously carried out on specimens from the index case. Relatively rapid techniques for diagnostic enzyme analysis performed on single cells have been described, but are not widely available.

If a pregnancy is terminated on the basis of information derived from pre-natal diagnostic investigations, the correctness of the diagnosis should be confirmed by further biochemical studies carried out on the aborted fetus.

Screening of neonates

Phenylketonuria (PKU) exemplifies many of the consequences of a genetic disorder. It is also one of the best examples of a potentially treatable condition that can be readily detected by neonatal screening programmes.

The first step in the major pathway of phenylalanine metabolism, its conversion to tyrosine, depends on hepatic phenylalanine hydroxylase (Fig. 21.1). The pathways leading to the deaminated and other metabolites ('phenylketones') of phenylalanine are normally only of minor importance. In the classical form of PKU, phenylalanine hydroxylase activity is either undetectable or very much reduced. It requires tetrahydrobiopterin (BH_4) as co-factor, BH_4 being oxidized to the quinonoid form of dihydrobiopterin ($q\text{-}BH_2$) at the same time as phenylalanine is converted to tyrosine. Dihydrobiopterin reductase (DHBR) normally reconverts most of the $q\text{-}BH_2$ that has been formed, but which is very unstable, back to BH_4. Another enzyme, dihydrobiopterin synthetase (DHBS) normally makes good any $q\text{-}BH_2$ that has been lost due to its instability. About 3% of patients with abnormalities of phenylalanine metabolism have a deficiency of DHBR or DHBS, or some other defect that is different from the deficiency of phenylalanine hydroxylase; these rarer forms of PKU must be differentiated from the classical form as they require different forms of treatment.

Normal metabolism of phenylalanine

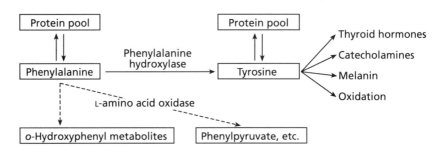

Altered metabolism of phenylalanine in classical phenylketonuria

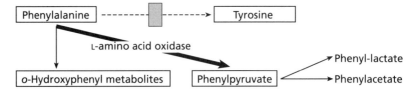

Fig. 21.1 The metabolism of phenylalanine. In the classical form of phenylketonuria (also by far the commonest form), the activity of phenylalanine hydroxylase is greatly reduced and normally minor metabolites of phenylalanine are excreted in much increased amounts.

Further discussion of PKU is restricted here to its classical form. It illustrates many of the principles that underlie the diverse effects of inherited metabolic disorders. The defect in PKU corresponds to a block at the first stage, A $\longrightarrow$ B, in the general reaction sequence (A $\longrightarrow$ R) shown on p. 323. The following effects may be observed:

1 *Accumulation of the substrate of the blocked reaction.* This occurs in the liver. Plasma [phenylalanine] and urinary phenylalanine excretion are much increased, unless dietary phenylalanine is restricted.

2 *Reduced formation of product.* Tyrosine formation is severely affected in patients, but tyrosine deficiency can be avoided if the diet is supplemented.

3 *Alternative paths of metabolism.* There is increased formation and urinary excretion of phenylpyruvate, phenyl-lactate and phenylacetate, and of various o-hydroxyphenyl metabolites. Dietary phenylalanine restriction reduces the output of these metabolites.

4 *Effects on other reactions.* Accumulation of phenylalanine and its metabolites inhibits the transport of other amino acids into the liver and brain and their concentrations in these tissues fall. The activity of enzymes involved in the metabolism of other amino acids (e.g. tyrosine, tryptophan) may also be inhibited.

Many inherited metabolic disorders give rise to blocks at later stages in the general metabolic sequence A $---\rightarrow$ R, and some may exhibit features additional to those exemplified by PKU. Reduced formation of an important product may interfere with a negative feedback control mechanism, e.g. failure to synthesize cortisol in normal amounts in congenital adrenal hyperplasia leads to increased output of ACTH, accumulation of precursors of the blocked reaction and over-production of the metabolites of these precursors (p. 286).

Screening for phenylketonuria

Almost the whole infant population in the UK is screened for PKU within a few days of birth. The most widely employed initial screening procedure, the *Guthrie test*, uses a mutant strain of *Bacillus subtilis*, spores of which are incorporated into agar that includes β-thienylalanine, an analogue of phenylalanine that prevents bacterial growth unless there is phenylalanine available. A few laboratories use a chromatographic procedure (the Scriver test) instead of the Guthrie test. Blood specimens from infants with PKU, and with hyperphenylalaninaemia due to other causes, enable the *B. subtilis* mutant to grow. Specimens for this test consist of drops of blood placed on to filter paper supplied by the laboratory that carries out the test.

The relative prevalence of classical PKU, and of hyperphenylalaninaemia due to other causes in the population under investigation, influences the predictive value for PKU of a positive result in the test used for measuring serum [phenyl-alanine] in the screening programme. The specificities of the Guthrie and Scriver tests are excellent, being over 99.5%. However, with the screening level set at a serum [phenylalanine] of 240 μmol/L, over 90% of positive tests are due to causes other than classical PKU (Table 3.5, p. 32); the commonest causes of false positives are transient tyrosinaemia and transient hyperphenylalaninaemia. Positive results require further investigation to determine whether the infant does indeed have PKU, in which case appropriate dietary treatment needs to be instituted and monitored. Additional tests may be needed to differentiate between classical PKU and the much rarer variants described above.

In the UK, blood specimens for PKU screening are collected from infants aged 6–14 days. In some countries, the specimens are collected earlier, but cases of PKU may be missed under these circumstances because the specimens are collected before infant feeding with protein has become established.

Interference in the screening tests (both Guthrie and Scriver) is liable to occur in neonates who are being treated with antibiotics. It is advisable to delay the screening test until the course of antibiotic treatment is finished, and to repeat the test if the laboratory reports that the test has been unsatisfactory.

Other screening programmes in infancy
Screening programmes require considerable organization. Before embarking on them, several questions need to be considered:
1 What is the incidence of the disease?
2 Is the disease life-threatening or liable to be severe?
3 Is acceptable treatment available?
4 Is a suitable screening test available?
5 Can abnormal results be followed up?
6 Are the costs acceptable?

Screening for PKU in the neonatal period fulfils these criteria. For other conditions, the question about costs is not difficult to answer if the disease for which a new screening programme is proposed can be included as an addition to a pre-existing programme (e.g. PKU screening) and without detriment to already established arrangements. Several inherited metabolic diseases can now be detected in the neonatal period by linking their performance to the PKU screening programme. They include tests for hypothyroidism, maple syrup urine disease, homocystinuria, tyrosinaemia and galactosaemia. However, the screening arrangements for PKU may be less than ideal for these other disorders. For example, many patients with galactosaemia will have life-threatening symptoms before the sixth day of life, and before biochemical investigation of such conditions can be completed (e.g. Gal-1-PUT (p. 179) assay cannot always be performed within this time).

The incidence of congenital hypothyroidism is about one in 4000 live births. As the condition is amenable to treatment, it is very important that the condition be diagnosed promptly and treatment thereafter initiated without delay. However, it can be very difficult to diagnose clinically in the neonatal period. As screening tests, serum [TSH] has been found to be more reliable than serum [total T4]; some programmes measure both serum [TSH] and [total T4] in blood spots collected on to filter paper.

Some biochemical problems in the neonatal period and infancy

Convulsions
Anoxia, infections and trauma are all relatively common causes of convulsions in

the neonatal period. These may all cause metabolic disturbances that give rise to convulsions. Sometimes, however, metabolic disturbances are the primary cause. Chemical investigations may prove helpful in the diagnosis and management of these conditions.

Glucose

Plasma [glucose] tends to be lower in the newborn than in adults (Table 21.1). Neonatal hypoglycaemia can be arbitrarily defined as a blood or plasma [glucose] less than 1.1 mmol/L in an underweight (small for gestational age) infant, and less than 1.6 mmol/L in an infant of normal weight. Blood [glucose] may fall as low as 0.5 mmol/L in the neonate without symptoms of hypoglycaemia developing, but such low concentrations can only be tolerated for short periods.

In the neonatal period, hypoglycaemia is most commonly due to decreased production of glucose; this often occurs in premature babies as a result of their inadequate glycogen stores. Neonatal hypoglycaemia is also quite often due to hyperinsulinism, e.g. in infants of diabetic mothers.

Hypoglycaemia giving rise to convulsions only affects about one in every 500 live births, usually between 24 and 72 hours after birth. Blood [glucose] can be monitored on the ward (p. 17). If a low reading is obtained on a ward glucose meter, this can be taken as an indication for treatment, and for the blood [glucose] to be confirmed by measurement in the laboratory. Hypoglycaemia in the neonatal period is often accompanied by ketosis, and urine tests for ketone bodies (p. 15) are then positive. However, urinary ketones may be low in patients with fatty acid beta-oxidation deficiency, one of the commoner metabolic causes of neonatal hypoglycaemia, and in hyperinsulinism.

Recurrent hypoglycaemia of infancy and childhood may be due to any of the causes listed in Table 11.5 (p. 177) as well as several other inherited metabolic disorders (e.g. dicarboxylic aciduria, maple syrup urine disease, tyrosinaemia), or Reye's syndrome (p. 338). One of the most important causes is hyperinsulinism of childhood (nesidioblastosis).

Functional hyperinsulinism of infancy usually develops before the infant is 6 months old. It is characterized by severe hypoglycaemia, as a rule accompanied by inappropriately high plasma [insulin] and [C-peptide]. About 50% of these infants show an excessive insulinaemic and hypoglycaemic response to L-leucine, produced by digestion of protein. There are diffuse lesions of the pancreas. Functional hyperinsulinism presenting in children over the age of 1 is usually due to an islet cell adenoma (p. 177).

Nutritional causes of hypoglycaemia in this age-group can be classified as ketotic hypoglycaemia or as hypoglycaemia secondary to malnutrition. Ketotic hypoglycaemia is associated with fasting and usually responds rapidly to administration of carbohydrate. Rarely, it is due to one of the glycogen storage diseases or other inherited metabolic disorders, or to deficiency of glucocorticoids, growth hormone or thyroid hormones.

Calcium and magnesium

Full-term infants have a reference range for plasma [calcium] that differs considerably from the corresponding range for adults (Table 21.1). Plasma [calcium] tends to fall by about 10–20% in the first 2–3 days of life; in normal full-term infants it then returns over the course of the next 3–4 days towards the value that was present at birth, as the infant begins to secrete parathyroid hormone.

Neonatal hypocalcaemia within the first 48 hours, sufficient to give rise to convulsions, occurs particularly in premature infants, in infants of diabetic mothers and in infants that have been asphyxiated; maternal vitamin D status may also be a factor. The mechanism is complex, but may relate to impaired mobilization of calcium in the presence of high neonatal plasma [calcitonin] and [cortisol], or it may be due to withdrawal of maternal calcium supplies via the placenta and slow development of the infant's normal physiological PTH response to the presence of hypocalcaemia. The hypocalcaemic tendency usually corrects itself spontaneously, but calcium gluconate may need to be given intravenously if convulsions occur, e.g. if plasma [calcium] falls to less than 1.50 mmol/L. Rarely, hypocalcaemic convulsions in the neonate are associated with maternal hyperparathyroidism, which may produce temporary hypoparathyroidism in the neonate due to the fetus having been exposed to maternal hypercalcaemia.

Late neonatal hypocalcaemia, between the fourth and tenth days of life, may occur in full-term as well as in premature infants. It is usually accompanied by signs of hyperexcitability of muscles. This is liable to occur in infants whose mothers had a low intake of vitamin D during pregnancy; these infants may also have low plasma [magnesium]. It may also be associated with hyperphosphataemia caused by the high phosphate content of cow's milk, or be due to renal disease presenting in the neonatal period. Treatment with intravenous calcium, and often magnesium, may be required.

Neonatal rickets. Hypocalcaemia and defective bone mineralization, sometimes giving rise to rickets, are liable to occur especially in premature infants because of their increased requirements for calcium, phosphate and vitamin D. It may present at any time during the neonatal period, or the next 2–3 months. This is an important condition, but is itself a very rare cause of convulsions or muscular hyperexcitability. Alkaline phosphatase activity in plasma is very high.

Hypomagnesaemia is an occasional cause of neonatal convulsions; it tends to occur in association with decreased plasma [calcium]. The primary defect is probably in the intestinal absorption of magnesium. In untreated infants, plasma [magnesium] may be as low as 0.1 mmol/L (reference range, 0.75–1.15 mmol/L).

Respiratory distress syndrome (RDS)

Any cause of hypoxia or marked acid–base disturbance may give rise to convulsions in the neonatal period.

Respiratory difficulty in neonates is most often due to RDS. This occurs mainly in premature infants of less than 38 weeks' gestation. There is atelectasis, probably due to deficiency of surfactant activity in the alveoli, a low arterial Po_2 and high Pco_2, and often an accompanying metabolic acidosis. Treatment should be monitored by measuring blood $[H^+]$, Pco_2 and Po_2. It is possible to predict the likelihood of RDS developing after birth by determining amniotic fluid [lecithin] late in pregnancy (p. 318).

Neonatal hyperbilirubinaemia

The definition of neonatal hyperbilirubinaemia is necessarily somewhat arbitrary. Over 90% of normal babies have plasma [bilirubin] exceeding 34 μmol/L (the upper reference value for adults) at some time during the first week of life. In some babies, plasma [bilirubin] may rise much higher, up to 200 μmol/L, without any apparent pathological cause. However, babies with plasma [bilirubin] greater than 200 μmol/L, especially if this persists after the first week of life or if it has a significant (over 20%) conjugated bilirubin component, must be regarded as having some additional cause for the hyperbilirubinaemia.

High concentrations of unconjugated bilirubin can cross the blood–brain barrier and cause kernicterus. The critical plasma [bilirubin] at which this occurs *in full-term infants* is about 340 μmol/L, but this depends on plasma [albumin], on the presence of drugs (e.g. sulphonamides) which occupy some of the binding sites on albumin, on acid–base disturbances that may affect the equilibrium between albumin-bound and unbound bilirubin, and on the integrity of the 'blood–brain barrier'. The critical level is much lower for severely ill infants. It is also much lower for premature infants, being approximately related to birthweight; it may, for instance, be as low as 200 μmol/L for very low birthweight infants.

Neonatal hyperbilirubinaemia is most often associated with increased plasma [unconjugated bilirubin]. It is useful, diagnostically, to be able to distinguish between increases in plasma [unconjugated or 'indirect' bilirubin], in which plasma [conjugated bilirubin] is normal, and increases in plasma [conjugated or 'direct' bilirubin]. 'Side-room' tests on urine specimens may not be practicable, but inspection of staining produced by urine and of the colour of any faecal material can be helpful. In jaundice due to increased plasma [unconjugated bilirubin], urine does not usually contain bilirubin; even when plasma [bilirubin] is over 340 μmol/L it only contains small amounts, unless there is concomitant glomerular damage and proteinuria.

Measurements of plasma [bilirubin] are valuable in following the progress of hyperbilirubinaemia and in determining when therapeutic measures (e.g. exchange transfusion) are required. In the neonatal period and infancy, separate measurements of conjugated and unconjugated bilirubin in plasma are of much more value than in adults. High concentrations of conjugated bilirubin often require further investigation before a diagnosis can be made.

Physiological unconjugated hyperbilirubinaemia

This occurs very frequently. Factors that contribute to its development include:

1 *Overproduction of bilirubin* from haemoglobin, due to shortened red cell lifespan and ineffective erythropoiesis.

2 *Immaturity of the hepatic processes* of bilirubin uptake from plasma and conjugation in the hepatocyte.

3 *Interference with hepatic transport functions* by compounds transferred across the placenta or present in human breast milk (e.g. progesterone and steroids with progesterone-like activity such as 3α, 20β-pregnanediol) or by drugs.

4 *Reabsorption of unconjugated bilirubin* from the intestine. In the neonate, β-glucuronidase in the small intestine releases bilirubin from its conjugates. Since the intestinal bacteria that normally then convert bilirubin to urobilinogen are not fully developed at this age, some unconjugated bilirubin can be reabsorbed and thus add to the load that the liver has to take up, conjugate and excrete.

Pathological causes of unconjugated hyperbilirubinaemia

In the neonate, these exacerbate the tendency for physiological hyperbilirubin-aemia, especially in premature infants. The groupings of pathological causes are:
1 *Increased haemolysis*, due to rhesus or ABO incompatibility, or to abnormalities within the red cell (e.g. glucose-6-phosphate dehydrogenase deficiency).
2 *Defective hepatic uptake or conjugation.* This may occur in prematurity or because of hypoglycaemia or hypothyroidism, or inherited disorders of bilirubin metabolism (Gilbert's syndrome, Crigler–Najjar syndrome, p. 111).

Conjugated hyperbilirubinaemia

Patients in this group have increased plasma [conjugated bilirubin], but this may nevertheless constitute only 20–30% of the total bilirubin in their plasma. Normally, most of the bilirubin in plasma is unconjugated. There are several causes of conjugated hyperbilirubinaemia in infancy. These may be grouped as follows:
1 *Developmental abnormalities of the biliary tree.* The most important of these is extrahepatic biliary atresia. Intrahepatic biliary atresia also occurs.
2 *Neonatal hepatitis.* This is an ill-defined group which includes patients with infective causes of hepatitis (e.g. cytomegalovirus), metabolic causes (e.g. α_1-protease inhibitor deficiency, p. 90), galactosaemia (p. 179) and endocrine causes (e.g. congenital hypopituitarism).

Chemical tests are of little help in distinguishing infants with jaundice due to extrahepatic biliary atresia (in whom surgery is indicated) from infants with intrahepatic lesions (in whom surgery is not indicated). The commonly performed 'liver function tests' usually show a predominantly cholestatic pattern, with large rises in plasma alkaline phosphatase activity and lipoprotein X detectable, but plasma aminotransferase (ALT and AST) activities are also increased.

Failure to thrive in childhood

There are many possible metabolic causes, but malnutrition is far the commonest. Of the many inherited metabolic diseases that can cause failure to thrive, only cystic fibrosis will be discussed here.

Malnutrition in children

Protein-energy malnutrition (PEM), in its severest forms, includes kwashiorkor and marasmus; there is a range of less severe clinical presentations. There may be other important factors, e.g. deficiency of essential fatty acids or the consequences of immune defence mechanisms impaired by malnutrition. Chemical tests are no substitute for serial measurement and recording of children's weights.

Measurement of plasma [albumin] is valuable in screening children at risk of developing malnutrition but in whom the disease is still at a subclinical stage; the rate of albumin synthesis is diminished when protein intake is deficient. The most consistent abnormality in severe kwashiorkor is a low plasma [albumin]. In practice, plasma [albumin] is not likely to be determined unless clinical impressions suggest the need; results greater than 34 g/L are taken as normal. Plasma [albumin] below 30 g/L should be regarded as abnormally low; values below 25 g/L are associated with increasing degrees of oedema. Other early indices of PEM include changes in plasma [pre-albumin] and [transferrin], both of which fall, but these measurements do not add much to the information gained from determining plasma [albumin].

Malnutrition severe enough to cause hypoglycaemia is encountered in children with kwashiorkor and in starvation (e.g. due to gross parental neglect). If malnutrition is severe enough to cause liver failure to develop, many other chemical tests become abnormal.

Vitamin deficiency diseases make up a potentially important group of nutritional causes of failure to thrive, since the growing child has relatively greater requirements for vitamins than the mature adult. Rickets (p. 209) due to inadequate nutrition continues to occur, even in developed countries.

Cystic fibrosis (CF)

This is the commonest inherited metabolic disease in Caucasians; it occurs in about one in 2000 live births. It is inherited as an autosomal recessive condition, usually affecting the exocrine glands. There are marked abnormalities in the ion-transporting functions of epithelial cells. The chloride ion-channels are normal, but fail to respond to cyclic AMP; the sodium ion-channels are also affected. Chemical investigations used for diagnostic purposes mostly depend on tests relating to sweat production or to pancreatic function.

The chances of heterozygous parents producing a child with cystic fibrosis are one in four, and the relatively high incidence of CF has focused attention on ways of achieving prenatal diagnosis. The new DNA technology can now be used to demonstrate linkage with a marker some distance from the defective CF gene (p. 360). These tests can be performed on fetal DNA prepared from chorion villus specimens obtained about the ninth week of pregnancy from women who have previously given birth to a CF-affected child.

Tests on sweat

The reference biochemical method for the diagnosis of CF is measurement of $[Na^+]$ and $[Cl^-]$ in sweat obtained by iontophoresis from a small area of skin under standardized conditions; sweating is induced by the intradermal injection of pilocarpine. The test demands close attention to detail, if reliable results are to be obtained, and should only be carried out by staff who are experienced in its performance. It should not be performed before 3 weeks of age, in full-term infants, as many very young infants fail to produce sweat fast enough, even in response to pilocarpine stimulation.

In healthy children and adults, in pilocarpine-stimulated sweat, $[Cl^-]$ and $[Na^+]$ are normally below 50 mmol/L. In patients with CF, the concentrations are nearly always above 70 mmol/L, sometimes being as high as 140 mmol/L.

Screening tests for cystic fibrosis

Sweat tests are too time-consuming and demanding of attention to detail to be used for this purpose. Screening tests are all based on the effects of CF on pancreatic function. They include:

1 *Immunoreactive trypsin* (IRT) concentration, measured in dried blood spots similar to those collected when screening for PKU. This is greatly increased in specimens collected from CF infants in the first month of life as compared with the IRT content in specimens from healthy infants. It is the best CF-screening method from among the tests so far evaluated, but it cannot be used after the first few weeks of life since IRT falls as pancreatic insufficiency develops.

2 *Faecal enzyme activity* has also been used to screen for pancreatic involvement in CF. Specimens are examined for tryptic or chymotryptic activity, using a synthetic substrate (benzoyl-arginine-*p*-nitroanilide); enzymic activity may be reduced or undetectable in these patients. The tests can be carried out on faecal specimens that have been smeared on a card and allowed to dry before being sent to the laboratory.

Short stature

Table 21.5 lists the principal categories of disordered growth, with examples. The endocrine causes of tall stature have been discussed elsewhere, as have several of the conditions that have a biochemical basis or which produce marked metabolic effects with short stature as one of their manifestations. Some of these metabolic causes of short stature can be identified by measuring, for instance, plasma [creatinine] or [TSH] to exclude renal disease and hypothyroidism, respectively.

Table 21.5 Disorders of growth

Growth abnormality and category	Examples
Short stature	
Genetic	Familial short stature, delayed development
Intra-uterine	Low birthweight dwarfism
Nutritional	Inadequate food supply, malabsorption (p. 158), coeliac disease,* infections
Systemic disease	Chronic renal disease, congenital heart disease
Endocrine disease	Growth hormone deficiency,* hypothyroidism, corticosteroid excess, precocious puberty
Miscellaneous	Emotional disturbance (battered children), Turner syndrome
Tall stature	
Genetic	Familial tall stature, advanced development
Endocrine disease	Growth hormone excess, hyperthyroidism, precocious puberty
Miscellaneous	Klinefelter (XXY) syndrome, XYY anomaly

* Growth hormone deficiency and coeliac disease are considered here.

In this section, we shall only consider the investigation of children for possible growth hormone deficiency and for coeliac disease.

Growth hormone deficiency

This may be an isolated defect, partial or complete, or it may be a component of panhypopituitarism. Growth hormone (GH) is released into the circulation in pulses, mainly at night. Measurements of basal plasma [GH] in specimens collected in the daytime are, therefore, of no diagnostic value since laboratory reports are likely to state that growth hormone cannot be detected, even in normal children. Consequently, GH provocation tests must be used.

Since the insulin-hypoglycaemia test is only safe in children if its performance can be properly supervised by staff who perform it on children regularly, it is usually preceded by other GH provocation tests such as collecting blood specimens for analysis after physical exercise, or after a meal, or soon after waking from a night's sleep. However, these tests are difficult to standardize, and the GH response to them is variable. The clonidine test is more reliable.

In the clonidine test, clonidine is given orally to stimulate GH release; blood specimens are collected before giving clonidine (0.15 mg/m^2 body surface area) and at 30-minute intervals for 2.5 hours afterwards. It may be considered advisable to 'prime' peri-pubertal children with the appropriate sex steroid, and the clonidine test can be combined with a TRH test and a Gn-RH test if a combined pituitary function test (p. 300) is to be performed.

Glucagon may also be used instead of insulin to provoke GH release. It is given by intramuscular injection (15 µg/kg of insulin-free glucagon) and blood specimens are collected similarly. As glucagon normally stimulates the release of both GH and ACTH from the pituitary, this test can be used to assess both the GH and cortisol responses to glucagon. However, whether the clonidine test or the glucagon test is used, in some children it may still be necessary to perform an *insulin-hypoglycaemia* test, but modified slightly from the test as used in adults (p. 297). Specimens are taken before an intravenous injection of soluble insulin (0.10 units/kg, or 0.05 units/kg if panhypopituitarism is suspected), and at 20, 30, 45, 60 and 90 minutes after the injection. Plasma [GH] and [glucose] are measured in all the specimens, and serum [cortisol] in the 20- and 45-minute specimens. The test may be combined with a TRH test and a Gn-RH test if a combined pituitary function test is to be performed. Whenever the insulin-hypoglycaemia test is performed, this should only be undertaken in a specialized unit with much experience of the test.

Coeliac disease

This is a common cause of growth retardation. The definitive method of diagnosis is small intestinal biopsy examination. Other diagnostic features include the improvement that is brought about by a gluten-free diet, both physically and in the severity of steatorrhoea, and the relapse that follows dietary relaxation.

Chemical tests can be valuable as preliminary investigations, intestinal biopsy being reserved for patients with abnormal results in preliminary tests such as faecal fat (p. 156) or xylose absorption (p. 154). Fat excretion may be greatly increased, and xylose absorption may be considerably impaired.

Patients with coeliac disease have abnormal secretin cells in the jejunal mucosa. They show a markedly reduced release of secretin and of glucose-dependent insulinotrophic peptide (GIP) in response to test stimuli, e.g. a protein-containing meal or intra-duodenal acid, but a greatly increased release of enteroglucagon from the ileum. This pattern of gut hormone release reflects the location of the intestinal lesion in coeliac disease; concentrations of hormones produced in areas unaffected by the disease (e.g. gastrin) remain normal. These gut hormone measurements are only performed by a few laboratories.

Miscellaneous conditions in Paediatrics

Abnormal calcium metabolism

Hypercalciuria in childhood may be due to increased intestinal absorption of calcium (e.g. due to excessive intake of vitamin D), renal tubular disorders and, rarely, primary hyperparathyroidism (alone or part of one of the MEN syndromes, p. 205). Children with hypercalciuria due to renal disease are best detected by measuring the urinary calcium : creatinine ratio (normally below 0.8); they have normal plasma [PTH]. Some children with hypercalciuria due to excessive intestinal absorption of calcium only have an abnormal urinary calcium : creatinine ratio after being given an oral load of calcium (1 g/1.73 m^2 body surface area).

Pseudohypoparathyroidism (PHP) has been discussed elsewhere (p. 211). For those children with suspected (i.e. not florid) PHP, a PTH-stimulation test can be performed. Normally, in response to the injection of PTH, plasma [cyclic AMP] rises but in patients with PHP there is little or no response.

Hypercalcaemia in childhood. In the neonatal period, phosphate depletion may lead to hypercalcaemia in premature neonates. In the infantile hypercalcaemia (Williams) syndrome, children usually present within the first 3 years with hypercalcaemia, characteristic facies and aortic stenosis. Hyperparathyroidism is rare in childhood.

Reye's syndrome

This is a rare, acute illness in which there are severe vomiting, drowsiness and behavioural changes; its onset is usually preceded by a viral illness (e.g. influenza, chickenpox). In the UK, most patients are under 6 and few are over 12 years old. The encephalopathy is often fatal, and 'liver function tests' reflect the severity of the general disturbance of mitochondrial functions.

Abnormal results of chemical investigations include increased plasma ALT and AST activities and blood [ammonia], hypoglycaemia and prolonged prothrombin time.

The cause of Reye's syndrome is unknown, but aspirin appears to have been a contributory factor in some cases. The differential diagnosis is wide, and includes several inherited metabolic disorders (e.g. urea cycle defects, fructosaemia and the organic acidurias).

Neuroblastoma and ganglioneuroma

Deaths due to malignant disease make up an important category of childhood mortality. Neuroblastoma and related tumours, although rare, account for approximately one-third of these deaths.

These are catecholamine-producing tumours and excessive formation of dopamine is a practically constant feature. However, dopamine overproduction is not associated with marked pharmacological effects because dopamine and the catecholamines derived from it (noradrenaline, adrenaline) are largely metabolized by the tumour tissue before inactive metabolites are released into the circulation. Only occasionally is there hypertension.

The following tests may be performed, the measurements usually being related to urinary [creatinine] because it is difficult to obtain complete 24-hour urine collections in children:

1 *Total metadrenalines* or other index of the output of noradrenaline and adrenaline (e.g. HMMA) are the tests most often performed initially. In children, abnormal excretion of these catecholamine metabolites nearly always points to a diagnosis of neuroblastoma or ganglioneuroblastoma; very occasionally, it signifies the presence of phaeochromocytoma.

2 *4-hydroxy, 3-methoxy phenylacetic acid* (homovanillic acid, HVA), is the metabolite of dopamine that is excreted in largest amount. Greatly increased excretion occurs in patients with neuroblastoma or ganglioneuroblastoma.

Clinical Biochemistry in Geriatrics

Many elderly patients admitted to hospital, for assessment and treatment, are suffering from more than one disease. Problems of diagnosis are often complex, and the interpretation of chemical investigations is more frequently affected by drug treatment than is usually the case with patients in younger age-groups. We shall consider a few aspects of Clinical Biochemistry particularly relevant to the specialty of Geriatrics. However, most of the other chapters in this book are also directly applicable to the investigation of elderly patients, so repetition will be avoided as far as possible.

Reference ranges in Geriatrics

There is no sharp distinction chemically between middle age and old age, such that each might have its own separate set of reference ranges. Instead, changes in reference ranges that are sometimes evident in those over 65 often merely represent the extension of changes that have been gradually occurring throughout adult life, and which may continue in the same direction with advancing age. The ideal would be to have different sets of reference ranges for age-bands such as 55–65, 65–75, 75–85 and 85–95. It is, however, very difficult to determine reference ranges for healthy subjects in the older age-groups. For individual patients, it is worth checking whether investigations have been carried out before; past records sometimes provide useful baseline data.

Examples of the effects of ageing

Creatinine clearance tends to fall, as a consequence of the progressive loss of

---

Case 21.1

A 68-year-old retired surgeon consulted his general practitioner on account of weight loss (12 kg in the last year), lethargy and poor appetite. He had noticed that his urine had been darker than usual, and his stools relatively pale. On examination, he was found to be slightly jaundiced and was tender in the right hypochondrium; his doctor thought that the liver was enlarged or that the gallbladder was palpable. 'Side-room' examination of urine showed the presence of bilirubin and a trace of urobilinogen; occult blood was detected in a specimen obtained on rectal examination. 'Liver function tests' were requested, and gave the following results:

Plasma analysis	Result	Reference range	Units
[Albumin]	37	36–47	g/L
Alkaline phosphatase activity	630	40–125	IU/L
ALT activity	35	10–40	IU/L
[Bilirubin, total]	90	2–17	μmol/L
GGT activity	150	10–55	IU/L

How would you interpret this pattern of results, and what would be your differential diagnosis? This patient is discussed on p. 344.

---

nephrons which starts in middle age. However, the reduction in muscle mass and the smaller dietary intake of protein, which tend to occur with older people, offset the effects of the loss of nephrons on plasma [creatinine]; this does not change with age.

Plasma [cholesterol], on average, increases progressively throughout adult life. In the UK, by the age of 65, mean values are 10–30% higher than in the 20–30 age-group.

Plasma [glucose] tends to increase with age, due to progressive impairment of glucose tolerance. Patients, however, do not necessarily go on to develop overt diabetes mellitus.

Plasma alkaline phosphatase activity is probably higher in healthy people over 65 than in younger adults, but not all agree about this. Some reports suggest that there is no difference between reference ranges for adults in the 20–65 age-range and those for apparently healthy adults over 65, if care is taken to exclude people with Paget's disease, or unsuspected liver disease, or malignancy (especially unsuspected malignant disease with secondary deposits in the liver or in bone). We consider that a plasma alkaline phosphatase activity more than 50% higher than the laboratory's upper reference value for younger adults should be regarded as abnormal in the elderly. High values are not necessarily serious, however, as they are often due to Paget's disease.

Some plasma constituents tend to decrease in concentration with increasing age (e.g. total protein, albumin), but these changes are unlikely to cause difficulties in interpretation.

Screening for disease in elderly patients

Illnesses often present differently in the elderly from in younger patients, and a logical ordered approach to the selection of investigations, based on the patient's history and the findings on clinical examination, may not always be appropriate. A common aim, in geriatric assessment units, is to identify the presence of treatable illness as quickly as possible, so as to be able to get the patient ambulant again and rehabilitated. Some diseases present so insidiously that the patient may not give a clear history. Also, multiple pathology may be present. These considerations at least partly justify the apparently blunderbuss approach to chemical investigations adopted by some geriatricians.

The choice of chemical tests to be incorporated into screening programmes for elderly patients (e.g. when first admitted to geriatric assessment units) has been much discussed. Table 21.6 lists tests that have been widely accepted. In addition to the laboratory measurements listed in the table, 'side-room' testing of urine specimens for glucose and protein, and faeces for occult blood, should form part of the initial investigation of all patients admitted to geriatric assessment units.

Inadequate nutrition

Old people living alone are particularly at risk of having an inadequate diet, especially if they are poor, or are unable or unwilling to feed themselves properly. Measurements of plasma [albumin] or [pre-albumin], for instance, may give low results. These tests may be helpful in the nutritional management of the patient, but there are other reasons why the results might be low in elderly patients (e.g. recent acute illness) and their diagnostic value is therefore limited.

Table 21.6 Admission screening of elderly patients, by means of chemical tests

Examination	Abnormalities commonly detected
'Side-room' tests	
(a) Urine	Glucosuria, proteinuria
(b) Faeces	Gastrointestinal tract blood loss (e.g. haemorrhoids, carcinoma of the colon or of the rectum)
Measurements on blood specimens	
Albumin, total protein	Evidence of poor nutrition
Creatinine, urea	Renal disease, post-renal uraemia
Glucose	Diabetes mellitus
Calcium (phosphate and alkaline phosphatase)	Hypocalcaemia (often due to osteomalacia)
Potassium	Hypokalaemia (often due to diuretic therapy)
Thyroid function tests	Hypothyroidism or hyperthyroidism (but see Tables 17.3 and 17.4, pp. 258, 259)
C-reactive protein (or erythrocyte sedimentation rate)	Non-specific indicator of the presence of organic disease

---

Case 21.2

A 73-year-old retired school-teacher had been admitted 1 month previously for an upper GI tract endoscopy. She gave a history of having moderately severe hypertension for which her general practitioner had been treating her with a combined preparation of atenolol and chlorthalidone for the last 2 years. Endoscopy confirmed that she had a benign gastric ulcer, and she was discharged home on treatment with ranitidine and carbenoxolone. Two weeks later, she was again seen by her general practitioner because her ankles had begun to swell, for which he prescribed frusemide. However, her ankle swelling persisted and she began to feel very weak. She was readmitted to hospital where examination of a blood specimen gave the following results:

Plasma analysis	Result	Reference range	Units
[Creatinine]	95	55–120	μmol/L
[Na$^+$]	148	132–144	mmol/L
[K$^+$]	1.9	3.3–4.7	mmol/L
[Total CO$_2$]	30	24–30	mmol/L

What do you think might be the explanation for this patient's hypokalaemia? She is discussed on p. 344.

Diabetes mellitus

The presence of diabetes mellitus may not be detected by 'side-room' testing of urine for glucose as the renal threshold for glucose tends to rise with age. Measurement of plasma [glucose] 2 hours after a 75 g load of anhydrous glucose (or 82.5 g glucose monohydrate) is a better screening test; the value should not exceed 11.0 mmol/L. Abnormal responses to this glucose load occur in about 25% of the population over 75 years. However, glucose tolerance tests are not normally required in this age-group; impaired glucose tolerance does not necessarily imply that an elderly patient will develop diabetes.

Management of elderly diabetics may need to depend on the help of relatives. Because of the higher renal threshold for glucose, home monitoring of blood [glucose] will probably be needed. In these patients, examination of records of home-monitoring measurements of blood [glucose] at the time of clinic attendances are usually adequate to assess treatment; there is little need for haemoglobin A$_1$ or plasma fructosamine to be measured.

Bone disease

The incidence of bone disease rises markedly in old age. Osteoporosis is the commonest cause, especially in women, but routinely available chemical investigations are not of value in its detection.

Paget's disease is very common. It is one of the first diagnoses to be considered when increased plasma alkaline phosphatase activity is found as an isolated abnormality in an elderly patient. It is occasionally necessary to determine whether the increased total enzymic activity is due to the bone isoenzyme, as would be the case in Paget's disease, or to the liver isoenzyme (e.g. due to secondary deposits of carcinoma in the liver).

Osteomalacia has an appreciable incidence in the elderly. It is usually due to lack of exposure to sunlight combined with nutritional deficiency. Plasma [calcium] and [phosphate] may both be reduced and alkaline phosphatase activity increased in many cases. However, there can be difficulties in interpreting the results of these measurements, due to lack of precise data for their reference ranges in the elderly. Plasma [25-HCC] is often normal, but it may be reduced due to inadequate intake of vitamin D or lack of endogenous synthesis, or both (p. 208).

Thyroid disease

Many geriatric assessment units have reported that screening for thyroid dysfunction is worthwhile. Using measurements of plasma [total T4] as a *screening* test, hitherto unsuspected hypothyroidism is said to have been detected in 2–6% of patients. If plasma [TSH] is measured, about 3% of patients admitted to these units may be found to have an undetectable plasma [TSH] without there necessarily being clinical or other biochemical evidence of hyperthyroidism.

In Chapter 17, we describe pitfalls in the use and interpretation of thyroid function tests, many of which are methodological in origin. The cautionary advice given there is particularly applicable to the use of thyroid function tests as screening investigations in elderly patients, many of whom are suffering from non-thyroidal illnesses (Table 17.3, p. 258) or are being treated with drugs that interfere with these tests (Table 17.4, p. 259), or both, at the time of their admission to geriatric assessment units.

Because abnormalities in the results of thyroid function tests are common in the elderly, and because these abnormalities can so often be explained by the high prevalence of non-thyroidal illnesses and drug treatment in these patients, we offer the following guidance on the use of these tests:

Case 21.3

A 78-year-old retired civil servant was admitted to a geriatric assessment unit with a recent history of rapidly progressing dementia. 'Side-room' tests and the results of admission screening investigations on blood were all normal apart from the results for thyroid function tests, which were as follows:

Analysis	Result	Reference range	Units
[TSH]	< 0.1	0.15–3.5	mU/L
[Free T4]	19	9–23	pmol/L
[Free T3]	3.0	3.0–9.0	pmol/L

How would you interpret these results? This patient is discussed on p. 345.

---

1 They should *not* be used indiscriminately as screening investigations. For instance, they should not be requested for elderly patients who are otherwise fit and well, and who have been admitted to hospital for surgery (e.g. herniorrhaphy). Also, they should not be requested for patients who are severely ill (e.g. myocardial infarction), unless there are clinical indications that thyroid disease, particularly hypothyroidism which is more common in the elderly, might be present.

2 Because hypothyroidism is relatively common, and often insidious in onset, it is reasonable to request thyroid function tests in patients with non-specific or vague symptoms, or who are for some other reason undergoing assessment in the absence of acute illness.

Measurements of plasma [TSH] provide the best screening test. The following conclusions can be drawn from its results:

1 A normal result excludes primary thyroid disease.

2 If, at the time the test is performed, the patient is not still recovering from a recent non-thyroidal illness, a plasma [TSH] greater than 10 mU/L indicates that the patient has hypothyroidism and may require treatment with thyroxine, or repetition of the test in a few weeks' time before deciding about the need for treatment.

3 If the plasma [TSH] is less than 0.1 mU/L, plasma [free T4] or [total T4] and plasma [total T3] should be measured. If the results for either of these measurements are raised, the patient should be referred for specialist advice as treatment for hyperthyroidism may be required. If, however, the results for the T4 and T3 measurements are normal or low, this suggests that the cause of the low plasma [TSH] is non-thyroidal illness.

Comments on Case 21.1 (p. 340)

The 'liver function tests' and side-room results of urine analysis indicated that the patient had cholestatic jaundice. Taken together with the finding of faecal occult blood, and the patient's history of loss of weight, a provisional diagnosis of carcinoma of the head of the pancreas was made. Ultrasound examination showed dilated bile ducts, but with no sign of gallstones, and the diagnosis was confirmed at laparotomy, when a cholecystjejunostomy was performed.

Comments on Case 21.2 (p. 342)

There are several drug-related reasons why this patient had developed marked hypokalaemia:

1 Chlorthalidone is a thiazide diuretic. It can cause modest K^+ depletion although not usually sufficient by itself to require potassium supplements.

2 Carbenoxolone has marked mineralocorticoid effects, causing retention of water and Na^+, and K^+ loss. Its use is contraindicated in elderly patients, and in patients who are hypertensive.

3 Frusemide causes K^+ loss. When using it for the treatment of oedema, it would be normal practice to use it in combination with a K^+-sparing diuretic. However, it is worth noting that amiloride and spironolactone (both K^+-sparing diuretics) antagonize the effects of carbenoxolone both on the kidney and on its ulcer-healing properties.

The drug treatment of this patient was changed in the light of these analytical results.

Comments on Case 21.3 (p. 343)

Undetectable plasma [TSH] is reported in 1–3% of patients admitted to geriatric assessment units if thyroid function tests are performed as part of a routine admission screening of all patients. Although undetectable plasma [TSH] is found in hyperthyroidism and in secondary hypothyroidism, in these elderly patients particularly 'non-thyroidal illness' and the effects of drug therapy are much commoner reasons for this finding.

In this patient, the normal plasma [free T4] and the low-normal plasma [free T3] excluded hyperthyroidism and secondary hypothyroidism. The final diagnosis was multiple cerebral infarctions caused by extensive atheromatous disease of the cerebral vessels, detected by CT scanning.

Chapter 22
Molecular Biology in Clinical Biochemistry

The purpose of this chapter is to review briefly some of the principles behind Molecular Biology, the methods which concern themselves with the analysis of the structure and function of DNA and RNA at the molecular level, and to illustrate how these principles can be applied to the investigation and diagnosis of human disease. The impact on therapy is already evident in the range of genetically engineered therapeutic products (e.g. insulin, growth hormone) and viruses for immunization (e.g. hepatitis B). The potential for 'gene therapy' is yet to be fully realized.

The potential contributions of Molecular Biology to the better understanding of the aetiology and pathogenesis and to improvements in the diagnosis of human disease are already clear. Enormous strides have been made in understanding the molecular pathology of single-gene disorders and the techniques have been applied to the antenatal diagnosis of an increasing number of these disorders. Common diseases (e.g. diabetes mellitus, ischaemic heart disease) which have an inherited component, but which are not classical single-gene defects, can also be investigated by these methods. In Microbiology the techniques of Molecular Biology are being increasingly used in the identification of pathogenic organisms.

Principles and applications

Several new techniques and discoveries have contributed to the developments in Molecular Biology. The details are beyond the scope of this chapter, but the outline of some of these techniques needs to be described.

One of the properties of nucleic acids that contributes to the analytical potential of Molecular Biology resides in the ability of complementary nucleotide sequences to hybridize with one another. Short pieces of DNA can thus act as specific probes to identify unique sequences in the genome. The genomic DNA can be dissociated by raising the temperature. Re-annealing to the probe is effected by subsequently dropping the temperature; careful attention to the temperature, ionic strength and other variables allows this process to be highly specific. Under stringent conditions, a suitable oligonucleotide probe of 20 base-pairs can bind to its complementary DNA sequence with complete fidelity. However, a change in a single base-pair in the genomic DNA in the complementary sequence will prevent hybridization. In other words, a mutation involving a single base-change in the genomic DNA can be detected with suitable oligonucleotide probes.

Restriction endonucleases and other enzymes

Restriction endonucleases. A major discovery, deriving from bacterial genetics, was the isolation of enzymes which cut DNA at specific sequences. Bacteria use these enzymes to degrade the DNA of invading viruses, preventing their replication in the host. By methylating bases in the host bacterial DNA, the same enzymes can be prevented from degrading host DNA. A battery of such enzymes is now available to cut human (or other) DNA at precisely defined sites. A useful feature of some of these endonucleases is their ability to recognize palindromic sequences in DNA and generate 'sticky ends' on the fragments produced; these fragments can then hybridize with other DNA pieces which have been generated by the same enzyme (Fig. 22.1). Other important enzymes include:

1 *Reverse transcriptase*. This allows single-stranded DNA to be synthesized from an RNA template. If the source of RNA is mRNA from a particular cell type, then it is possible to generate copy DNA (cDNA) from all the representative mRNA species that are being expressed in that cell type.

2 *DNA ligases*. These allow pieces of DNA to be covalently inserted at specific locations. For example, circular DNA from a plasmid may be opened at a discrete location, using a restriction endonuclease, and then closed with a ligase enzyme. If the closure is carried out in the presence of linear pieces of foreign DNA which can hybridize with the open ends of the plasmid DNA, some recombinant plasmids will

Segment of nucleic acid being acted upon by *Eco*R1

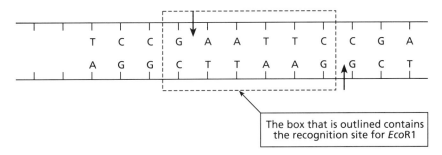

The box that is outlined contains the recognition site for *Eco*R1

Products of enzymic cleavage

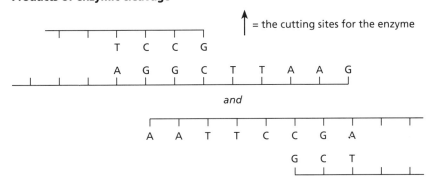

= the cutting sites for the enzyme

Fig. 22.1 The action of a restriction endonuclease, *Eco*R1. Note how *Eco*R1 recognizes a palindromic nucleotide sequence, producing daughter molecules with 'sticky ends'. In this and later figures: A, adenine; C, cytosine; G, guanine; and T, thymine.

be produced containing the inserted DNA. The hybridization is made possible if the same restriction endonuclease is used to open the plasmid and to cleave the foreign DNA, provided the endonuclease also produces 'sticky ends'.

3 *DNA polymerase 1*. This enzyme can be used to label a DNA probe by synthesizing a complementary labelled strand from ^{32}P-labelled nucleotides, provided short oligonucleotides are provided as primers.

4 *Taq polymerase*. This DNA polymerase, isolated from a bacterial species thriving at high temperature, *Thermus aquaticus*, is the basis of a method which *repeatedly* replicates defined segments of DNA by using oligonucleotide primers to each complementary strand of DNA. This is the polymerase chain reaction (PCR, p. 359).

Gene cloning

This is a method for isolating and amplifying the DNA sequence corresponding to a particular gene. There are two types of clone, the so-called genomic clone and the copy DNA (or cDNA) clone.

A *genomic clone* consists of the true genomic sequence of nucleotides corresponding to the cloned gene. It therefore includes non-coding regions of the gene (introns) as well as the coding regions (exons) which are ultimately responsible for mRNA formation. The precise functions of the introns, which are a feature of eukaryotic genes, are unknown. Both the introns and exons are transcribed as RNA during gene expression, but the intron sequences are cleaved from the resultant product, splicing the exon sequences together in the mRNA product. Further modification to the mRNA occurs before translation; it is 'capped' and a series of adenine (A) residues added to its tail. A genomic clone may also contain 'upstream' sequences (before the 5' end of the gene) and 'downstream' sequences (beyond the 3' end of the gene) which may be important in understanding the regulation of gene expression.

cDNA clones are DNA copies of the mRNA coding for a specific protein. In this regard, they contain only the corresponding coding regions of the gene and lack sequence information upstream or downstream of the gene.

Cloned genes are powerful analytical tools. The genomic clone provides detailed sequence information about the gene itself and enables characterization of a mutant gene, from simple point-mutations to deletions and mutations in regulatory elements. This probe, or specific oligonucleotide sequences directed at the mutation site, can be used to identify the mutant gene by specific DNA–DNA hybridization using a method called Southern blotting (p. 354). Although cDNA clones may be less informative, they can be used as probes to isolate the genomic clone. The cDNA clone will also specifically hybridize to cytoplasmic mRNA, and can be used to quantify gene transcription in another technique, known as 'Northern' blotting.

The cloned gene can be expressed from within the genomic DNA of foreign hosts, whether bacteria, yeasts or higher animals. The gene-product can be made available in large quantities (e.g. for therapeutic purposes) if a rapidly growing bacterial culture, for example, is used to express it. A cloned gene can be injected into a single fertilized egg or the early embryo stage of a foreign species. The cloned DNA is injected as a 'construct' which guides its insertion into the foreign host's DNA; it may include a suitable promoter which enables the gene to be expressed in specific cell types in the developing embryo. At least some of the germ cells of the developing embryo contain the foreign gene, allowing the gene to be transferred to the next generation, thereby producing a true transgenic animal. Such animals can serve as models of human disease and for gene therapy.

Sequence information about mRNA also allows the construction of 'anti-sense' oligonucleotides. These are single-stranded lengths of DNA (15–30 nucleotides in length) complementary to part of the specific mRNA under study. If these oligonucleotides can be made to enter cells, they hybridize there with the specific mRNA. The double-stranded regions thereby formed cannot be translated and, furthermore, they initiate degradation of the mRNA. By this means it is possible to suppress the synthesis of a particular protein uniquely, and to examine the consequences.

How are genes cloned?
The DNA sequence, whether genomic DNA or cDNA, must be part of a conveniently sized recombinant DNA that has the ability to replicate. Several suitable vectors have been extensively characterized and widely used for this purpose. Plasmids are simple, self-replicating organisms which infect bacteria. In clinical practice, they are important in carrying genes for antibiotic resistance in the host bacterium. One of the best characterized plasmid-cloning vehicles is pBR322, a circular double-stranded DNA carrying antibiotic-resistance sites and known endonuclease restriction enzyme sites. One of the limitations of these plasmids is that the size of the foreign DNA insert cannot be much more than 10 kb (1 kb = 1000 nucleotide bases). Bacteriophage vectors (e.g. lambda) have also been widely used in cloning, and artificially engineered cosmids (consisting of plasmid DNA packaged into a phage) allow cloning of fragments of DNA up to 50 kb.

Many ingenious strategies for cloning have been used and it is beyond the scope of this chapter to consider these in detail. Inevitably, there is a hit-and-miss component to cloning. In general, the more abundant the protein and the more that is known about the protein the gene of which is to be cloned, the more straightforward the procedure. On the other hand, many years of patient endeavour may be required to clone the gene of a low abundance protein. It is even possible to clone the gene before anything is known about the protein. This has been the case in cystic fibrosis (CF), for example, where the structure and properties of the mutant protein have been inferred from the cloned gene for CF.

A cloning technique using a plasmid is illustrated in Fig. 22.2. A cell type is first chosen on the basis that the gene is expressed in that particular cell; for instance, to clone the gene coding for an enzyme of the urea cycle, liver cells would be chosen. The mRNA is extracted from liver cells and cDNA synthesized using reverse transcriptase; included amongst the cDNA formed will be one which codes for the protein of interest. Reverse transcriptase creates a double-stranded cDNA–RNA hybrid from which the RNA is removed by alkaline digestion. The single-stranded cDNA is then rendered double-stranded using DNA polymerase and the product treated with another endonuclease, designated S1, to destroy the 'hairpin loop'

(a)

Step 1: Selection of the cell type and isolation of mRNA

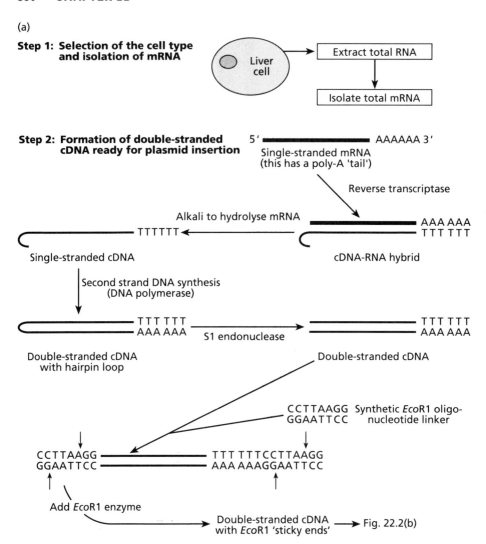

Step 2: Formation of double-stranded cDNA ready for plasmid insertion

Fig. 22.2 (a) An example of a cloning stategy for preparing cDNA for a liver-specific protein. In the final stage, the *Escherichia coli* restriction endonuclease 1 (*Eco*R1) enzyme cleaves the double-stranded cDNA at the points indicated by the arrows, thereby generating 'sticky ends'. The double-stranded cDNA is then ready for insertion into a plasmid. (b) The remaining stages in the example of a cloning stategy for preparing cDNA for a liver-specific protein. ●, clones with required cDNA insert; ○, other clones.

which is present. Finally, a short oligonucleotide linker sequence is added to each end of the duplex, creating 'sticky ends' which hybridize with the corresponding 'sticky ends' created when the plasmid vector is opened using a specific restriction enzyme (in the example, *Eco*R1 was used, Fig. 22.2). The cut plasmid and cDNA are then mixed together and ligated. This procedure results in the re-formation of intact plasmid, and in the formation of recombinant plasmids containing inserts of

(b)

Step 3: Insertion of cDNA into plasmid

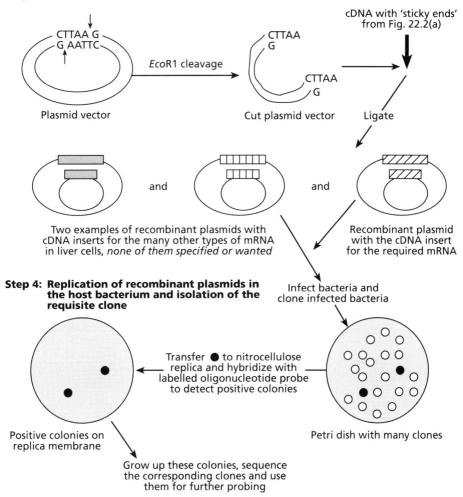

Two examples of recombinant plasmids with cDNA inserts for the many other types of mRNA in liver cells, *none of them specified or wanted*

Recombinant plasmid with the cDNA insert for the required mRNA

Step 4: Replication of recombinant plasmids in the host bacterium and isolation of the requisite clone

Infect bacteria and clone infected bacteria

Transfer ● to nitrocellulose replica and hybridize with labelled oligonucleotide probe to detect positive colonies

Positive colonies on replica membrane

Petri dish with many clones

Grow up these colonies, sequence the corresponding clones and use them for further probing

cDNA. Included among the recombinant plasmids should be some which contain cDNA synthesized from the relevant message.

The recombinant plasmids which result can be replicated in the host bacterium; infected bacteria can be specifically isolated by their antibiotic resistance conferred by the infecting phage. The collection of recombinant plasmids, containing portions of cDNA derived from liver cell mRNA, is known as a 'liver cell cDNA library'. This is the starting point for screening for the particular cDNA; in practice, it is often possible to obtain commercially such a cDNA library. It is also possible to construct genomic libraries in which the recombinant organism is constructed, not with cDNA but with suitably sized fragments of genomic DNA. Fragments of about 20 kb can be generated with an appropriate endonuclease, isolated, and inserted into a cosmid or lambda phage which can then be replicated. By producing a suitably large number of recombinants, the statistical probability that the library will contain almost the whole of the genome, distributed among the recombinants, can be made very high.

A method has to be devised to isolate plasmid recombinants which contain the relevant cDNA. At this stage, it is a great help to have some information about the primary amino acid sequence of the corresponding protein. If a sequence of six amino acids (or more) is known, it is possible to predict (from the genetic code) the corresponding sequence of bases in DNA which would code for this amino acid sequence. The precise oligonucleotide sequence (18 bases in length) cannot be known because of redundancy in the genetic code (e.g. the triplets -CCC-, -CCA-, and -CCG- all code for proline in mRNA), so it is necessary to synthesize a number of oligonucleotide probes to cover these various permutations; the number can be reduced by choosing residues such as phenylalanine or tyrosine, which use only two different triplet codons.

By plating out bacteria infected with the cDNA phage library at an appropriate dilution, individual bacterial colonies develop. These are clones, derived from a single bacterium ancestor, and therefore containing only one unique plasmid, which also confers antibiotic resistance. After replica transfer to a nitrocellulose membrane and denaturing the DNA, the radiolabelled oligonucleotide probe(s) can be incubated under appropriately stringent conditions to 'light up' (by auto-radiography) colonies which contain the complementary DNA sequence. At least some of these clones should contain recombinant plasmids which contain some cDNA sequence corresponding to the protein studied. The chosen clones can be isolated, grown and the DNA sequence of the recombinant phage determined. It is possible to use the DNA from these plasmids to screen the library further to obtain eventually a clone (or clones) which cover the full length of the appropriate gene. Knowing the primary amino acid sequence is also a great help in identifying the correct cDNA clones.

It must be emphasized that other strategies can be used, and indeed must be used, if there is no sequence information about the protein.

DNA sequencing (Fig. 22.3)

The ability to sequence DNA is fundamental to the success of much of Molecular Biology. Two methods are used, the Maxam–Gilbert method and the Sanger method; both depend upon an initial fractionation of the DNA into manageable pieces. In the Sanger method, DNA synthesis occurs from the cloned DNA template and is carried out in the presence of chemically modified nucleotides, radiolabelled, the incorporation of which leads to chain termination. Four incubations are set up; each contains tracer amounts of only one of the four possible nucleotide analogues (the other three nucleotides are present, but unmodified). If the analogue is incorporated, then the newly synthesized strand fails to elongate further. Since the unmodified counterpart of the analogue is also present, all possible lengths of newly synthesized strand, terminating at the selected base, occur. All four incubations are then subjected to electrophoresis, using a poly-acrylamide gel system which separates the fragments on the basis of mol mass

Aim: To determine the nucleotide sequence, the structure of which is eventually shown to be:

3′end of the sequence: –ATCGATCG– : 5′end of the sequence

'Tools': Chemically modified nucleotides that are also radioactively labelled and which act as *chain-terminators*. Also required are DNA polymerase (Klenow) and a primer

Method: Four sets of incubations with DNA polymerase, each using a different chain-terminator

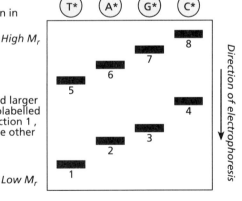

1 –ATCGATCG– $\xrightarrow[\text{+ primer}]{\text{+ DNA polymerase}}$ –T* and –TAGC T*

2 –ATCGATCG– $\xrightarrow[\text{+ primer}]{\text{+ DNA polymerase}}$ –T A* and –TAGCT A*

3 –ATCGATCG– $\xrightarrow[\text{+ primer}]{\text{+ DNA polymerase}}$ –TA G* and –TAGCTA G*

4 –ATCGATCG– $\xrightarrow[\text{+ primer}]{\text{+ DNA polymerase}}$ –TAG C* and –TAGCTAG C*

Electrophoresis on polyacrylamide gel and then identify the radioactive products by autoradiography

The products of each reaction are run in separate lanes

T* A* G* C*

High M_r

and = the smaller and larger of the two radiolabelled products of Reaction 1, and so on for the other reactions

1   5

Low M_r

Direction of electrophoresis

Radiolabelled base	Adenine*	Cytosine*	Guanine*	Thymine*
Complementary base	Thymine	Guanine	Cytosine	Adenine

Fig. 22.3 The Sanger method of DNA sequencing. Read the *complementary* nucleotide sequence 5′-TAGCTAGC-3′ from the gel, in ascending numerical order of the radiolabelled products.

(and, therefore, length). The sequence of nucleotides can then be read directly from the gel.

Southern blotting (Fig. 22.4)

The Southern blot is a method for detecting DNA fragments by hybridization to a suitable probe. If genomic DNA is cut using a restriction enzyme, a series of fragments is produced; the number depends upon the frequency with which the particular restriction endonuclease recognition site occurs throughout the DNA. A

Step 1: DNA extraction and cleavage

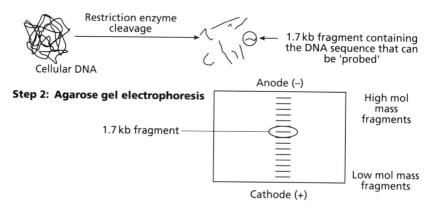

Step 2: Agarose gel electrophoresis

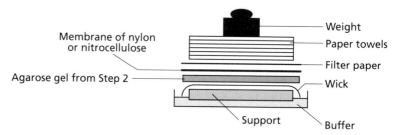

Step 3: Transfer to nitrocellulose ('blotting')

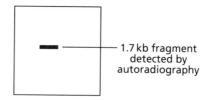

Step 4: Hybridization with radiolabelled probe and autoradiography

Fig. 22.4 Steps in the technique of Southern blotting. The 'blot' is a replica on nitrocellulose or nylon of the DNA fragments that have been separated by electrophoresis on an agarose gel. Specific DNA sequences of interest are identified by hybridization to a specific radiolabelled probe. Fragment(s) containing the particular sequence are identified by autoradiography.

cDNA probe or a genomic DNA probe might therefore hybridize with a number of fragments if, for example, the complementary stretch of DNA has been internally cut by the restriction enzyme. In this technique, the cleaved DNA fragments are first separated on the basis of size, using agarose gel electrophoresis. After alkaline denaturation, the DNA fragments are replica-transferred to a nitrocellulose membrane (the blot). This is achieved by layering the nitrocellulose membrane over the gel (which rests in buffer) and overlaying the membrane with absorbent paper which acts as a wick to encourage DNA transfer to the membrane. The membrane is much easier to handle then the fragile agarose and allows the hybridization to be carried out in a stringent fashion. The labelled probe identifies those fragments of DNA which contain sufficient complementary sequence; the labelled fragments are detected by autoradiography.

In the clinical laboratory, this method is very important in the diagnosis of single-gene defects. The precise way in which it can be applied depends upon how much detailed knowledge is available about the mutation event. Where this is known in detail, the technique can be made highly specific. In sickle cell anaemia, for example, the single amino acid substitution of valine for glutamic acid is the result of a single-base change in which thymine (T) replaces adenine. This single base-change leads to the loss of the recognition sequence for a restriction endonuclease termed *Mst*III in the mutant gene. When the genomic DNA is cut with this enzyme and subjected to Southern blotting using a probe specific for the β-globin gene, the length of DNA containing the appropriate complementary sequence differs between the sickle cell and normal specimens; this is readily detected on the Southern blot.

An alternative method uses labelled oligonucleotide probes to detect normal and mutated sequences. Labelled oligomers of about 19 nucleotides in length are constructed, one complementary to the normal sequence and the other to the mutated sequence. Under strict hybridization conditions the 'normal' oligomer will hybridize only with the normal gene and vice versa. The technique has been applied to the detection of α_1-protease inhibitor (α_1-antitrypsin) variants. In the example shown (Fig. 22.5) α_1-protease inhibitor (API) deficiency results from homozygosity of the Pi^Z allele.

Restriction fragment length polymorphisms (Fig. 22.6)

Even if the particular gene responsible for a single-gene defect is unknown, the Southern blot technique can still be used to follow the segregation of the mutated gene.

At the molecular level, inherited differences in the structure of DNA will be reflected in changes in the nucleotide sequence. Where these changes involve a coding region of DNA or a region which regulates gene expression, the consequences may be serious. Nevertheless, about 50% of the human genome consists of repetitive sequences of uncertain function. If the introns and non-coding flanking sequences are included, there is clearly the possibility of inherited differences in DNA structure which have no known serious clinical consequences. These individual differences lead to altered patterns of DNA fragments when the genome is subjected to digestion by specific restriction endonucleases. It is these

Coding sequences in a segment of the polynucleotide chains of the M and Z genes

1 M-sequence: (5'end)---ACC ATC GAC $\boxed{\text{G}}$AG AAA GGG A---(3'end)

2 Z-sequence: (5'end)---ACC ATC GAC $\boxed{\text{A}}$AG AAA GGG A---(3'end)

Note the single base change between the M-gene and the Z-gene. This change makes possible the synthesis of two oligonucleotide probes, one that is M-specific and the other Z-specific

Oligonucleotide probes, each composed of 19 nucleotides

1 M-specific probe, complementary to
the *coding sequence*: (3'end), TGG TAG CTG CTC TTT CCC T (5'end)

2 Z-specific probe, complementary to
the *anti-coding sequence*: (5'end), ACC ATC GAC AAG AAA GGG A (3'end)

Investigation of a family carrying the Z gene

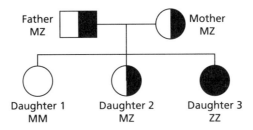

Southern blots

| M-specific oligonucleotide labelled probe, followed by autoradiography | Z-specific oligonucleotide labelled probe, followed by autoradiography |

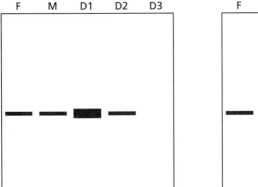 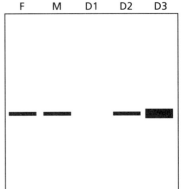

Fig. 22.5 Detection of homozygous ZZ α_1-protease inhibitor (α_1-antitrypsin) deficiency by means of Southern blots, using specific oligonucleotide probes and autoradiography.

Normal gene

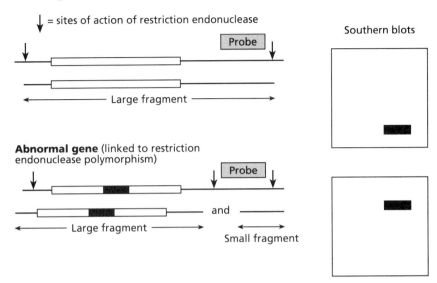

Investigation of a family carrying the mutant gene

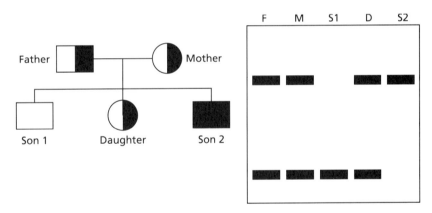

Fig. 22.6 Restriction fragment length polymorphism (RFLP) analysis. An additional restriction endonuclease site linked to the mutant gene is present in affected individuals. When the DNA is cut using the appropriate restriction endonuclease, fragments of different size are produced from normal and affected individuals. Although the probe is not directed at the gene itself, it is able to detect the different fragments thereby produced.

inherited differences in the size of fragments produced by restriction endonuclease digestion that are known as restriction fragment length polymorphisms (RFLP).

If a particular RFLP is closely linked to a mutant gene of interest, it can be used to follow the segregation of that gene across different generations. As with all linkage analysis, the method is not fool-proof since crossing-over between the mutant gene and the RFLP site will destroy the linkage and potentially lead to misdiagnosis. By choosing RFLP sites that are very close to the mutant gene, this probability can be kept as low as possible. Moreover, several linked RFLP, generated using different restriction endonucleases, can be used to follow the segregation of the gene (Fig. 22.6).

If the mutant gene is unknown, 'random' genomic DNA probes must be used initially to search for any RFLP. The method can be made less hit-and-miss by using genomic probes that do not contain repetitive sequences and presumably detect structural loci. If the chromosomal location of the mutant gene is known, then probes derived from libraries made exclusively from the DNA of this chromosome can be used. In this way it is possible to refine the analysis progressively to obtain probes closer and closer to the mutant gene. The technique is such that it is possible eventually to obtain genomic probes which contain the coding region of the mutant gene itself, even before knowledge of the gene-derived polypeptide product is available. In this way, it has been possible to clone the gene responsible for cystic fibrosis (CF).

In studies of CF, random screening techniques located the gene to chromosome 7. Once the general location of the gene was known, further refinements with different batteries of probe produced polymorphic markers with progressively closer linkage, based on family studies, to the putative gene. Eventually, it was possible to obtain sequence information on the gene itself. As a result of this work, it is now known that a number of mutations within the CF gene occur, although about 70% of cases of CF are accounted for by deletion of a single base in codon 507 and two bases in codon 508. This results in a deletion of phenylalanine at position 508 of the CF gene-product, a membrane protein which is involved in cellular chloride transport.

Hypervariable regions and RFLP

Another application of RFLP is in connection with the so-called hypervariable regions of DNA present in the genome of mammals, other animals and plants. These regions are made up of short DNA sequences, perhaps six to eight base-pairs in length and often rich in guanine (G) and cytosine (C), which are repeated in tandem. Polymorphism arises because the number of tandem repeats of the core DNA sequence varies between individuals. Moreover, the same tandem repeat can be found scattered throughout the genome in hypervariable regions of different lengths. The repeat structure of these regions has led to their being described as 'mini-satellite' DNA. If a restriction enzyme digest is used to cut on each side of the hypervariable region, a Southern blot analysis can be carried out to identify the different lengths of hypervariable region using the appropriate mini-satellite probe. The 'DNA fingerprint' obtained is unique to a particular individual. Although there is considerable variability in the lengths of these segments of DNA, it is not so great as to prevent the pattern being used in segregation studies. A band which appears to segregate with a disease in a large pedigree study, for example, can be isolated and cloned to search for a locus-specific probe. One application of this technique has been in paternity disputes and in other forensic work.

Polymerase chain reaction (PCR) (Fig. 22.7)

This reaction is a means of greatly amplifying selected portions of DNA. Its specificity for the particular length of DNA (usually from 100 to several thousand nucleotides in length) depends upon the use of two oligonucleotide probes (each typically 20 nucleotides in length) that are complementary to the two ends of the sequence to be amplified; the probes are also made to hybridize to opposite strands. In PCR, the template DNA to be amplified is first heated to 90–95°C, to cause strand separation, and then cooled to 50–65°C in the presence of the two primers to allow annealing of the primers to their respective DNA sequences. The reaction temperature is then adjusted to 60–75°C in the presence of heat-stable *Taq* polymerase. The *Taq* polymerase leads to a primer-mediated extension of both strands of the template DNA, in the region between the two primers. The three reactions of denaturation, primer-annealing and primer-directed extension

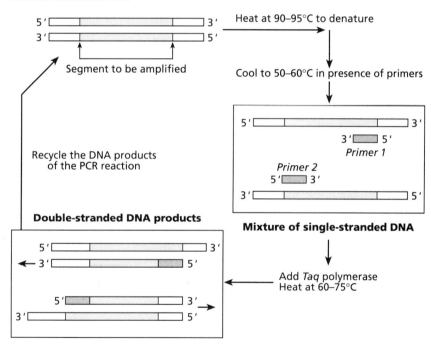

Directions of chain-lengthening of the two
Taq polymerase products is shown by arrows

Fig. 22.7 The polymerase chain reaction (PCR). The two double-stranded products of the first PCR cycle are subjected to a repeat cycle of denaturation, primer annealing and primer-directed extension and these processes are then repeated again and again. After three of these cycles, one-quarter of the DNA is present as short products and thereafter these products begin to accumulate exponentially. After 30 or more cycles, the vast majority of the DNA is present as short products. Amplification is sufficient to allow direct visualization of the product on a gel after staining with ethidium bromide.

are then repeated, leading to a *geometric* increase in the DNA between the two primers whereas the single-stranded long products accumulate arithmetically (Fig. 22.7). The theoretical amplification achieved is 2^n, where n is the number of cycles of denaturation–annealing–extension, though the amplification is usually somewhat less as the reaction is less then 100% efficient. Using this reaction, specific lengths of DNA can be amplified a million-fold, to an extent that the amplified product can be directly visualized on an agarose gel without the need for a Southern blot to be carried out using a labelled probe. The amplified DNA band is visualized on the gel by staining with ethidium bromide, a compound which binds avidly to DNA and fluoresces.

The PCR is a very powerful diagnostic and research tool. In Microbiology, for example, it can be used to pick out and amplify DNA sequences which are unique to invading organisms and enable their identification. It can also be used to amplify DNA for the purposes of 'DNA fingerprinting' in the forensic laboratory. In Clinical Biochemistry and Molecular Biology it is used, like Southern blotting, in the antenatal diagnosis of single-gene mutations and in studying structural gene polymorphisms. Thus, an amplified DNA sequence can be subject to digestion by a restriction enzyme which recognizes an allele which is linked to, or causes, an inherited disorder. The interested reader is referred to the article in the list (p. 421) on the applications of PCR to the antenatal diagnosis of various disorders including CF, Duchenne and Becker muscular dystrophies, and phenylketonuria. Its use in the detection of the commonest mutation responsible for CF is illustrated in Fig. 22.8, in which a modification of the PCR is used, the so-called amplification refractory mutation system (ARMS).

Oligonucleotides with a single 3'-mismatched residue fail to act as primers so fail to amplify a particular segment of DNA by PCR, and the ARMS is based on this fact. For example, in screening for the ΔF_{508} mutation in CF, one primer is constructed which matches the normal nucleotide sequence at this site and a second primer is constructed which matches the mutated sequence at this site. Amplification by PCR is then tested, in turn, with each primer (the primer on the other strand remains the same in both incubations). Provided this mutation alone is responsible for the CF gene defect, it can be used successfully in antenatal diagnosis (Fig. 22.8).

Molecular genetics of single-gene and polygenic disorders

The diagnostic aspects of single-gene defects are mostly carried out in molecular genetics units. Clinical biochemistry departments in the UK as yet undertake only a limited amount of diagnostic work on single-gene defects (e.g. API deficiency, monogenetic apolipoprotein abnormalities). It is likely that, as these newer techniques are applied to diseases such as diabetes mellitus and cardiovascular disease, there will be an increasing use of DNA-based tests in the routine diagnostic laboratory. The application of these methods to research and development in Clinical Biochemistry will also increase.

Single-gene disorders

Several examples of the way in which Molecular Biology has been used in the

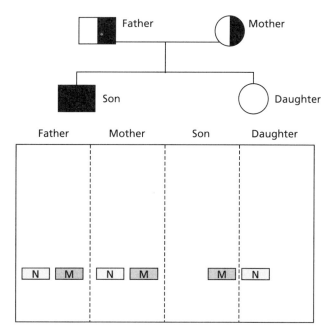

Fig. 22.8 Detection of the mutation in cystic fibrosis by an amplification-refractory mutation system. Each individual is tested in a PCR with a 'normal' (N) and with a 'mutant' (M) primer; these symbols denote the PCR products in the members of the family. They are visualized on the gel with ethidium bromide. Mismatches prevent PCR amplification, and are shown by the absence of a band from the gel.

The designation of the mutation in cystic fibrosis is ΔF_{508}.

diagnosis of single-gene defects have already been mentioned. These techniques have greatly improved our understanding of the molecular events underlying many of these single-gene defects.

Point-mutations within the coding region of a protein can lead to defective protein formation. The best known example of this is haemoglobin S, but the two most important allelic variants for API deficiency, Pi^Z and Pi^S (p. 90), are also point-mutations; these mutations probably interfere with the teriary folding of the newly synthesized protein and this, in turn, prevents the processing of the enzyme which is needed for secretion to occur. As a consequence, the protein accumulates in the liver cell.

Several point-mutations associated with defective receptor function have been described. In the case of the LDL receptor, these mutations can lead to reduced transport from the endoplasmic reticulum to the Golgi apparatus, to reduced LDL binding, and to a failure of the receptor–LDL ligand complex to cluster in coated pits. Some point-mutations lead to defective enzymes with the accumulation of toxic precursors or metabolic by-products (e.g. PKU, Tay–Sachs disease) and others to defective membrane proteins (e.g. hereditary spherocytosis).

Molecular biology techniques have characterized the basis of other types of mutation. Genes or portions of genes may be deleted or fused with other genes.

Regions of DNA can become inverted or additional DNA can become inserted into coding regions. These types of mutation may be associated with a failure of transcription or lead to defective products. More unusual mutations may involve the promoter site, or recognition sites for splicing, or the initiation or termination codons of the gene. More details can be obtained from the reference list (p. 421).

Polygenic disorders

The analytical and diagnostic power of Molecular Biology has been maximally exploited in single-gene defects. Some of these defects are relatively common, notably the haemoglobinopathies and cystic fibrosis; many are rare. However, most common diseases, those which have the greatest impact on morbidity and mortality, are not the result of single-gene defects. Nevertheless, serious public health problems such as ischaemic cardiovascular disease, hypertension, diabetes mellitus and cancer do run in families. Environmental factors undoubtedly exert an important effect in the development of these diseases (e.g. smoking and cancer, diet and cardiovascular disease) but, at the same time, inherited factors clearly contribute.

The genetic study of disorders where multiple-gene (polygenic) inheritance contributes is complex. One approach is to make a calculated guess that particular genes might influence susceptibility to a disease. For example, in the study of cardiovascular disease due to atheroma, where epidemiological studies indicate a clear association between plasma [cholesterol] and ischaemic heart disease (Fig. 12.1, p. 188), and where cholesterol is known to be a major component of the atheromatous plaque, a study of polymorphism among the apolipoproteins would be a rational approach. Remnant hyperlipoproteinaemia (p. 191) is an example of an association of an apolipoprotein polymorphism with environmental factors in the genesis of atheroma. These studies may also reveal monogenetic contributions to the susceptibility to atheroma, as in familial defective apoB in which an abnormal $apoB_{100}$ is produced that reduces the binding of LDL to its receptor, leading to elevated plasma [LDL-cholesterol].

If probes exist to putative candidate genes, they can be used in RFLP analysis either to investigate large families over several generations or to compare affected with unaffected sibs; alternatively, a range of probes can be used to look for RFLP in these groups. Whichever method is chosen, the aim is to discover RFLP that segregate with the disease, as any such RFLP linkage would indicate a potentially important gene, or gene-cluster, that influences the development of the disease under investigation.

Inheritance is known to be important in the development of diabetes mellitus, contributing more in type II than type I (p. 168). RFLP polymorphism in a hypervariable region upstream of the insulin gene has been described for both types of diabetes mellitus, but it is not yet known whether there is a gene close to the insulin gene that influences susceptibility to diabetes mellitus. In the case of type I diabetes mellitus, where auto-immune factors are important, RFLP analysis has shown linkage of polymorphisms within the class II (or DR) major histocompatibility complex, which is involved in cell-surface antigen recognition by helper T cells, with both susceptibility and resistance to type I diabetes mellitus.

Table 22.1 Examples of single-gene and of polygenic disorders which impinge upon the practice of Clinical Biochemistry

Single-gene defects		Polygenic disorders
Acute intermittent porphyria	Homocystinuria	Cancer susceptibility
α_1-Protease inhibitor deficiency	Hurler disease	Coronary heart disease
Congenital adrenal hyperplasia	Hyperlipidaemias*	Diabetes mellitus
Cystic fibrosis	Multiple endocrine	Epilepsy
Galactosaemia	neoplasia	Hypertension
Gaucher's disease	Phenylketonuria	Manic-depressive psychosis
Growth hormone deficiency	Tay–Sachs disease	Schizophrenia
Haemochromatosis	Wilson's disease	

* Examples include LDL-receptor defects and familial defective apoB.

Future applications

At the time of writing, over 2000 single-gene defects with an established mode of inheritance have been described. Although many of these are rare, there is no reason why the techniques of Molecular Biology should not be applied to their antenatal diagnosis and carrier detection; this has already been achieved with the commoner disorders such as cystic fibrosis, the haemoglobinopathies, Huntington's disease, etc. Table 22.1 lists some of the single-gene defects associated with biochemical abnormalities which have been discussed elsewhere in this book. In all cases, these defects have been mapped to particular chromosomal locations and, in most of the examples, carrier detection and antenatal screening is feasible. Also listed in Table 22.1 are some of the more common polygenic diseases which are amenable to study using the techniques described in this chapter. For most of the polygenic diseases listed, the risk for a first-degree relative contracting the disorder is broadly in the region 5–15%.

Chapter 23
The CNS and CSF

Many neurological disorders would appear to have a biochemical basis or to be associated with disturbances of metabolism. Several metabolic disorders with neurological manifestations have been discussed elsewhere and the control of treatment for epilepsy and manic-depressive states, for example, has been greatly improved now that therapeutic drug monitoring (TDM) of anticonvulsant and of lithium therapy is widely available, but it is debatable whether routine TDM for 'tricyclic' antidepressant drugs is cost-effective (Chapter 24). However, neurochemistry is a specialized subject that is beyond the scope of this book, and chemical tests, such as lysosomal studies on leucocytes needed for the precise characterization of the lipidoses and the mucopolysaccharidoses, for instance, are only performed in a few laboratories.

Metabolic disorders affecting the CNS

Many inherited metabolic disorders are associated with mental retardation. As a rule, the enzymic defect is general, affecting other organs besides the CNS, especially the liver. The defect can often be characterized by measuring the activity of the affected enzyme, or by investigating the pattern of abnormal metabolites, but the way in which the defective enzyme or the accumulation of metabolites affects mental function is not clear. Examples discussed elsewhere include galactosaemia (p. 179), Hartnup disease (p. 134), Lesch–Nyhan syndrome (p. 248) and phenylketonuria (PKU, p. 328).

Mass screening for neurometabolic disease is of value for a few conditions (e.g. PKU). For the rest, the main diagnostic effort is applied to family studies. Many of these disorders have an inevitably fatal outcome at present, and specialized chemical determinations are needed to identify the biochemical defect precisely. However, with some (e.g. congenital hypothyroidism, PKU, galactosaemia), early diagnosis and institution of appropriate treatment can prevent deterioration in mental function.

Wilson's disease is an example of a treatable degenerative metabolic disorder that affects the CNS, the liver and other organs, and one which can be diagnosed by chemical tests (p. 121). The porphyrias (p. 220) constitute another group of metabolic disturbances, some of which exhibit neuropsychiatric abnormalities.

Cerebrospinal fluid

The CSF approximates to an ultrafiltrate of plasma. There are, however, differences between the relative concentrations in plasma and CSF of low mol mass substances, and between the relative concentrations of high mol mass substances.

For example:
1 *Low mol mass substances*:
   (a) *Differential rates of diffusion*. Dissolved CO_2 diffuses into CSF more rapidly than HCO_3^-, so CSF $[H^+]$ (which depends on the $HCO_3^- : H_2CO_3$ ratio) may be significantly different from plasma $[H^+]$.
   (b) *Effects of ultrafiltration*. Bilirubin is nearly all protein-bound in plasma, and normally very little crosses the blood–brain barrier. Calcium is only partly protein-bound, and Ca^{2+} readily cross into the CSF.
2 *High mol mass substances*:
   (a) *Differential rates of diffusion*. Albumin is present in CSF in relatively higher concentration than larger proteins. However, because of the blood–brain barrier, plasma [total protein] is about 200 times greater than CSF [total protein].
   (b) *Secretion of proteins*. Some proteins, e.g. immunoglobulins, are secreted into the CSF.

Examination of CSF

CSF is normally clear and colourless. Turbidity is usually due to leucocytes, but it may be due to micro-organisms. Blood-stained CSF may indicate recent haemorrhage, or damage to a blood vessel during specimen collection. Xanthochromia (yellow colour) is most often due to previous haemorrhage into the CSF, but it may be an indication that CSF [protein] is very high. The CSF may be yellow in jaundiced patients.

CSF glucose

Lumbar CSF [glucose] is normally 0.5–1.0 mmol/L lower than plasma [glucose], whereas CSF [glucose] in specimens obtained from the cerebral ventricles and from the cisterna magna normally differs little from plasma [glucose]. In hypoglycaemia, CSF [glucose] may be very low; it is raised when there is hyperglycaemia.

CSF [glucose] may be low or undetectable in patients with acute bacterial, cryptococcal or carcinomatous meningitis, probably due to consumption of glucose by leucocytes or other rapidly metabolizing cells. In patients with tuberculous meningitis or cerebral abscess, it may also be markedly reduced or undetectable. In meningitis or encephalitis due to viral infections, it is often normal.

CSF total protein

Lumbar CSF [protein] (reference range, 100–400 mg/L) is normally almost all albumin. Ventricular and cisternal CSF [protein] is lower than lumbar CSF [protein]. Much higher CSF [protein] may have no pathological significance in the neonatal period, e.g. lumbar CSF [protein] may then be as much as 900 mg/L.

CSF [protein] is increased in a large number of pathological conditions. Whenever it is increased, organic disease of the CNS is probably present. In *infections of the CNS*, the increase may be very marked; capillary permeability is increased in acute inflammatory conditions of the CNS and in many chronic inflammatory conditions.

In the *demyelinating disorders*, the increase in CSF [protein] is often only moderate, usually in the range 500–1000 mg/L.

Primary and secondary neoplasms involving the brain or the meninges can cause very large increases in lumbar CSF [protein], if spinal block occurs. Values over 5000 mg/L may be observed. These specimens may be xanthochromic, and a protein clot may form on standing.

CSF immunoglobulins

CSF normally contains small amounts of IgG (reference range, 8–64 mg/L), a trace of IgA and minute amounts of IgM. Increases in CSF [Ig], particularly CSF [IgG], may be due to increased ultrafiltration of plasma immunoglobulins into the CSF, or to increased local synthesis of immunoglobulins.

Whenever there is increased local synthesis of IgG, the ratios CSF [IgG] : CSF [albumin] and CSF [IgG] : CSF [total protein] are higher than normal. This occurs in multiple sclerosis, neurosyphilis, subacute sclerosing panencephalitis and some other conditions. In all these conditions, limited numbers of clones of B-cells produce immunoglobulins and discrete, oligoclonal bands are demonstrable by isoelectric focusing of CSF.

Multiple sclerosis. It can be difficult to confirm a diagnosis of multiple sclerosis in its early stages. The following tests may help in this respect:

1 *CSF [IgG].* This test lacks specificity. Any cause of increased CSF [total protein] will also tend to cause an increase in CSF [IgG].

2 *CSF [IgG] : CSF [albumin].* This ratio renders the CSF [IgG] measurement more specific for CNS immunoglobulin synthesis, but is only abnormal in about 60–70% of clinically definite cases of multiple sclerosis.

3 *Isoelectric focusing* for the presence in CSF of oligoclonal bands that are not present in serum. This test is abnormal in over 90% of cases of clinically definite multiple sclerosis. However, the method is not widely available, and results require skill for their proper interpretation.

Chapter 24
Therapeutic Drug Monitoring and Chemical Toxicology

Clinical biochemistry departments play an important part in monitoring the therapeutic use of certain drugs, in investigating patients when drugs and poisons may have been taken in overdose, and in screening for drugs of abuse. Some departments are also involved in monitoring the environment, and in investigating certain industrial and occupational hazards.

Therapeutic drug monitoring

The control of several forms of drug treatment can be substantially improved if steady-state drug concentrations in blood specimens collected from individual patients are known. However, therapeutic drug monitoring (TDM) is no substitute for careful clinical assessment and surveillance. With some drugs, the dosage can be satisfactorily controlled by other means, e.g. the pharmacological actions of anticoagulants and of antihypertensive drugs can be assessed, and dosage adjusted, on the basis of prothrombin time and blood pressure measurements, respectively. Plasma (or serum) drug concentrations can be used to guide the treatment of individual patients if the following are known:

1 *Therapeutic ranges*. Published ranges are often little more than guidelines. They indicate inter-individual variation in the clinical response to drugs, usually under the ideal conditions of single-drug therapy. When applied to individual patients, because several factors can contribute to intra-individual variation (e.g. age, sex, diet, nutritional state), their shortcomings become apparent.

2 *Clinical pharmacokinetics*. Most drugs circulate partly bound to erythrocytes or plasma proteins, the bound drug being in equilibrium with unbound drug. For most drugs, the size of the pharmacological response is determined by the tissue concentration, which, in turn, is related to the plasma [unbound drug]. However, plasma [free drug] is difficult to measure and TDM mostly depends on measurements of plasma [total drug].

3 *Timing of blood specimen collection*. If specimens are collected too soon after the start of treatment, or after dosage has been changed (i.e. before a steady-state concentration of drug has been achieved), TDM results will be misleading. Adjusting the dosage on the basis of such results could have adverse effects (e.g. increasing the dose prematurely might lead to toxic effects). Also, if specimens are collected too long after the drug was administered, results will be misleadingly low.

The times taken for many drugs to establish steady-state concentrations in plasma, when given at regular intervals, are known as are their elimination half-times. Based on these data, it is usual to allow a sufficient period to elapse following a change in treatment before measuring plasma drug concentrations. It is also advisable to adhere to recommended times for collecting blood specimens for TDM, these depending on the requirements appropriate for a particular drug.

4 *Clinical information.* Published therapeutic ranges cannot make allowance for the possible effects of hepatic or renal disease in individual patients, nor for the consequences of drug interactions that might stem from particular prescribing combinations. The use of therapeutic ranges, when interpreting TDM results, has to be the responsibility of the doctor who is looking after the patient. In this context, the possibility of non-compliance (see below) is often highly relevant.

Indications for therapeutic drug monitoring

Where there is a satisfactory (sensitive, specific and reliable) method of assay available, TDM can be of great value in the following circumstances:

1 *Drugs with a low therapeutic ratio*, if their effects cannot be gauged precisely by clinical observation or by other laboratory measurements. Lithium is a good example. Regular measurements of serum [lithium], or plasma [lithium] using EDTA as anticoagulant, are essential if toxicity is to be avoided. Blood should be collected 12–18 hours after the last dose, as trough concentrations are particularly important for therapeutic control of lithium treatment.

2 *Checking for non-compliance*, as a possible explanation for therapeutic failure in a patient, especially if this occurs unexpectedly when drug treatment has previously been adequate. This is particularly true with psychiatric disorders as these are mostly heterogeneous in their aetiology and clinical manifestations. Patients' compliance may be imperfect, and clinical assessment of therapeutic response is liable to be at least partly subjective. Low plasma [drug], e.g. 'tricyclic' antidepressants, may help to explain the apparent lack of a treatment's clinical effectiveness. However, to use TDM routinely for all or most patients being treated with 'tricyclic' antidepressants would be very expensive, and studies have shown that this would not be cost-effective; TDM should be reserved for those patients in whom the need to check for possible non-compliance is indicated.

3 *Signs of drug toxicity.* Some drugs (e.g. digoxin) may produce toxic manifestations (e.g. nausea, cardiac arrhythmias) that can be difficult to distinguish from the symptoms and signs of the diseases for which they were prescribed. Blood for digoxin measurements should be collected 6–18 hours after the last dose, since plasma [digoxin] then mirrors most closely the myocardial [digoxin].

4 *Hepatic or renal function impaired.* Close monitoring of treatment is needed especially when potentially toxic drugs are being given, as with anti-arrhythmic drugs (e.g. procainamide) or aminoglycoside antibiotics (e.g. gentamicin).

The importance of drug metabolites

Most drugs are metabolized to inactive products (e.g. by oxidation, conjugation) and then excreted. Some drugs, however, are inactive when taken and are first rendered active (e.g. in the GI tract, liver) before exerting their actions, and later inactivated by further metabolism and excreted. Specific analytical methods are required if active drugs and structurally closely related but nevertheless inactive compounds are to be differentiated. Such methods are essential for TDM, since results from methods that fail to differentiate between active drugs and related but inactive compounds are of little or no value.

Amitryptiline and imipramine, and similar 'tricyclic' antidepressants, are examples of drugs that undergo *in vivo* metabolism to active demethylated metabolites (nortryptiline, desipramine, etc.). Some methods provide results for plasma [amitryptiline + nortryptiline], whereas a specific measure of plasma [nortryptiline] is what is required. Other methods show similar shortcomings in respect of plasma [desipramine]. Primidone is another drug that acts after conversion to active metabolites, principally phenobarbitone. If primidone therapy is to be monitored, plasma [phenobarbitone] is the measurement required.

Therapeutic drug monitoring in clinical practice

TDM is essential for the management of patients treated with digoxin, lithium, phenytoin and aminoglycoside antibiotics. Table 24.1 lists examples of drugs where TDM is either essential or very helpful. The frequency with which TDM is required for a particular drug is very variable. To recapitulate, the indications include:

Table 24.1 Therapeutic drug monitoring: the principal drugs for which TDM is essential

Drug	Therapeutic range of the drug in plasma*		Time to collect blood	Reason for TDM†
	Mass units	Molar units		
Carbamazepine	4–10 mg/L	17–42 µmol/L	Just before next dose	3
Digoxin	0.8–2.0 ng/mL	1.0–2.6 nmol/L	6–18 h after last dose	1,2,3,4
Gentamicin (a) Peak	5–10 mg/L		30–60 min after last dose	2,3,4,5
(b) Trough	< 2 mg/L		Just before next dose	2,3,4,5
Lithium	416–694 mg/100 mL	0.6–1.0 mmol/L	12–18 h after last dose	1,2,5
Phenytoin	10–20 mg/L	40–80 µmol/L	Long half-life — not critical	1,3
Procainamide	4–10 mg/L	17–42 µmol/L	18–24 h after last dose	2,4
Theophylline	10–20 mg/L	55–110 µmol/L	2–4 h after oral dose‡	1,2,3,4

* For conversion factors for numerical values from mass units into molar units, see p. 411.
† Key to the reasons for performing therapeutic drug monitoring:
  1 Wide inter-individual variation.
  2 Low therapeutic index.
  3 Therapeutic effect or signs of toxicity difficult to recognize.
  4 Administration of a potentially toxic drug to a seriously ill patient.
  5 Very toxic in overdose.
‡ Longer for slow-acting preparations.

1 Failure to achieve therapeutic control, although dosage is apparently adequate.

2 Loss of control in a patient previously stabilized on treatment.

3 To check for toxicity, especially if several drugs are being given.

4 To confirm that plasma [drug] remains acceptable when the dosage of the drug is changed, or the accompanying therapy is altered.

More frequent TDM may be needed in pregnancy or in children, and in patients with hepatic or renal disease, as metabolism or excretion might be impaired.

Units of measurement

The practice of referring to numerical values of drug measurements without mentioning the units cannot be condoned since it can lead to serious, sometimes fatal, mistakes.

Plasma drug concentrations may be expressed in mass (gravimetric) or molar units of concentration. Table 24.1 includes examples of both types of unit. Whatever the units of measurement adopted locally, doctors must note the units used for expressing the results of measurements of drug concentrations. Special care is needed when considering results reported from a laboratory other than the one with which the doctor is accustomed to work.

Chemical toxicology

Self-poisoning and accidental poisoning with drugs normally prescribed for therapeutic purposes, or with other substances, are common causes of emergency admission to hospital. Occasionally such admissions are due to deliberate (felonious) poisoning.

Where the diagnosis is drug overdosage, in most cases clinical management is based on clearly defined criteria (e.g. those relating to the management of an unconscious patient). Frequently, there is no specific treatment to help with the elimination of drug(s) thought or known to have been taken in overdose, or to counteract their effects. However, active forms of treatment now exist for some potentially lethal drugs.

Emergency chemical toxicology

Investigation of blood specimens for the possible presence of toxic agents, and determination of their concentration are particularly useful if a specific treatment is available or if the rate of elimination of the toxin can be increased (Table 24.2). Three of the drugs most commonly ingested in overdose will be considered.

1 *Paracetamol* is often taken in overdose. It is converted in the liver to a toxic metabolite that binds covalently to proteins inside the hepatocyte. If paracetamol overdose is diagnosed sufficiently quickly, specific treatment is available (e.g. intravenous N-acetylcysteine).

The diagnosis of paracetamol overdose depends on measurement of plasma [paracetamol]. The time when the possible overdose was taken needs to be known, since the blood specimen should be collected not less than 4 hours and not more than 12–16 hours later. If blood is collected too early, the result for

Table 24.2 The principal examples of substances that cause acute poisoning in the UK

Examples of substances	Active treatment of overdose or toxin
Drugs commonly taken as overdose	
Benzodiazepines	Flumazenil
Ethanol	No specific treatment available
Paracetamol	N-acetylcysteine, intravenously
Salicylates	Forced alkaline diuresis, haemodialysis
Tricyclic antidepressants	No specific treatment available
Drugs less commonly taken as overdose	
Carbamazepine	Activated charcoal
Iron	Desferrioxamine
Lithium	Saline, intravenously
Phenobarbitone	Activated charcoal
Phenytoin	Activated charcoal
Quinine	Activated charcoal
Toxic substances	
Carbon monoxide	Oxygen
Cyanide (non-fatal dose)	Cobalt edetate, hydroxycobalamin
Ethylene glycol	Ethanol, haemodialysis
Methanol	Ethanol, haemodialysis
Organophosphorus agents	Pralidoxime, atropine
Paraquat	No specific treatment available

plasma [paracetamol] is liable to be misleadingly low as the drug may not have been fully absorbed. If the specimen is not collected until 12–16 hours after the overdose, toxic damage to the liver will already have occurred and treatment is usually ineffective.

2 *Salicylates* are often taken in overdose. The effects of overdosage are very varied, especially in children. Dehydration is frequently severe, due to vomiting, and acid–base balance is often markedly affected. If vomiting is severe, a metabolic alkalosis develops, but otherwise a mixed disturbance (respiratory alkalosis and metabolic acidosis) usually develops.

The diagnosis of salicylate overdose is confirmed by measuring plasma [salicylate], and the nature of the acid–base disturbance can be determined from the clinical features plus the results of blood-gas analyses (p. 60). Although there is no specific antidote, the rate of excretion of salicylates can be increased by forced alkaline diuresis; this is often employed if the plasma [salicylate] exceeds 3.6 mmol/L in adults, or 2.2 mmol/L in children. Haemoperfusion or haemodialysis may also be employed, particularly if there is evidence of severely impaired renal function or if other treatments have proved ineffective.

3 *Ethanol*. The acute effects of over-indulgence in ethanol sometimes lead to admission to hospital. If the diagnosis is in doubt, plasma [ethanol] should be measured. Some patients may have drunk methylated spirits rather than ethanol, and rapid identification of both methanol and ethanol is then needed.

Ethanol is taken together with other drugs in more than half of the cases of self-poisoning attempts, and may have an important potentiating effect on the pharmacological actions of these other drugs. It may be worthwhile, therefore, to make a practice of measuring plasma [ethanol] in these patients. Determining plasma [ethanol] urgently may also help in managing patients after road traffic accidents, especially if they have suffered head injuries.

Non-urgent drug analyses

Other specimens and materials, obtained at the time of emergency admission, may help in the fuller, non-urgent investigation of patients in whom poisoning is a possible cause, especially if such patients fail to respond to conventional support-ive medical treatment. Examination of these specimens may serve to exclude drug toxicity, when the diagnosis is uncertain. Many of the investigations required for this purpose are either too complex, or needed too infrequently, to be included in the laboratory's 24 hours/day repertoire of emergency chemical toxicology inves-tigations. The following specimens should be collected, labelled carefully, and kept for later examination, should this be required:

1 *Any tablets or medicine* found near the patient, however small in amount. Pharmacy departments can often identify tablets and drug residues, but chemical analysis may be needed.

2 *Vomit, stomach aspirate and the first portion of gastric lavage.* Stomach contents sometimes contain large quantities of undigested and unmetabolized drug or poison, so can prove very helpful for drug-identification purposes in difficult cases. However, these specimens can give no indication of the amount of drug that has been absorbed.

3 *Urine, the first specimen passed.* 'Side-room' tests for glucose and ketone bodies (p. 14) should be carried out immediately on a sample. The rest of the specimen should be stored in a refrigerator in case non-urgent screening for drugs and their metabolites is required later.

4 *Blood.* A specimen should be collected, in addition to any specimens for emergency toxicology; the plasma or serum should be separated and stored frozen for possible later drug analysis.

Drug screening

Screening for drugs and poisons may be of value:

1 To exclude drugs or poisons as the cause of illness when the diagnosis is uncertain or the patient is not responding to conventional therapy.

2 In suspected poisoning or drug administration to children.

3 In suspected brain death.

4 To investigate suspected solvent or drug abuse.

When drug screening is being performed, interference by drugs given as treatment may sometimes lead to a failure by the laboratory to detect other drugs in samples from patients with symptoms thought to be due to poisoning. This effect is called *masking*. Specimens for toxicological analysis should, if possible, be taken *before* any medication is started. If this is not possible, details of *all* drugs administered in treatment should be given to the laboratory.

Poisoning in children

The diagnosis of poisoning in childhood presents difficulties not usually encountered in adults. The differential diagnosis may be wider, and the range of substances that may have been taken or administered is very large. Also, some compounds (e.g. salicylates) may produce much more marked toxic effects in young children than in adults. The position is further complicated by the inability of the patient, as a rule, to give useful information. The history obtained from the parent(s) may be vague or misleading, especially if one or both have been responsible for unauthorized drug administration.

Non-accidental poisoning in children or child abuse, i.e. the deliberate administration of a potentially toxic compound with intent to poison a child, is an increasingly common and very serious problem. Its recognition and management, which may include treatment directed specifically against the poison, require rapid and definitive methods of analysis, sometimes extending to include a full drug screen.

Suspected brain death

In cases of suspected brain death, where the cause is unknown, a drug screen is considered mandatory before life-support systems can be removed. With the widespread availability of life-support systems, and the growing demand for firm information on which to base difficult decisions (e.g. relating to possible organ transplantation), requests for drug screening are increasing. The investigations to be performed require specific methods of analysis sufficiently sensitive to prove that drug effects (including therapeutic drugs) are no longer operative. The analyses to be performed on specimens from these patients may require the best available modern techniques and considerable expertise.

Social problems

Over-indulgence in ethanol is a widespread and serious social problem; it can give rise to various pathological effects, especially alcoholic liver disease and cirrhosis (p. 120). Solvent abuse and drug addiction are other problems of great social importance. Confirmation of the diagnosis may require chemical investigations:

1 *Solvent abuse*: A wide range of volatile substances, many of them found in glues or in aerosol sprays or fuel gases, have been reported as being involved in cases of volatile solvent abuse, 'glue sniffing', etc. Gas chromatographic analysis of blood specimens provides a rapid and specific means of detecting the volatile compounds, and liquid chromatography of urine extracts enables identification of organic acids formed by the metabolism of toluene and xylene.

2 *Drugs of abuse*: The marked growth in drug misuse in the UK, USA and elsewhere has resulted in increasingly frequent requests, from drug clinics and from general practitioners, for the screening of urine specimens for the possible presence of opiates and related drugs. Many of these specimens come from patients for whom treatment with dihydrocodeine or methadone has been prescribed, to alleviate the symptoms associated with heroin withdrawal.

It is essential to be able to distinguish between opioids given as treatment and morphine derived from heroin metabolism. Immunoassay and chromatographic procedures are widely used for these analyses, and it is now possible for hospital laboratories to identify specifically minute amounts of many drugs of addiction, including morphine and its derivatives, cocaine and its derivatives, tetrahydrocannabinol, lysergic acid diethylamide (LSD), amphetamine, benzodiazepines, methadone, and buprenorphine. *It is important to screen for drugs of abuse:*

1 To corroborate claims that drugs are being misused when these claims are made by patients requesting maintenance therapy.

2 To determine if prescribed drugs (e.g. methadone) are being taken.

3 To determine if drug abuse is continuing.

4 To monitor changing patterns of drug abuse.

Most drug-screening procedures are performed on urine specimens. It is essential to obtain a sample which has not been substituted by the patient (i.e. been passed by someone else), and it is just as important to ensure that the urine specimen has not been adulterated. Some patients may adulterate their urine with salt, bleach, bicarbonate, or detergents to obtain a negative result in a drug-screening test. Others may add codeine, methadone or morphine preparations to obtain a positive result. The laboratory can determine if adulteration has taken place by testing to see whether drug metabolites are also present; absence of these metabolites indicates that adulteration has occurred.

The preliminary drug screen uses immunoassays that are sensitive but may lack specificity due to cross-reaction with related compounds. Confirmatory tests using specific chromatographic methods are required as a follow-up to positive results because of the possibly very serious implications for patients that can stem from being identified, correctly or incorrectly, as abusers of drugs.

Industrial and occupational hazards

There is a formidable list of potentially toxic compounds used in industry. In Britain, their use is controlled by Acts of Parliament, including the Factories Acts and the Health and Safety at Work, etc., Act. Concern arises when the provisions of these Acts are not observed or when faulty equipment leads to a breakdown in precautions. Hospital laboratories may be involved in investigating these problems, but more often they are the responsibility in the UK of the Health and Safety Executive.

Metal poisons

Mercury, cadmium and lead are all highly toxic to man. Their effects depend partly on the type of compound involved, whether inorganic or organometallic, and partly upon the route of absorption. In all cases the kidney is liable to be severely damaged, and other organs that may be affected include the liver and the nervous system.

Blood and urine measurements of the metal are important for the specific identification of the toxic agent. In blood, these metals are predominantly associated with erythrocytes so it is essential for toxicological analyses to be carried out on specimens of whole blood, not on plasma or serum. In some cases there is lack of agreement as to the concentration of the toxic agent to be regarded as potentially dangerous; this applies particularly in the case of blood [lead].

Chemical investigations also provide valuable information about the severity of organ damage. Intoxication with mercury, lead or cadmium can all give rise to an overflow amino aciduria (p. 132). Lead poisoning causes abnormalities in porphyrin metabolism (p. 226).

Trace element toxicity

Excessive quantities of the essential but potentially toxic trace elements (p. 230) may be ingested as a result of industrial exposure, and these accidents have sometimes proved fatal. Workers exposed to these elements should have their blood or urine concentrations, or both, monitored regularly. Toxic effects may also occur if excessive amounts of any of the trace elements are given as excessive supplements in total parenteral nutrition regimes, or other form of therapeutic overdose, and in some instances as a result of deliberate self-poisoning.

Aluminium

Chronic renal failure patients who are being maintained on haemodialysis regimens are particularly at risk from poisoning by dialysis fluid constituents. Aluminium toxicity leading to dialysis dementia and to metabolic bone disease has been described. Prevention of toxicity requires periodic checks of aluminium content in the water supply and in the effluent from deionizers used with dialysers.

Organic solvents

Many organic solvents used in industry are toxic (e.g. chlorinated hydrocarbons, ethylene glycol). Toxicity may be due to accidental exposure, or sometimes to solvent abuse. The toxic agent can usually be identified specifically (e.g. by gas chromatography). Other chemical investigations may be needed, to assess hepatic and renal function.

Pesticides and herbicides

Organophosphates (e.g. parathion, malathion) may cause poisoning among farm-workers by inhibiting acetyl cholinesterase; plasma cholinesterase (ChE) is also inhibited. Other causes of low plasma ChE activity are summarized in Table 6.3 (p. 81).

Measurements of plasma ChE or erythrocyte acetyl cholinesterase activity can help in the recognition of excessive exposure to organophosphates, especially if tests are repeated at intervals. Serial determinations provide comparative data and enhance the value of the tests; there is a wide variation between individuals in the baseline levels of cholinesterase activity. These measurements are also useful when following the progress of patients recovering from organophosphorus poisoning.

Paraquat and diquat are extremely dangerous herbicides, if ingested. Paraquat has severe effects, especially on the lungs and kidneys. Clinical features usually suggest the diagnosis, before the onset of complications, and the diagnosis can be confirmed by chemical examination of blood or urine for the presence of these herbicides or their metabolites. These measurements may help determine the prognosis.

Chapter 25
Revision: Examination Questions

Multiple choice questions

The acceptability of multiple choice questions (MCQ) to medical students and doctors preparing for higher professional qualifications depends partly upon their objectivity, when used in examinations, and partly on the ease and rapidity with which they can be used to assess knowledge when revising for examinations. However, it can be difficult to set questions that are both testing and unambiguous. Also, some subjects do not lend themselves to the MCQ format.

Ambiguities in the wording of MCQ may only become apparent after they have been repeatedly used in examinations. Most of the questions in this book have been tested in this way. They are, in general, set at a level of difficulty considered appropriate for medical students nearing the end of their clinical course and junior hospital doctors or trainee general practitioners preparing for postgraduate professional qualifications. Many are also suitable for medical laboratory scientific officers or technologists preparing for their examinations. In setting the questions for examination purposes, we were able to assume that the candidates would possess the knowledge of Medicine that they could reasonably be expected to have acquired by the time of first qualifying as doctors.

Marking systems

The method of scoring answers is not important when the questions are being used simply for self-assessment, although we would advise against adopting a simple system that encourages guessing since areas of lack of knowledge might then be missed. In a real-life examination, information about the marking system (especially if it involves penalty marks) can be very important in deciding whether or not to answer a question. Any system that involves the award of penalty marks for wrong answers offers a more exacting test of knowledge.

All the questions in the MCQ section are of the independent true–false (multiple true–false) type. Each consists of an initial statement, or stem, followed by five completions or items identified by the letters A, B, C, D and E. Each completion is either True or False. For example:

Insulin-induced hypoglycaemia normally produces an increase in the plasma concentration of:
A adrenaline (True)
B cortisol (True)
C gastrin (False)

D glucagon (True)
E growth hormone (True)

In every question, any number (0–5) of completions may be True (T) or False (F). In the above example, a correct set of answers could be recorded as TTFTT.

It is for the reader to determine *whether* to award one mark for every correct answer and to score nothing for abstentions and wrong answers, *or* to make the test of knowledge and confidence harder by, for instance, awarding one penalty mark for every wrong answer and, possibly also, half a penalty mark for every abstention.

Practice examinations

For practice examination purposes, we recommend that readers should decide in advance to allow themselves 90 minutes to answer not more than 50 questions. Furthermore, as the questions in Part 1 are grouped on a chapter-by-chapter basis (Table 25.1), we suggest that in any one 'examination session', the reader should only *attempt alternate questions* so as to avoid a feeling of possible duplication between some of the questions.

Terminology

Much information obtainable from chemical investigations helps to establish a diagnosis, without at the same time necessarily always being a constant feature of a particular clinical condition. We have, therefore, been compelled in drafting questions to use words such as 'usually', 'often', 'occasionally' or 'rarely'. The context of the questions will, in most instances, make the intention clear.

Multiple choice questions, Part 1

The questions in this first part, questions 1–100, are all based entirely, or almost entirely, on biochemical information contained in the corresponding single chapters (Table 25.1). The key to the answers is given on p. 409, but this *should not be consulted* during an 'examination session'.

Table 25.1 Chapters to which MCQ relate

Chapter	Questions	Chapter	Questions	Chapter	Questions
1	1–3	9	32–38	17	76–80
2	4–8	10	39–44	18	81–85
3	9	11	45–48	19	86–87
4	10–13	12	49–51	20	88–94
5	14–17	13	52–61	21	95–98
6	18	14	62–67	22	—
7	19–24	15	68–70	23	99
8	25–31	16	71–75	24	100

Questions 1–100 each relate entirely, or almost entirely, to information contained in the corresponding chapters, as listed in this table. Questions 101–150 are almost all concerned with information contained in two or more chapters.

1 **Case-finding and screening surveys:**
  A involve screening a definable population group for a particular condition or group of conditions
  B yield an unacceptable number of false-negative results if the sensitivity of the test(s) is set too low
  C for malnutrition in old age can be carried out satisfactorily by measuring plasma [albumin]
  D for phenylketonuria in neonates are performed by measuring blood [phenylalanine]
  E for poisoning by organophosphate pesticides should be performed by measuring urinary cholinesterase excretion

2 **Changes that occur in urine specimens on standing at room temperature include:**
  A conversion of urea to ammonia, with consequent fall in pH
  B utilization of glucose by bacteria
  C oxidation of urobilinogen to urobilin
  D precipitation of phosphate
  E conversion of porphobilinogen to porphyrins

3 **Significant differences in plasma concentrations between blood samples collected from ambulant and from recumbent patients might be expected with:**
  A calcium
  B cortisol
  C potassium
  D cholesterol
  E urea

4 **Blood specimens deteriorate in the following ways, despite proper specimen collection, if plasma (or serum) is left overnight in contact with cells:**
  A plasma [glucose] rises
  B plasma prostatic acid phosphatase activity falls
  C plasma [total CO_2] falls
  D plasma [phosphate] falls
  E plasma lactate dehydrogenase activity rises

5 **'Side-room' tests for glucosuria using glucose oxidase test strips are likely to be positive in:**
  A lactating females
  B idiopathic haemochromatosis
  C cystinuria
  D diabetes insipidus
  E primary gout

6 **In the 'side-room' investigation of ketonuria, urine test strips:**
   A detect acetoacetic acid in urine
   B detect 3-hydroxybutyric (β-hydroxybutyric) acid in urine
   C detect lactic acid in urine
   D give a semi-quantitative assessment of the severity of ketonuria
   E are used also to test for ketones in plasma

7 **When carrying out 'side-room' tests with test strips for proteinuria, the tests:**
   A detect all proteins normally detectable in plasma with about equal sensitivity
   B often fail to detect Bence Jones protein when it is present
   C are not sensitive enough to detect the 'microalbuminuria' of diabetic nephropathy
   D often give false-positive results in patients with glycosuria
   E often give false-positive results if the patient has recently had a pyelogram

8 **'Side-room' tests for glycosuria using a reductive method give positive results in the presence of:**
   A galactose
   B creatinine, in high concentration
   C fructose
   D acetoacetic acid
   E sucrose

9 **For substances with concentrations in plasma that show a normal (Gaussian) distribution in a reference healthy population:**
   A the values for that population are distributed symmetrically about the mean
   B the reference ranges are independent of the accuracy of the analytical methods used
   C the reference ranges are independent of the precision of the analytical methods used
   D about 50% of the results obtained in other healthy people will be within two standard deviations of the mean of the corresponding reference range
   E over 99% of the results obtained in other healthy people will be within three standard deviations of the mean of the corresponding reference range

10 **In assessing fluid and electrolyte balance:**
   A in adults, about 50% of the total body water is extracellular
   B in infants, about 60% of the total body water is extracellular
   C in adults, insensible fluid losses are normally less than 250 mL/day
   D most of the normal daily loss of K^+ occurs in the urine
   E losses of Na^+ via the skin are normally less than 5% of the total daily loss

11 Water depletion, unaccompanied by sodium depletion:
   A results in a fall in plasma osmolality
   B stimulates release of arginine-vasopressin
   C causes fluid to transfer from the extracellular to the intracellular compartment
   D is a cause of hypernatraemia
   E causes a fall in glomerular filtration rate

12 As a result of the severe loss of isosmotic Na^+-containing fluid:
   A patients become thirsty
   B ADH secretion is stimulated
   C plasma [creatinine] rises
   D plasma [renin] falls
   E aldosterone secretion decreases

13 Potassium tends to move from the ECF to the ICF in patients:
   A with metabolic alkalosis
   B treated with adrenaline
   C who are dehydrated
   D treated with insulin
   E following a major operation

14 The undernoted results for arterial blood-gas analyses (reference ranges in parentheses) might be expected in the following conditions:
$[H^+]$ = 60 nmol/L (36–44 nmol/L)
Plasma $[HCO_3^-]$ = 8 mmol/L (21.0–27.5 mmol/L)
Pco_2 = 3.9 kPa (4.4–6.1 kPa)
Po_2 = 13.1 kPa (12.0–15.0 kPa)
   A chronic obstructive airways disease
   B diabetic ketoacidosis
   C hysterical overbreathing
   D methanol poisoning
   E chronic nephritis

15 Which of the following results obtained on an arterial blood specimen collected at the time of emergency admission of a 40-year-old man would be expected if the patient had been vomiting repeatedly due to pyloric stenosis (reference ranges in parentheses)?
   A $[H^+]$ = 30 nmol/L (36–44 nmol/L)
   B Pco_2 = 4.0 kPa (4.4–6.1 kPa)
   C plasma $[HCO_3^-]$ = 18 mmol/L (21.0–27.5 mmol/L)
   D [total CO_2]   = 34 mmol/L (24–30 mmol/L)
   E $[K^+]$ = 2.8 mmol/L (3.3–4.7 mmol/L)

16 When assessing the blood-gas status of a patient with chronic respiratory insufficiency:

A the acid–base disturbance can be fully characterized by measuring plasma $[H^+]$ or pH, P_{CO_2} and blood [haemoglobin]

B plasma $[HCO_3^-]$ principally reflects changes in the 'respiratory component' of the Henderson equation

C arterialized venous blood is the most suitable specimen for analysis

D laboratory measurements should be made at the temperature of the patient at the time of specimen collection

E blood P_{O_2} and per cent oxygen saturation need to be measured in addition to the tests listed in A

17 **A metabolic acidosis is an expected consequence of:**

A pyloric obstruction

B common bile duct obstruction

C ureterosigmoidostomy

D unilateral ureteric obstruction

E colonic obstruction

18 **In a patient with a severe but uncomplicated myocardial infarction, in the absence of thrombolytic treatment:**

A plasma total creatine kinase (CK) activity becomes abnormal within 4–8 hours after the onset of chest pain

B plasma CK-MB isoenzyme activity becomes abnormal within 30–60 minutes after the onset of chest pain

C peak plasma total CK activity occurs about 12 hours after the onset of chest pain

D peak plasma activities of total CK and aspartate aminotransferase (AST) occur at about the same time

E 'heart-specific' lactate dehydrogenase activity is likely to remain raised for about 3 weeks

19 **Plasma proteins:**

A are all synthesized in the liver

B are the principal blood buffers

C have hormone-transport functions

D are important components of the body's defence mechanisms

E turn over more rapidly than normal in untreated hyperthyroidism

20 **A low plasma α_1-protease inhibitor (α_1-antitrypsin) concentration is of diagnostic value in patients with:**

A carcinoma of the lung

B juvenile cirrhosis

C myocardial infarction

D polyarteritis nodosa

E pulmonary emphysema

21 In an untreated patient in whom the diagnosis of multiple myeloma has been made by radiology:

A the plasma concentration of one of the immunoglobulin classes (IgG, IgA, etc.) is usually increased

B immunoglobulin light chains are usually demonstrable in urine in excess

C plasma [calcium] is often increased

D plasma alkaline phosphatase activity is often increased

E plasma [β_2-microglobulin] provides a good indication of prognosis

22 In the diagnosis and management of patients with carcinoma of the colon, plasma carcinoembryonic antigen (CEA) is:

A a tumour marker with high specificity for carcinoma of the colon

B used as a screening test for early detection of carcinoma of the colon in people over 40 years

C a sensitive and specific indicator of spread of colonic carcinoma prior to operation to remove the primary tumour

D a useful post-operative confirmatory test that the tumour has been removed completely at operation

E a sensitive indicator of tumour recurrence

23 The following plasma measurements are used for the early detection of recurrence of tumours following their treatment:

A acid phosphatase activity

B C-reactive protein concentration

C α_2-macroglobulin concentration

D chorionic gonadotrophin (hCG) concentration

E placental-like alkaline phosphatase activity

24 The following plasma protein concentrations are likely to be increased a few days after severe injury:

A albumin

B transferrin

C C-reactive protein

D fibrinogen

E α_1-protease inhibitor (α_1-antitrypsin)

25 In a 45-year old man with a three weeks' history of obstructive jaundice, uncomplicated by cholangitis, chemical investigations would usually show:

A normal plasma [albumin]

B plasma ALT activity below 100 IU/L and alkaline phosphatase activity above 250 IU/L

C plasma AST activity below 100 IU/L and plasma GGT activity above 150 IU/L

D increased plasma [conjugated bilirubin]

E increased plasma [bile salts]

Reference ranges

Alanine aminotransferase (ALT)	= 10–40 IU/L
Alkaline phosphatase	= 40–125 IU/L
Aspartate aminotransferase (AST)	= 10–35 IU/L
Gamma-glutamyl transferase (GGT)	= 10–55 IU/L

26 In a 40-year-old man who has alcoholic cirrhosis but who is not clinically jaundiced:

A plasma [ammonia] is likely to be increased

B serum protein electrophoresis is not indicated

C plasma [bilirubin] might nevertheless be as high as 70 μmol/L (reference range 2–17 μmol/L)

D plasma [urea] is likely to be below 2.5 mmol/L (reference range 2.5–6.6 mmol/L)

E plasma GGT activity is likely to be normal

27 In the pre-icteric stage of infection with hepatitis A virus, there is often:

A increased urinary urobilinogen excretion

B decreased plasma [albumin]

C increased plasma [bilirubin]

D decreased plasma [Na^+]

E increased plasma aminotransferase activity

28 An 11-year-old girl with a predominantly cholestatic form of infective hepatitis is likely to have:

A greatly increased plasma alkaline phosphatase activity

B normal plasma alanine aminotransferase activity

C normal plasma gamma-glutamyl transferase activity

D lipoprotein X detectable in plasma

E increased plasma [conjugated bilirubin]

29 Unconjugated bilirubin:

A is mostly derived from the breakdown of haemoglobin

B is rendered more water-soluble by binding to albumin

C is conjugated with glucuronic acid in the hepatocytes

D is re-formed in the intestine by bacterial action on conjugated bilirubin

E undergoes an enterohepatic circulation in adults

30 The following plasma enzyme activities are often increased when the corresponding forms of liver disease are present:

A alanine aminotransferase and Gilbert's syndrome

B copper oxidase (ceruloplasmin) and hepatolenticular degeneration (Wilson's disease)

C aspartate aminotransferase and acute viral hepatitis

D alkaline phosphatase and extrahepatic cholestasis

E gamma-glutamyl transferase and intrahepatic cholestasis

31 **In patients with alcoholic cirrhosis:**

A a prolonged prothrombin time usually fails to revert to normal in response to parenteral vitamin K

B plasma [albumin] provides a good index of severity in the later stages of the disease

C plasma [IgG] tends to be increased to a greater extent than [IgA] or [IgM]

D plasma cholinesterase activity is often increased

E plasma gamma-glutamyl transferase activity, if high, provides a sensitive means of confirming the diagnosis

32 **Plasma [creatinine]:**

A is a useful screening test for the presence of renal tubular disease

B is often reduced in patients with hepatic failure

C is unaffected by changes in diet

D increases whenever plasma [amino acids] increase

E rises in acute renal failure in proportion to the rate of tissue catabolism

33 **In patients who are found to have proteinuria:**

A urine formed while the patient is lying flat does not contain detectable amounts of protein if the patient has orthostatic proteinuria

B urine protein electrophoresis should be performed if multiple myeloma is suspected

C transient proteinuria occurring only after severe physical exercise is rarely of pathological significance

D the amount of protein excreted, if proteinuria is persistent, indicates the severity of the underlying renal disease

E due to the nephrotic syndrome, this is likely to respond to steroid treatment if the proteinuria is selective

34 **Creatinine clearance determinations:**

A provide a useful measure of the total number of functioning glomeruli

B correlate poorly with inulin clearance in patients with chronic renal failure

C are unaffected by a high-protein diet

D are usually imprecise if the urine collection period is short (e.g. 2 hours)

E are more precise (have a lower coefficient of variation) than plasma creatinine measurements

35 **Results for creatinine clearance measurements may be considerably reduced (below 80 mL/min) in patients:**

A with persistent hypotension

B with prostatic obstruction

C treated with cimetidine
D taking salicylates
E whose urine collections are incomplete

36 Renal calculi may be composed of:
A calcium oxalate
B cholesterol
C cystine
D uric acid
E hypoxanthine

37 In acute renal failure, in the oliguric phase:
A chemical investigations help to determine the aetiology
B plasma [urea] rises more rapidly in patients with acute
  glomerulonephritis than when renal failure follows major surgery
C the urine usually has a high osmolality, relative to plasma
D plasma $[K^+]$ is usually high
E plasma $[Na^+]$ is often low

38 Low threshold (renal) amino aciduria occurs in:
A acute hepatic necrosis
B cystinuria
C Hartnup disease
D heavy metal poisoning
E cystinosis

39 Plasma amylase activity is often raised to more than five times the upper reference value in:
A acute pancreatitis
B perforated peptic ulcer
C acute parotitis
D macro-amylasaemia
E carcinoma of the pancreas

40 The pentagastrin test is used:
A to investigate suspected Zollinger–Ellison syndrome
B to help establish a diagnosis of pernicious anaemia
C to differentiate between benign and malignant gastric ulcers
D to confirm that vagotomy has been complete
E to differentiate between giant hypertrophic gastritis and hypersecretory gastropathy

41 A diagnosis of chronic pancreatitis is supported by the following findings:
A a decreased urinary PABA/^{14}C excretion index in the BT-PABA/[^{14}C]-PABA test

B a decreased urinary excretion of fluorescein after fluorescein dilaurate administration in the pancreolauryl test

C a decreased fasting serum [immunoreactive trypsin]

D a normal faecal fat excretion

E a normal response to a Lundh test meal

PABA = p-aminobenzoic acid, BT = N-benzoyl-L-tyrosyl-

42 **In bacterial colonization of the small intestine:**

A breath $^{14}CO_2$ excretion is often increased after oral administration of [^{14}C]-triolein

B breath $^{14}CO_2$ excretion is often increased after oral administration of [^{14}C]-glycocholate

C breath $^{14}CO_2$ excretion is often decreased after oral administration of [^{14}C]-xylose

D urinary indican excretion is often increased

E faecal fat excretion is often increased

43 **Malabsorption of fat occurs in patients with:**

A Zollinger–Ellison syndrome

B carcinoid tumours

C biliary cirrhosis

D Crohn's disease affecting the terminal ileum

E Hartnup disease

44 **A normal result in a xylose absorption test that is based on urinary xylose measurements depends on:**

A gastric H^+ production being normal

B pancreatic amylase secretion being normal

C absorption of hexoses (e.g. galactose, fructose) from the small intestine being normal

D metabolism of monosaccharides by the liver being normal

E renal function (e.g. plasma [creatinine]) being normal

45 **A 20-year-old woman was admitted to hospital in diabetic precoma. Her urine contained glucose and ketones and the following abnormal results were obtained for investigations in plasma at the time of admission: [glucose], 50 mmol/L; [Na$^+$], 164 mmol/L; [K$^+$], 5.3 mmol/L; [total CO$_2$], 5 mmol/L; [urea], 12 mmol/L. In this patient:**

A the plasma [Na$^+$] indicates that there has been no net loss of body sodium

B the plasma [K$^+$] will begin to fall as soon as insulin and fluid replacement treatment are started

C plasma [free fatty acids] are likely to be low

D Kussmaul (deep sighing) respiration is likely to be the main reason for the low plasma [total CO$_2$]

E the increased plasma [urea] probably indicates the presence of renal damage

Reference ranges:
Na^+, 132–144 mmol/L; K^+, 3.3–4.7 mmol/L
Total CO_2, 24–30 mmol/L; urea, 2.5–6.6 mmol/L

46 **In the performance of an oral glucose tolerance test:**
   A the patient's carbohydrate intake should be restricted to 75 g/day for 3 days prior to the test
   B nervous patients may be allowed to smoke during the test
   C during the test, the patient must not lie on the left side
   D the test should be prolonged to 6 hours if reactive hypoglycaemia is suspected
   E the test should not be performed while the patient is recovering from another illness

47 **Hypoglycaemia:**
   A should be investigated using an enzymic technique for measuring plasma [glucose]
   B is defined as a plasma [glucose] below 3.0 mmol/L
   C in a patient not treated with insulin, is due to insulinoma if fasting plasma [insulin] is increased
   D stimulates the production of glucagon
   E often occurs in galactosaemia

48 **Impaired glucose tolerance in an oral glucose tolerance test tends to occur in association with:**
   A normal pregnancy
   B hypopituitarism
   C previous gastric surgery (e.g. gastroenterostomy)
   D chronic pancreatitis
   E intestinal malabsorptive disease

49 **Lipoproteins have the following properties:**
   A chylomicrons are the largest of the lipoproteins
   B HDL are the smallest of the lipoproteins
   C chylomicrons and VLDL are the main carriers of cholesterol
   D LDL and HDL are the main carriers of triglycerides
   E VLDL are formed from LDL by the incorporation of cholesterol

50 **A specimen of blood from a fasting patient is found to have increased plasma [cholesterol] and [triglycerides]. This pattern of results:**
   A is consistent with a diagnosis of remnant hyperlipoproteinaemia
   B indicates that the patient carries an increased risk of developing ischaemic heart disease

C can usually be explained by an increase in LDL alone

D may occur in primary hypothyroidism

E is caused by abnormal conversion of LDL to VLDL

51 **Plasma [low-density lipoproteins] are often abnormally high in:**

A primary hypothyroidism

B diabetes mellitus

C primary biliary cirrhosis

D nephrotic syndrome

E familial hypercholesterolaemia

52 **The following chemical abnormalities are often present in patients with osteoporosis:**

A increased plasma [calcium]

B increased plasma alkaline phosphatase activity

C decreased fasting plasma [phosphate]

D decreased urinary calcium excretion

E increased serum [parathyroid hormone]

53 **The active form of vitamin D_3 (cholecalciferol):**

A can be synthesized in the body from cholesterol

B is 1 : 25-dihydroxycholecalciferol (1 : 25-DHCC or calcitriol)

C has its formation promoted by hypercalcaemia

D is the main metabolite of vitamin D in the blood

E exerts a local feedback effect on renal 1α-hydroxylase

54 **Osteomalacia (untreated) may be due to:**

A inadequate intake of cholecalciferol

B diseases causing steatorrhoea

C inadequate endogenous synthesis of ergocalciferol

D impaired 25-hydroxylation of 1α-hydroxycholecalciferol in the liver

E impaired 24-hydroxylation of 25-hydroxycholecalciferol in the kidney

55 **Parathyroid hormone increases the:**

A synthesis of a calcium-binding protein in the intestinal mucosa

B release of calcium from bone

C renal tubular reabsorption of calcium

D renal clearance of phosphate

E activity of kidney 1α-hydroxylase

56 **Hypocalcaemia is a feature of:**

A pseudohypoparathyroidism

B chronic renal failure

C hysterical over-breathing

D acute haemorrhagic pancreatitis

E nephrotic syndrome

57 Plasma alkaline phosphatase activity is often increased in patients with:
   A osteomalacia
   B hypoparathyroidism
   C Paget's disease of bone
   D multiple myelomatosis
   E tertiary hyperparathyroidism

58 In a 30-year-old man with a plasma [calcium] of 3.17 mmol/L (reference range, 2.12–2.62 mmol/L) and a normal plasma [albumin], the following results would support a diagnosis of primary hyperparathyroidism:
   A decreased fasting plasma [phosphate]
   B decreased urinary phosphate excretion
   C normal serum [parathyroid hormone]
   D normal plasma alkaline phosphatase activity
   E increased plasma acid phosphatase activity

59 Hypercalcaemia is a recognized feature of:
   A primary hyperparathyroidism
   B secondary hyperparathyroidism
   C thyrotoxicosis
   D sarcoidosis
   E Paget's disease of bone

60 Magnesium deficiency should be suspected as the cause of tetany in patients:
   A with post-operative ileus that fails to respond to treatment with potassium salts
   B with hypocalcaemia that fails to respond to treatment with calcium gluconate
   C with normal plasma [magnesium] but low urinary magnesium excretion
   D with renal tubular defects
   E on maintenance haemodialysis in districts where the water is hard

61 Plasma [magnesium]:
   A is influenced by parathyroid hormone
   B is occasionally reduced in patients with chronic renal failure
   C may be affected by changes in plasma [protein]
   D provides a sensitive index of the body's content of magnesium
   E is unaffected by haemolysis

62 A 25-year-old man with recurrent attacks of abdominal pain is found to have greatly raised urinary 5-aminolaevulinate and porphobilinogen. The differential diagnosis includes:

A lead poisoning
B porphyria cutanea tarda
C carcinoid syndrome
D acute intermittent porphyria
E variegate porphyria

63 In chronic lead poisoning:
A ferrochelatase activity is reduced
B erythrocyte [zinc protoporphyrin] is reduced
C urinary porphobilinogen (PBG) excretion is greatly increased
D urinary 5-aminolaevulinic acid (ALA) excretion is greatly increased
E measurements of erythrocyte ALA dehydratase activity provide a sensitive index of exposure to lead

64 In acute intermittent porphyria:
A there is a deficiency of hepatic steroid 5α-reductase
B faecal excretion of porphyrins is usually normal
C urinary excretion of 5-aminolaevulinic acid is greatly increased
D urinary excretion of porphyrins is usually increased
E the basic defect is deficiency of porphobilinogen deaminase

65 Plasma iron:
A shows diurnal variation, with higher values in the morning
B usually increases in women taking oestrogen-containing oral contraceptives
C constitutes about 5% of total body iron
D has a higher reference range in men than in women
E mainly circulates as a ferritin–iron complex

66 Plasma total iron-binding capacity (TIBC):
A is often low in idiopathic haemochromatosis
B consists mainly of transferrin
C is usually reduced in iron deficiency
D often falls in chronic infections
E is normally about 70% saturated

67 When investigating possible iron deficiency:
A plasma [ferritin] is a good index of the body's iron stores
B ferritin is the most sensitive measurement for use in case-finding programmes
C plasma [iron] and the percentage saturation of TIBC are both reduced, if deficiency is present
D plasma [ferritin] is reduced and plasma TIBC increased, if deficiency is present
E plasma [transferrin] is usually increased, if deficiency is present

68 **The active form of vitamin D$_3$:**
  A is synthesized in the body from cholesterol
  B requires sunlight for its formation from dietary cholecalciferol
  C has its formation in the kidney promoted by parathyroid hormone
  D is the main circulating metabolite of vitamin D
  E exerts a feedback effect on renal 24-hydroxylase

69 **For patients who are receiving long-term total parenteral nutrition (TPN):**
  A the daily requirement for sodium, in the absence of excessive losses or retention, will be 80–120 mmol in adults
  B the energy will be mostly provided as carbohydrate
  C the previous day's nitrogen loss can be estimated by measuring the 24-hour urinary excretion of creatinine
  D chromium and selenium both need to be provided as trace metal supplements
  E each day's nutrients can conveniently be combined and administered in a single big bag

70 **The following tests may help in the investigation of the corresponding conditions:**
  A erythrocyte aminotransferase activity and beri-beri
  B plasma [25-hydroxycholecalciferol] and rickets
  C erythrocyte transketolase activity and pellagra
  D leucocyte [ascorbate] and scurvy
  E pentagastrin test and megaloblastic anaemia

71 **Hyperuricaemia tends to occur in patients:**
  A with essential hypertension
  B with xanthinuria
  C treated with thiazide diuretics
  D treated with high doses of salicylates
  E with deficiency of hypoxanthine-guanine phosphoribosyl transferase (Lesch–Nyhan syndrome)

72 **Plasma [urate] tends to be:**
  A higher in alcoholics than in teetotallers
  B higher in social classes IV–V than in social classes I–II
  C higher in men than in women of the same age-group
  D increased in the obese
  E increased by treatment with cytotoxic drugs

73 **Increased renal excretion of urate is associated with:**
  A low-dose salicylate treatment
  B treatment with thiazide diuretics
  C allopurinol treatment

   D probenecid treatment
   E indomethacin treatment

74 In patients with primary gout:
   A acute attacks can usually be shown to follow a sudden increase in plasma [urate]
   B there is usually a defect of urate excretion
   C there is usually gross overproduction of urate
   D formation of renal tract stones is less likely if the urine is alkaline
   E joint fluid crystals show negative birefringence

75 An abnormally high plasma [urate] is associated with:
   A chronic renal failure
   B glycogen storage disease, type I (von Gierke's disease)
   C polycythaemia rubra vera
   D psoriasis
   E starvation

76 Thyroid function tests should not be performed unless clinically indicated until after patients have recovered from non-thyroidal illnesses because, although euthyroid:
   A plasma [TSH] is occasionally increased
   B plasma [TSH] is occasionally decreased
   C plasma [free T4] is occasionally increased
   D plasma [total T3] is occasionally increased
   E plasma [total T3] is often decreased

77 Plasma [total T3]:
   A is influenced by changes in plasma [thyroxine-binding globulin]
   B is normal in patients who are clinically hyperthyroid whenever plasma [total T4] is normal
   C is often high in elderly patients who have a non-thyroidal illness
   D is often low in middle-aged patients soon after a myocardial infarction
   E is nearly always low in patients with primary hypothyroidism

78 Plasma [total T4] tends to fall in euthyroid patients treated with:
   A salicylates
   B cortisol in high dosage
   C potassium iodide
   D phenytoin
   E lithium

79 A clinical diagnosis of primary hypothyroidism would be supported by:
   A a low plasma [free T4]
   B a greatly increased basal plasma [TSH]
   C little or no TSH response to TRH injection

D increased plasma [triglycerides] in a fasting specimen

E increased plasma [HDL-cholesterol]

80 **In primary hyperthyroidism:**

A there are increased numbers of available (free) thyroxine-binding sites on thyroxine-binding globulin

B basal plasma [TSH] is usually increased

C TSH cannot be detected in plasma even by sensitive immunometric assay methods

D plasma [total T3] is nearly always increased

E plasma [cholesterol] is frequently increased

81 **A diagnosis of pituitary-dependent Cushing's syndrome is supported by finding:**

A an increased urinary cortisol : creatinine ratio

B loss of nychthemeral rhythm for plasma [cortisol]

C an increased plasma cortisol response in an insulin-hypoglycaemia test

D an increased plasma [ACTH]

E absence of a response in the high-dose dexamethasone test

82 **In patients with severe depressive illness:**

A the nychthemeral rhythm of plasma [cortisol] is often lost

B urinary cortisol excretion is often increased

C the cortisol response to tetracosactrin tests is nearly always normal

D the cortisol response to insulin-hypoglycaemia tests is nearly always normal

E cortisol production in response to a low-dose dexamethasone test is often maintained

83 **A child with congenital adrenal hyperplasia due to 21-hydroxylase deficiency, before treatment, would be likely to have:**

A high plasma [ACTH]

B high plasma [17α-hydroxyprogesterone]

C high plasma [11-deoxycortisol]

D greatly increased urinary pregnanetriol excretion

E marked hypokalaemia

84 **A patient with untreated adrenal insufficiency is liable to have:**

A hyponatraemia

B hypokalaemia

C hypocalcaemia

D hypomagnesaemia

E fasting hypoglycaemia

85 **When investigating patients for primary hyperaldosteronism as the possible cause of hypertension:**

A plasma $[K^+]$ should be performed as a screening test
B hypokalaemia is often due to laxatives
C patients with normal plasma $[K^+]$ should be put on a low Na^+ diet to see if they develop hypokalaemia
D if plasma renin activity is low and [aldosterone] is high, this confirms the diagnosis
E if plasma [angiotensin II] is low and urinary aldosterone excretion is high, this supports the diagnosis

86 **Increased production of ADH:**
A occurs in response to a fall in plasma osmolality
B occurs in response to a fall in ECF volume
C in excess of physiological requirements causes hyponatraemia
D occurs in some patients following head injury
E occurs in patients with psychogenic diabetes insipidus

87 **The response to the TRH test is:**
A exaggerated in primary hypothyroidism
B normal in mild hyperthyroidism
C impaired in secondary hypothyroidism
D used to measure anterior pituitary reserve
E usually assessed by measuring plasma [total T4] or [free T4]

88 **Chorionic gonadotrophin is:**
A produced in the third trimester by the fetal liver
B measured in maternal urine as a test for pregnancy
C useful in the diagnosis of seminoma
D useful in the diagnosis of tumours of the trophoblast
E useful in the management of testicular teratoma

89 **In the third trimester of a normal pregnancy:**
A plasma [total T4] is often increased
B plasma [free T4] is often reduced
C plasma total alkaline phosphatase activity is often increased
D plasma [urea] is often increased
E plasma [albumin] is often reduced
'Increased' and 'reduced' refer to the concentration or activity of these analytes that would be found in the same woman in the non-pregnant state, and not taking any form of contraceptive pill.

90 **Women taking oestrogen-containing oral contraceptives are likely to have increased plasma concentrations of:**
A albumin
B LDL-cholesterol
C fasting triglycerides

D cortisol

E copper

91 During pregnancy:

A plasma [Na$^+$] tends to be lower than in non-pregnant women

B plasma [transferrin] usually increases

C the renal threshold for glucose often rises

D plasma [human placental lactogen] peaks at about 20 weeks' gestation, and then falls progressively

E maternal serum [α-fetoprotein] peaks at about 20 weeks' gestation, and then falls progressively

92 In infertile women of child-bearing age:

A plasma [progesterone] should be measured about the 21st day, if menstrual periods are occurring

B plasma [FSH] and [LH] are both high in patients with primary gonadal failure

C patients with secondary amenorrhoea often have low plasma [prolactin]

D plasma [TSH] and [free T4] should be measured

E a Gn-RH stimulation test should be performed in patients with secondary gonadal failure

93 In women carrying a singleton fetus with an open neural tube defect:

A maternal serum [AFP] is nearly always significantly increased at 16–18 weeks' gestation

B amniotic fluid [AFP] is nearly always increased at 18–20 weeks' gestation

C amniotic fluid [AFP] should not be requested if the fluid is blood-stained

D amniotic fluid acetylcholinesterase activity measurements should not be requested if the fluid is blood-stained

E serum [free β subunit of hCG] is often increased

94 In the polycystic ovary syndrome:

A plasma [FSH] is often increased

B plasma [LH] is often increased

C serum [testosterone] is usually increased

D plasma [prolactin] is usually increased

E plasma [oestradiol-17β] is usually reduced

95 Neonatal hypocalcaemia is a recognized complication or manifestation of:

A prematurity

B poorly controlled maternal diabetes mellitus

C feeding with high phosphate-containing foods (e.g. cow's milk)

D pseudohypoparathyroidism

E maternal hyperparathyroidism

96 Diagnosis of the following tumours in childhood is supported by the finding of an increased urinary excretion of 4-hydroxy, 3-methoxymandelic acid (HMMA):
A hepatoma
B medullary carcinoma of the thyroid
C nephroblastoma
D neuroblastoma
E phaeochromocytoma

97 A diagnosis of cystic fibrosis in children would be supported by finding:
A an increased meconium [albumin]
B a decreased faecal trypsin activity
C an increased sweat $[K^+]$
D an increased sweat $[Na^+]$
E an increased blood [immunoreactive trypsin]

98 Phenylketonuria:
A is always associated with reduced phenylalanine hydroxylase activity
B is often detectable in heterozygotes, by the phenylalanine loading test
C is usually screened for, in neonates, by measuring blood [phenylalanine]
D is associated, in homozygotes on a low phenylalanine diet, with reduced plasma [tyrosine]
E has treatment monitored by measuring urinary phenylpyruvate excretion

99 Lumbar CSF [protein]:
A is normally lower in the neonatal period than in childhood
B is normally higher than ventricular CSF [protein]
C normally consists almost entirely of albumin
D is often increased, predominantly as IgM, in patients with multiple sclerosis
E is greatly increased in patients with spinal block

100 Therapeutic drug monitoring is cost-effective and should be performed routinely on patients being treated with:
A digoxin
B lithium
C phenytoin
D salicylates
E 'tricyclic' antidepressants

Multiple choice questions: Part 2

The questions in this part, 101–150, are almost all concerned with biochemical information contained in two or more chapters. The key to the answers (p. 410) should not be consulted during an 'examination session'.

101 As a result of the metabolic response to major surgery, in the first two days after operation:

A ADH secretion is suppressed

B urinary excretion of Na^+ is usually increased

C gluconeogenesis is increased

D plasma [urea] is usually increased

E a metabolic acidosis tends to develop

102 In a patient who has been maintained for 4 days on parenteral fluids following right hemicolectomy, a fall in plasma [urea] is likely to be:

A due to a fluid intake that has consisted solely of intravenous glucose–saline solutions

B a sign of early hepatic failure

C due to decreased catabolism of body proteins

D partly caused by the normal post-operative release of antidiuretic hormone

E partly caused by the normal post-operative release of adrenal steroids

103 Increased plasma $[K^+]$ may be caused by or be a prominent feature of:

A storing blood specimens in a refrigerator

B delay in separation of plasma from leukaemic cells

C secondary hyperaldosteronism

D diabetic ketoacidosis

E renal tubular acidosis

104 The following plasma enzyme activities are frequently abnormal in acute viral hepatitis in young adults:

A alanine aminotransferase

B alkaline phosphatase

C cholinesterase

D creatine kinase

E gamma-glutamyl transferase

105 In a patient with pyloric stenosis who has been vomiting for 3–4 days:

A plasma [total CO_2] is often raised

B plasma [calcium] is often reduced

C plasma $[H^+]$ is usually reduced

D plasma $[K^+]$ is often raised

E plasma [albumin] is often reduced

106 In the first 2–3 days after major surgical operations:

A the rate of protein catabolism is increased

B plasma [cortisol] is usually reduced

C there is often fluid retention

D plasma [C-reactive protein] is often decreased

E plasma creatine kinase activity is often increased

107 In patients presenting with a clinical diagnosis of acute pancreatitis:
    A greatly increased plasma amylase activity confirms the diagnosis
    B plasma [calcium] is often raised
    C urinary amylase activity should be measured urgently
    D glycosuria is often present
    E methaemalbumin is often detectable in plasma

108 Water retention and a reduced plasma [Na$^+$] are liable to occur in:
    A nephrogenic diabetes insipidus
    B the metabolic response to trauma
    C AVP-secreting tumours
    D psychogenic diabetes insipidus
    E acute renal failure

109 Urinary osmolality as a measure of renal concentrating power:
    A should be measured on an early morning specimen
    B should always be measured if urinary sp. gr. is more than 1.020
    C is usually inappropriately low in patients with SIADH
    D is usually increased in uncontrolled diabetes mellitus
    E is usually increased in patients with the nephrotic syndrome

    SIADH = syndrome of inappropriate secretion of ADH (or AVP)

110 Plasma alkaline phosphatase acitivity is often increased in patients with:
    A osteomalacia
    B hypoparathyroidism
    C acute viral hepatitis
    D post-menopausal osteoporosis
    E tertiary hyperparathyroidism

111 The following conditions are likely to be associated both with hyponatraemia and with water and sodium depletion prior to the start of treatment:
    A severe vomiting and diarrhoea
    B alcoholic liver disease
    C primary hyperaldosteronism
    D Addison's disease
    E diabetes insipidus

112 In the following conditions, both plasma alkaline phosphatase and gamma-glutamyl transferase activities are likely to be much increased:
    A normal pregnancy
    B alcoholic cirrhosis
    C carcinoma of the head of the pancreas

D Paget's disease of bone

E metastatic carcinoma of the prostate

113 Gamma-glutamyl transferase activity in plasma is often significantly increased in:

A chronic nephritis

B chronic alcoholism

C hepatoma causing partial biliary obstruction

D acute nephritis

E congestive cardiac failure

114 Impairment of renal tubular function occurs in:

A Fanconi syndrome

B primary hyperparathyroidism

C lithium toxicity

D Wilson's disease

E multiple myelomatosis

115 Plasma cortisol concentration is normally:

A higher at 2200 h than at 0800 h

B often increased in women taking oestrogen-containing oral contraceptives

C often increased in women with simple hirsutism

D altered in parallel with changes in plasma [albumin]

E decreased in response to betamethasone administration

116 Abnormally high urinary 'total metadrenalines' excretion supports a diagnosis of:

A neuroblastoma

B Verner–Morrison syndrome

C multiple endocrine neoplasia IIa (Sipple syndrome)

D Conn's syndrome (primary hyperaldosteronism)

E Zollinger–Ellison syndrome (gastrinoma)

117 A previously healthy 22-year-old woman was admitted to hospital 3 hours after a self-administered overdose of thirty 300 mg aspirin tablets. The following results, measured on arterial (A–D) and venous (E) blood samples, taken at the time of admission and before any treatment was instituted (reference ranges in parentheses), are consistent with this history:

A H^+ = 60 nmol/L (36–44 nmol/L)

B P_{CO_2} = 7.0 kPa (4.4–6.1 kPa)

C plasma $[HCO_3^-]$ = 40 mmol/L (21.0–27.5 mmol/L)

D P_{O_2} = 14.5 kPa (12–15 kPa)

E AST = 850 IU/L (10–40 IU/L)

118 A 57-year-old man was admitted to hospital having collapsed after a meal at work. He is a heavy smoker but takes little alcohol. Pulse and blood pressure were normal with no signs of shock. Chest X-ray detected a 3 cm shadow in the left lung. Emergency investigations (reference ranges in parentheses) gave plasma Na^+, 116 (132–144) mmol/L; urea, 1.8 (2.5–6.6) mmol/L; calcium, 2.80 (2.12–2.62) mmol/L; albumin, 33 (36–47) g/L. Which of the following statements are likely to be true and which false?

    A the findings indicate that the patient has sodium and water depletion

    B the plasma calcium result would be explicable on the basis of the albumin result

    C the likely diagnosis is an ACTH-secreting bronchial tumour

    D the plasma osmolality at the time of admission was found to be 265 (reference range, 280–290) mmol/kg

    E measurement of urine osmolality should prove of considerable diagnostic value

119 Presence of the following tumours may be suspected if increased amounts of the corresponding tumour markers are found in plasma:

    A osteosarcoma and acid phosphatase activity

    B recurrent carcinoma of the cervix and CA 125

    C medullary carcinoma of the thyroid and calcitonin

    D recurrent carcinoma of the colon and carcinoembryonic antigen

    E hepatoma and prolactin

120 The following inborn errors, when untreated and severe, are characteristically associated with the corresponding metabolic abnormalities:

    A familial hypercholesterolaemia and increased plasma [LDL]

    B congenital adrenal hyperplasia (11β-hydroxylase defect) and increased urinary pregnanetriol excretion

    C galactosaemia and glycosuria

    D phenylketonuria and increased plasma [tyrosine]

    E iodotyrosyl coupling enzyme defects and decreased plasma [TSH]

121 Haemolytic anaemia, in an 11-year-old boy, is likely to:

    A cause increased plasma lactate dehydrogenase activity

    B give rise to bilirubinuria in the absence of proteinuria

    C be accompanied by impaired enterohepatic circulation of urobilinogen

    D cause a fall in plasma [haptoglobin]

    E be accompanied by a decreased plasma [ferritin]

122 In the neonate:

    A partially defective bilirubin conjugation is a recognized cause of jaundice

B plasma [IgM] is normally very low compared with adult concentrations

C feeds based on unmodified cow's milk are a recognized cause of hypocalcaemia

D a low plasma [Na$^+$] is one of the main biochemical features of congenital adrenal hyperplasia due to 21-hydroxylase deficiency

E glycogen of normal structure accumulates when there is deficiency of phosphorylase kinase

123 Low threshold (renal) amino aciduria:

A occurs in association with vitamin D-resistant rickets

B sometimes affects the excretion of amino acids selectively

C is usually due to disease confined to the distal renal tubule

D is sometimes associated with similar abnormalities affecting amino acid transport across the intestinal mucosa

E is nearly always accompanied by tubular proteinuria

124 The parenchymal cells of the liver:

A convert bilirubin to urobilinogen

B incorporate triglycerides into very low density lipoproteins

C hydroxylate 25-hydroxycholecalciferol

D catabolize chylomicron remnants

E convert lactate to glucose

125 In the carcinoid syndrome, urinary excretion of the following is likely to be increased:

A 4-hydroxy-3-methoxymandelic acid (HMMA)

B 5-hydroxytryptophan

C 5-hydroxyindoleacetic acid (5-HIAA)

D dopamine

E N'-methyl nicotinamide

126 An insulin-induced hypoglycaemia test normally causes increased plasma concentrations of:

A cortisol

B C-peptide

C growth hormone

D gastrin

E prolactin

127 A low fasting plasma [phosphate] is a feature of:

A chronic renal failure

B chronic pancreatitis

C primary hyperparathyroidism

D vitamin D deficiency

E Fanconi syndrome

128 Rickets is likely to occur in association with:
A renal 1α-hydroxylase deficiency
B protein-energy malnutrition
C coeliac disease
D hypophosphatasia
E idiopathic hypercalciuria

129 In multiple myelomatosis:
A plasma [normal immunoglobulins] are usually decreased
B Bence Jones protein is detectable in urine in most cases
C plasma acid phosphatase activity is often increased
D plasma [urate] is often increased
E renal function should be periodically assessed by measuring plasma [creatinine]

130 Greatly increased excretion of total metadrenalines often occurs in:
A Cushing's syndrome
B congenital adrenal hyperplasia
C essential hypertension
D multiple endocrine neoplasia I (Werner's syndrome)
E phaeochromocytoma

131 Which of the following results, obtained on blood specimens at the time of emergency admission of a 25-year-old woman, might be expected if the patient has diabetic ketoacidosis? (Reference ranges in parentheses):
A plasma amylase activity, 500 IU/L (50–300 IU/L)
B plasma [total CO_2], 35 mmol/L (24–30 mmol/L)
C plasma [K^+], 6.0 mmol/L (3.3–4.7 mmol/L)
D plasma [urea], 15 mmol/L (2.5–6.6 mmol/L)
E plasma [Na^+], 130 mmol/L (132–144 mmol/L)

132 Hypokalaemia is likely to occur in:
A Bartter's syndrome
B acute renal failure, diuretic phase
C patients treated with corticosteroids
D patients treated with thiazide diuretics
E primary hyperaldosteronism (Conn's syndrome)

133 Metabolic acidosis:
A is often accompanied by hypokalaemia
B often develops when there is ketosis
C is compensated by falls in plasma [total CO_2] and P_{CO_2}
D occurs in patients with severe diarrhoea
E is a common cause of a decreased anion gap

134 An increased arterial plasma $[HCO_3^-]$ is liable to develop in:
   A acute hyperventilation due to hysteria
   B respiratory failure due to neuromuscular paralysis
   C ammonium chloride ingestion
   D patients with ectopic ACTH-secreting tumours
   E vomiting due to pyloric stenosis

135 Patients with chronic renal failure usually have:
   A an increased solute load per functioning nephron
   B a high plasma [phosphate] and a low plasma [calcium]
   C an impaired ability to hydroxylate 25-hydroxycholecalciferol
   D an increased plasma [magnesium]
   E an inability to excrete an acid urine

136 Overflow amino aciduria is liable to occur in patients with:
   A acute hepatic necrosis
   B hepatolenticular degeneration
   C diabetic nephropathy
   D renal glucosuria
   E phenylketonuria

137 The following plasma enzyme activities are often increased when
   the corresponding disease states are present:
   A acetyl cholinesterase and scoline apnoea
   B alkaline phosphatase and osteolytic secondary deposits
   C acid phosphatase and osteoblastic secondary deposits
   D amylase and chronic pancreatitis
   E gamma-glutamyl transferase and chronic alcoholism

138 A 30-year-old woman presents with hypertension and
   glycosuria. The following conditions might account for
   these findings:
   A primary hyperaldosteronism (Conn's syndrome)
   B Cushing's syndrome
   C phaeochromocytoma
   D adrenogenital syndrome
   E Bartter's syndrome

139 Hypokalaemia is liable to develop in the absence of treatment in:
   A 'non-endocrine' ACTH-producing tumours
   B patients who abuse laxatives
   C excessive sweating
   D diabetic ketoacidosis
   E renal tubular acidosis

140 The long-term management of a 25-year-old woman with insulin-dependent diabetes mellitus, as an out-patient, can be satisfactorily based on results of:

A urine tests for glucose, ketones and protein performed regularly at home, as instructed, and properly recorded

B urine tests (as in A) and random plasma [glucose] at times of clinic attendance

C capillary blood [glucose] measured regularly at home, as instructed and properly recorded, and random plasma [glucose] at times of clinic attendance

D blood tests (as in C) and blood [haemoglobin A_1] measured at times of clinic attendance

E blood tests (as in C) and plasma [fructosamine] measured at times of clinic attendance

141 A plasma [creatinine] of 250 μmol/L (reference range 55–120 μmol/L) is likely to be reported in patients with:

A secondary hyperparathyroidism

B proximal renal tubular acidosis

C porphyria cutanea tarda

D pyloric stenosis

E acute glomerulonephritis

142 In a 30-year-old nulliparous woman, the combination of findings of increased plasma [FSH] and [LH], normal plasma [prolactin] and low plasma [oestradiol-17β] is consistent with a diagnosis of:

A primary ovarian failure

B polycystic ovary syndrome

C primary hypothyroidism

D premature menopause

E carcinoma of the ovary

143 An increased plasma [testosterone] is likely to be found in men with:

A congenital adrenal hyperplasia

B testicular feminization syndrome

C prolactinoma

D seminoma

E a recent history of taking anabolic steroids

144 A diagnosis of Wilson's disease (hepatolenticular degeneration) is supported by:

A increased plasma [ceruloplasmin]

B increased plasma [copper]

C increased urinary copper excretion

D increased liver [copper]

E a generalized (overflow) amino aciduria

145 **In the primary hyperlipoproteinaemias:**
   A plasma [fasting triglycerides] is much increased in lipoprotein lipase deficiency
   B plasma [cholesterol] and [fasting triglycerides] are both increased in remnant hyperlipoproteinaemia
   C LDL is the lipoprotein class mainly affected in familial hypertriglyceridaemia
   D VLDL is the lipoprotein class mainly affected in familial hypercholesterolaemia
   E plasma [HDL-cholesterol] and [LDL-cholesterol] are both increased in familial combined hyperlipidaemia

146 **The insulin-hypoglycaemia test is used to:**
   A stimulate calcitonin release when investigating relatives of a patient with medullary carcinoma of the thyroid
   B assess gastric H^+ production before vagotomy for peptic ulcer
   C assess the effects of vagotomy
   D confirm a diagnosis of Cushing's syndrome
   E stimulate growth hormone release as a test of anterior pituitary function

147 **Lactic acidosis:**
   A is usually one of the features of diabetic coma
   B is often one of the features of galactosaemia
   C is a common complication of severe myocardial infarction
   D is a common feature of hyperchloraemic acidosis
   E is a common consequence of severe dehydration

148 **Plasma [fasting inorganic phosphate]:**
   A increases if a blood specimen is left unseparated over a weekend
   B is often low in primary hyperparathyroidism
   C is usually low in pseudohypoparathyroidism
   D is usually increased in renal osteodystrophy
   E is occasionally increased in patients with steatorrhoea (20 g fat/day; normally less than 5 g/day)

149 **It is possible to make the following general statements about the activities of enzymes in tissues and in plasma (where 'high' is stated, this is equivalent to tissue activity more than 100 times the activity in plasma):**
   A creatine kinase (CK) is high in the liver
   B CK-MM isoenzyme in the heart is greater than CK-MB isoenzyme in the heart
   C aspartate aminotransferase is high in the liver
   D lactate dehydrogenase is high in the heart, liver and erythrocytes
   E gamma-glutamyl transferase is higher in the kidney than in the liver

150 A plasma [Na$^+$] of 126 mmol/L (reference range 132–144 mmol/L) could be due to:

A fasting hypertriglyceridaemia, if marked

B mineralocorticoid deficiency

C acute renal failure

D macroglobulinaemia

E psychogenic diabetes insipidus

Short answer questions

The initial enthusiasm of examiners and candidates for examinations consisting mainly or solely of multiple choice questions soon waned, as the shortcomings of MCQ as tests of both knowledge and understanding became apparent, whatever marking system or type of question was adopted.

Essay papers, requiring candidates to answer four questions out of five in 3 hours, for instance, fell out of favour because of occasional ambiguities in the wording of questions as well as difficulties with the marking of answers and because they could usually only test a fraction of the material comprised by the subject that was being examined. Also, inevitably, some examiners' assessments of essays were and are influenced by poor presentation such as illegibility of hand-writing, bad grammar and frequent spelling mistakes, even though the meaning intended by the candidates might be clear.

Short answer questions have been adopted by some medical schools, in an attempt to overcome the criticisms of essay examinations and the perceived deficiencies of multiple choice questions. In one kind of pathology examination, for instance, 12 of these questions might require to be answered in 1 hour, three questions each being allocated to a clinical biochemistry, a haematology, a microbiology and a pathology examiner. This section contains examples of such questions. The average time that should be allocated to answering any of the questions listed below is 5–6 minutes each, and we suggest that not more than five questions be attempted in any one practice examination session. This should suffice to set down the salient points and to write one or two short sentences amplifying each of these points. Alternatively, a table or a simple illustration should help to formulate a satisfactory answer in the limited time available.

1 By means of a diagram or a table, show the time-course following a myocardial infarction for two plasma enzyme activity measurements that are widely used in the investigation of these patients. Also state, for a patient admitted within 3 hours of an infarction:

(a) Which enzyme test(s) you would routinely request, and the time(s) when you would collect the blood specimen(s) for examination.

(b) What enzyme test(s) you would request if you suspected that the patient had had an extension of the infarct 4 days after the initial episode.

2 Define osteomalacia and briefly describe the biochemical basis underlying the various causes of this condition. List the chemical investigations you would request in order to help establish a diagnosis.

3 List the investigations you would request in order to confirm a clinical diagnosis of primary hypothyroidism. State in qualitative terms the type of result (e.g. high, normal, low) that would support this diagnosis, and indicate where a different type of result would be obtained in patients with secondary hypothyroidism.

4 What chemical tests ('side-room' and laboratory) should be performed on a 40-year-old woman who has been clinically jaundiced for the last week? Indicate which of these investigations you would expect to be normal (N), high (H) or low (L) depending on whether the patient has intrahepatic (hepatocellular) or extrahepatic jaundice. Answers may be given in the form of a table.

5 List the chemical investigations that you consider to be important in the investigation of patients with chronic renal failure. For each test listed, indicate the nature of the abnormality and explain briefly the reason for its occurrence.

6 Describe briefly the collection of specimens required for the determination of a patient's creatinine clearance. List the principal reasons for clearance results being reduced. State briefly why plasma creatinine measurements are to be preferred as an index of the GFR.

7 List the biochemical abnormalities which may be found in a patient with multiple myeloma. Briefly explain the possible reason(s) for each abnormality you list.

8 Discuss briefly the selection and interpretation of chemical investigations, other than glucose measurements, in the out-patient management of diabetes mellitus.

9 A 24-year-old sales executive is found to be hypertensive (BP 260/105 mmHg) at an insurance medical examination, and to have a fasting plasma cholesterol of 8.9 mmol/L (reference range 3.6–6.7 mmol/L). Urinalysis reveals glucosuria. She is overweight, smokes about 20 cigarettes daily and consumes about 35 units of alcohol per week. List the chemical tests you would request on this patient, giving your reasons for each test requested.

10 Describe the place of tumour markers in the diagnosis and management of carcinoma of the colon.

11 Describe briefly the information to be derived from haemoglobin A_1 and from urinary albumin measurements in the management of patients with diabetes mellitus.

12 What nutritional components need to be included when formulating a standard 'big bag' for patients maintained on long-term total parenteral nutrition (TPN)? Indicate which chemical investigations you would request, and how frequently, in order to help you formulate patients' TPN intake.

13 A 30-year-old man is found to have a severe metabolic acidosis. Indicate what this would mean in terms of the results of blood-gas measurements. List the further chemical investigations that you would request, stating briefly the reasons for each request.

14 Briefly describe how the results of 'side-room' tests and chemical investigations on blood can help to differentiate between infectious hepatitis and pre-hepatic jaundice in a 15-year-old boy. Which of these tests would you choose to monitor the course of infectious hepatitis, and why?

15 List the endocrine causes of hypertension and indicate, for each condition listed, the chemical investigations you would select in order to confirm the diagnosis.

16 List the chemical investigations that you would request in order to confirm a clinical diagnosis of thyrotoxicosis in a 25-year-old woman who is 3 months pregnant. Indicate in qualitative terms the type of result (e.g. high, low) for each test listed. Which two tests would you select as the best combination for diagnostic purposes?

17 Which chemical investigations would you request in order to confirm a clinical diagnosis of Cushing's syndrome? Explain briefly which of the results would indicate that the patient had Cushing's disease rather than one of the other causes of the syndrome.

18 List the chemical investigations that you would request in a 30-year-old man with a history of recurrent renal calculi and who is suspected of having primary hyperparathyroidism. Indicate whether you would expect the result of each test that you have listed to be increased, decreased or within the reference range if the result is to be interpreted as supporting the diagnosis of hyperparathyroidism. Mark with asterisks the two most important investigations from among those you have listed.

19 List the chemical measurements that you regard as necessary for the management of a patient in the diuretic phase of acute renal failure. Briefly explain why you think each of the measurements you have listed is necessary.

20 List the chemical investigations you would request in order to confirm a clinical diagnosis of . . . in a 60-year-old woman. Indicate in descriptive terms (e.g. high, normal, low) the type of result you would expect for each of the tests you have listed, assuming that the diagnosis is correct. State which result or combination of results for the tests listed would serve to confirm the diagnosis.

This question is able to be modified in several ways. For instance, the age or the sex of the patient, or both, can be altered. Examples of conditions that might be entered in the blank include primary or secondary hypothyroidism, primary or secondary hypogonadism, secondary or tertiary hyperparathyroidism, and chronic hepatitis.

Appendix A
Multiple Choice Questions: Key to the Answers

Question	A	B	C	D	E	Question	A	B	C	D	E
1	T	F	T	T	F	38	F	T	T	F	F
2	F	T	T	T	T	39	T	F	T	F	F
3	T	T	F	T	F	40	T	T	F	F	T
4	F	T	T	F	T	41	T	T	T	F	F
5	F	T	F	F	F	42	F	T	F	T	T
6	T	F	F	T	T	43	T	F	T	T	F
7	F	T	T	F	F	44	F	F	F	T	T
8	T	T	T	F	F	45	F	T	F	F	F
9	T	F	F	T	T	46	F	F	T	T	T
10	F	T	F	F	T	47	T	F	T	T	T
11	F	T	F	T	T	48	T	F	F	T	F
12	F	T	T	F	F	49	T	T	F	F	F
13	T	T	F	T	F	50	T	T	F	F	F
14	F	T	F	T	T	51	T	T	T	T	T
15	T	F	F	T	T	52	F	F	F	F	F
16	T	T	F	F	T	53	T	T	F	F	T
17	F	F	T	F	F	54	T	T	F	F	F
18	T	F	F	T	F	55	F	T	T	T	T
19	F	F	T	T	T	56	T	T	F	T	T
20	F	T	F	F	T	57	T	F	T	F	T
21	T	T	T	F	T	58	T	F	T	F	F
22	F	F	F	T	T	59	T	F	F	T	F
23	T	F	F	T	T	60	T	T	T	T	F
24	F	F	T	T	T	61	T	F	T	F	F
25	T	T	T	T	T	62	F	F	F	T	T
26	F	T	F	F	F	63	T	F	F	T	T
27	T	F	T	F	T	64	T	T	T	T	T
28	T	F	F	T	T	65	T	T	F	T	F
29	T	T	T	T	F	66	T	T	F	T	F
30	F	F	T	T	T	67	T	T	T	T	T
31	T	T	F	F	F	68	T	F	T	F	F
32	F	F	F	F	T	69	T	F	F	T	T
33	T	T	T	F	T	70	F	T	F	T	T
34	T	T	F	T	F	71	T	F	T	F	T
35	T	T	T	T	T	72	T	F	T	T	T
36	T	F	T	T	F	73	F	F	F	T	F
37	F	F	F	T	T	74	F	T	F	T	T

Continued on p. 410

Question	A	B	C	D	E	Question	A	B	C	D	E
75	T	T	T	T	T	113	F	T	T	F	T
76	T	T	T	F	T	114	T	T	T	T	T
77	T	F	F	T	F	115	F	T	F	F	T
78	T	T	T	T	T	116	T	F	T	F	F
79	T	T	F	F	F	117	T	F	F	T	F
80	F	F	T	T	F	118	F	F	F	T	T
81	T	T	F	T	F	119	F	F	T	T	F
82	T	T	T	T	T	120	T	F	T	F	F
83	T	T	F	T	F	121	T	F	F	T	F
84	T	F	F	F	T	122	T	T	F	F	T
85	T	T	F	T	T	123	T	T	F	T	F
86	F	T	T	T	F	124	F	T	F	T	T
87	T	F	T	T	F	125	F	T	T	F	F
88	F	T	F	T	T	126	T	F	T	T	T
89	T	T	T	F	T	127	F	F	T	T	T
90	F	F	T	T	T	128	T	T	T	T	F
91	T	T	F	F	T	129	T	T	F	T	T
92	T	T	F	T	T	130	F	F	F	F	T
93	T	T	T	F	F	131	T	F	T	F	T
94	F	T	T	F	F	132	T	T	T	T	T
95	T	F	T	T	T	133	F	T	T	T	F
96	F	F	F	T	T	134	F	T	F	T	T
97	T	T	F	T	T	135	T	T	T	T	F
98	T	T	T	F	F	136	T	F	F	F	T
99	F	T	T	F	T	137	F	F	T	F	T
100	T	T	T	F	F	138	F	T	T	F	F
101	F	F	T	T	T	139	T	T	F	F	T
102	T	F	F	F	F	140	F	F	F	T	T
103	T	T	F	T	F	141	T	F	F	T	T
104	T	T	F	F	T	142	T	F	F	T	F
105	T	F	T	F	F	143	F	T	F	F	F
106	T	F	T	F	T	144	F	F	T	T	T
107	F	F	F	T	T	145	T	T	F	F	F
108	F	T	T	T	T	146	F	T	T	T	T
109	T	F	F	T	F	147	F	F	T	F	T
110	T	F	T	F	T	148	T	T	F	T	F
111	T	F	F	T	F	149	T	T	F	F	T
112	F	T	T	F	F	150	T	T	T	T	F

Appendix B
SI Units and 'Conventional' Units

Système International (SI) units express concentrations for substances of known atomic or molecular mass in molar units. In 1974, SI units were adopted in the UK for reporting the results of chemical investigations, and many other countries worldwide have likewise made the change from 'conventional' to SI units for these analyses. Mass units continue to be used for the results of analyses of mixtures and

Table 1 Examples of reference ranges in SI and equivalent 'conventional' units

Plasma constituent	SI units	'Conventional' units
Albumin	36–47 g/L	3.6–4.7 g/100 mL
Bilirubin (total)	2–17 μmol/L	0.1–1.0 mg/100 mL
Blood urea nitrogen (BUN) (males below 50)	2.5–6.6 mmol/L	7.0–18.5 mg/100 mL
Calcium	2.12–2.62 mmol/L	8.5–10.5 mg/100 mL
Cholesterol (total)	3.6–6.7 mmol/L	140–260 mg/100 mL
Copper	12–26 μmol/L	76–165 μg/100 mL
Cortisol (total)	160–565 nmol/L at 0800–0900 h < 205 nmol/L at 2200–2400 h	5.8–20.3 μg/100 mL at 0800–0900 h < 7.4 mg/100 mL at 2200–2400 h
Creatinine	55–120 μmol/L	0.6–1.3 mg/100 mL
Glucose (fasting)	3.6–5.8 mmol/L	65–105 mg/100 mL
Iron (males)	14–32 μmol/L	80–180 μg/100 mL
Iron (females)	10–28 μmol/L	60–170 μg/100 mL
Iron-binding capacity (total)	47–72 μmol/L	250–400 μg/100 mL
Magnesium	0.7–1.0 mmol/L	1.6–2.4 mg/100 mL
Phosphate (fasting, as P)	0.8–1.4 mmol/L	2.5–4.5 mg/100 mL
Protein (total)	63–83 g/L	6.3–8.3 g/100 mL
Triiodothyronine (total T3)	1.2–2.8 nmol/L	78–182 ng/100 mL
Thyroxine (total T4)	70–150 nmol/L	5.5–11.7 μg/100 mL
Urate (males)	0.12–0.42 mmol/L	2.0–7.0 mg/100 mL
Urate (females)	0.12–0.36 mmol/L	2.0–6.0 mg/100 mL
Urea (males below 50)	2.5–6.6 mmol/L	15–40 mg/100 mL
Zinc	10–20 μmol/L	650–1300 μg/100 mL
Blood constituent (arterial blood)	**SI units**	**Other units**
Hydrogen ion	36–44 nmol/L	7.35–7.45 pH units
P_{CO_2}	4.5–6.1 kPa	34–46 mmHg
P_{O_2}	12–15 kPa	90–112 mmHg

proteins, and some clinical pharmacologists in the UK retain a preference for mass units. The litre (L) is the systematic SI unit of volume in Medicine.

The introduction of SI units into Medicine came much later in the USA. There, such serious problems of acceptability have been encountered that the *New England Journal of Medicine* has reverted to 'conventional' or mass units; 100 mL is the most frequently used volume, when expressing concentrations in 'conventional' units. Parts of Germany and Italy also continue to use

Table 2 Examples of conversion factors between SI units and 'conventional' units

Plasma constituent	Relative mol mass (Da) Column A	Multiplication factor (approx.) to convert numerical values of results expressed in:	
		SI units to 'conventional' units Column B	'conventional' units to SI units Column C
Albumin	66 000	0.1	10
Bilirubin	584.67	0.06	17
Blood urea nitrogen (BUN)	28.01	2.8	0.38
Calcium	40.08	4	0.25
Carbamazepine	236.26	0.24	4.2
Cholesterol (unesterified)	386.66	39	0.026
Copper	63.54	6.4	0.16
Cortisol	362.47	0.036	28
Creatinine	113.12	0.011	88
Digoxin	780.92	0.78	1.28
Glucose	180.16	18	0.055
Iron	55.84	5.6	0.18
Iron-binding capacity (total)		5.6	0.18
Lead	207.19	21	0.048
Lithium	6.939	694	0.0014
Magnesium	24.31	2.4	0.41
Phenytoin	252.26	0.25	4
Phosphate (as P)	30.97	3.1	0.32
Protein (total)	A mixture	0.1	10
Theophylline	180.17	0.18	5.55
Tri-iodothyronine (T3)	650.98	65	0.015
Thyroxine (T4)	776.87	0.078	12.9
Urate	168.11	17	0.06
Urea	60.06	6	0.17
Zinc	65.38	6.5	0.15

Blood constituent (arterial blood)	SI units to mmHg Column B	mmHg to SI units Column C
P_{CO_2}	7.5	0.13
P_{O_2}	7.5	0.13

'conventional' units, and some direct read-out chemical equipment for 'side-room' use presents results in these units.

It is unsatisfactory to report results in two different sets of units, whether in SI units (with the corresponding result in 'conventional' units in parentheses) or in 'conventional' units (with the corresponding result in SI units in parentheses). Because of this, we had intended that the previous edition of this book would be the last to present reference ranges both in SI units and in 'conventional' units. However, in view of the difficulties experienced in gaining universal acceptance for SI units, we provide guidance here to enable readers to carry out interconversions of results expressed in one or other system of units.

Table 1 lists the reference ranges for most of the analytes for which data in SI units are given elsewhere in this book, together with the corresponding values for these reference ranges expressed in 'conventional' units. Table 2 gives examples of conversion factors for the analyses listed in Tables 1 and 24.1 (p. 369). The general formulae governing these numerical interconversions are as follows:

1 X (result expressed in mmol/L) × factor in column B = Y (result expressed in mg/100 mL).

2 Y (result expressed in mg/100 mL) × factor in column C = X (result expressed in mmol/L).

The factors in column C are the reciprocals of the factors in column B. The data for relative mol mass are given in column A for use by those who want to work out multiplication factors that are more exact than those given in columns B and C of Table 2.

Appendix C
References

Chapter 1

Asher R. Straight and crooked thinking in medicine. *British Medical Journal* 1954; **2**: 460–2.

Flynn FV. Screening for presymptomatic disease. *Journal of Clinical Pathology* 1991; **44**: 529–38.

Fraser CG. *Interpretation of Clinical Chemistry Laboratory Data.* Oxford: Blackwell Scientific Publications, 1986.

Gama R, Nightingale PG, Broughton PMG *et al.* Feedback of laboratory usage and cost data to clinicians: does it alter requesting behaviour? *Annals of Clinical Biochemistry* 1991; **28**: 143–9.

Hopkins A (Editor). *Appropriate Investigation and Treatment in Clinical Practice.* London: The Royal College of Physicians, 1989.

Hopkins A, Costain D (Editors). *Measuring the Outcomes of Medical Care.* London: The Royal College of Physicians, 1990.

Kaplan EB, Sheiner LB, Boeckmann AJ *et al.* The usefulness of preoperative laboratory screening. *Journal of the American Medical Association* 1985; **253**: 3576–81.

Peters M, Broughton PMG. The role of expert systems in improving the test requesting patterns of clinicians. *Annals of Clinical Biochemistry* 1993; **30**: 52–9.

Chapter 2

Anderson JR, Linsell WD, Mitchell FM. Guidelines on the performance of chemical pathology assays outside the laboratory. *British Medical Journal* 1981; **282**: 743.

Bachorik PS, Rock R, Cloey T, Treclak E, Becker D, Sigmund W. Cholesterol screening: comparative evaluation of on-site and laboratory-based measurements. *Clinical Chemistry* 1990; **36**: 255–60.

Burtis CA. Advanced technology and its impact on the clinical laboratory. *Clinical Chemistry* 1987; **33**: 352–7.

Leading article. Is routine urinalysis worthwhile? *Lancet* 1988; **i**: 747.

Marks V. Essential considerations in the provision of near-patient testing facilities. *Annals of Clinical Biochemistry* 1988; **25**: 220–5.

Marks V. Stick testing. *British Medical Journal* 1991; **302**: 482–3.

Pearson TA, Bowlin S, Sigmund, WR. Screening for hypercholesterolemia. *Annual Reviews in Medicine* 1990; **41**: 177–86.

Stott NCH. Desktop laboratory technology in general practice. *British Medical Journal* 1989; **299**: 579–80.

UKCCR. *Faecal Occult Blood Testing: Report of United Kingdom Coordinating Committee on Cancer Research Working Party.* London: UKCCR, PO Box 123, Lincoln's Inn Fields, WC2A 3PX, 1989.

Whitehead TP, Garvey K. *Quality Assessment of Tests Performed Outside the Laboratory.* Association of Clinical Pathologists Broadsheet **114**. London: British Medical Association, 1985.

Chapter 3

Fraser CG. *Interpretation of Clinical Chemistry Laboratory Data*. Oxford: Blackwell Scientific Publications, 1986.

Friedman RB, Young DS. *Effects of Disease on Clinical Laboratory Tests* (Second Edition. Washington DC: AACC Press, 1989.

McQueen MJ. *SI Unit Pocket Guide*. Chicago: ASCP Press, 1990.

Pocock SJ, Ashby D, Shaper AG, Walker M, Broughton PMG. Diurnal variations in serum biochemical and haematological measurements. *Journal of Clinical Pathology* 1989; **42**: 172–9.

Solberg HE, Grasbeck R. Reference values. *Advances in Clinical Chemistry* 1989; **27**: 2–79.

Chapter 4

Beck LH (Editor). Symposium on Body Fluid and Electrolyte Disorders. *Medical Clinics of North America* 1981; **65**, 247–451.

Gill GV, Flear CTG. Hyponatraemia. In: Price CP, Albert KGMM (Editors) *Recent Advances in Clinical Biochemistry* **3**. Edinburgh: Churchill Livingstone, 1985: 149–76.

Jamieson MJ. Hyponatraemia. *British Medical Journal* 1985; **290**: 1723–8.

Penney MD, Walters G. Are osmolality measurements clinically useful? *Annals of Clinical Biochemistry* 1987; **24**: 566–71.

Seckl J, Dunger D. Postoperative diabetes insipidus. *British Medical Journal* 1989; **298**: 2–3.

Chapter 5

Kurtzman NA, Batlle DC (Editors). Symposium on Acid–Base Disorders. *Medical Clinics of North America* 1983; **67**: 753–932.

Lolekha PH, Lolekha S. Value of the anion gap in clinical diagnosis and laboratory evaluation. *Clinical Chemistry* 1983; **29**: 279–82, and the addendum by Natelson S.

Relman AS. 'Blood gases': arterial or venous? *New England Journal of Medicine* 1986; **315**: 188–9.

Weil MH, Rackow EC, Trevino R, Grundler W, Falk JL, Griffel MI. Differences in acid–base state between venous and arterial blood during cardiopulmonary resuscitation. *New England Journal of Medicine* 1986; **315**: 153–6.

Winters RW. Terminology of acid–base disorders. *Annals of the New York Academy of Sciences* 1966; **133**: 211–24.

Chapter 6

Bowman JE. Screening newborn infants for Duchenne muscular dystrophy. *British Medical Journal* 1993; **306**: 349.

Bradley DM, Parsons EP, Clarke AJ. Experience with screening newborns for Duchenne muscular dystrophy in Wales. *British Medical Journal* 1993; **306**: 357–60.

Evans RT. Cholinesterase phenotyping: Clinical aspects and laboratory applications. *CRC Critical Reviews in Clinical Laboratory Sciences* 1986; **23**: 35–64.

Lewis F, Jishi F, Sissons CE, Baker JT, Child DF. Value of emergency cardiac enzymes: audit in a coronary care unit. *Journal of the Royal Society of Medicine* 1991; **84**: 398–9.

Moss DW. *Isoenzymes*. London: Chapman & Hall, 1982.

Schmidt E, Schmidt FW. Enzyme release. *Journal of Clinical Chemistry and Clinical Biochemistry* 1987; **25**: 525–40.

Sherman KE. Alanine aminotransferase in clinical practice. *Archives of Internal Medicine* 1991; **151**: 260–5.

Smith AF. Multiple forms of alkaline phosphatase. *Clinical Chemistry and Enzymology Communications* 1989; **2**: 1–22.

Timmis AD. Early diagnosis of acute myocardial infarction. *British Medical Journal* 1990; **301**: 941–2.

Wu AHB. Creatine kinase isoforms in ischemic heart disease. *Clinical Chemistry* 1989; **35**: 7–13.

Chapter 7

Beastall GH, Cook B, Rustin GHS, Jennings J. A review of the role of established tumour markers. *Annals of Clinical Biochemistry* 1991; **28**: 5–18.

Duffy MJ. New cancer markers. *Annals of Clinical Biochemistry* 1989; **26**: 379–87.

Oesterling JE. Prostate specific antigen. *Journal of Urology* 1991; **145**: 907–23.

Roulston JE, Leonard RCF. *Serological Tumour Markers: An Introduction*. Edinburgh: Churchill Livingstone, 1992.

Spickett GP, Misbah SA, Chapel HM. Primary antibody deficiency in adults. *Lancet* 1991; **337**: 281–4.

Thompson D, Milford-Ward A, Whicher JT. The value of acute phase protein measurements in clinical practice. *Annals of Clinical Biochemistry* 1992; **29**: 123–31.

Whicher JT, Spence CE. Serum protein zone electrophoresis — an outmoded test? *Annals of Clinical Biochemistry* 1987; **24**: 133–9.

Whicher JT, Spence CE. When is serum albumin worth measuring? *Annals of Clinical Biochemistry* 1987; **24**: 572–80.

Whicher JT, Calvin J, Riches P, Warren C. The laboratory investigation of paraproteinaemia. *Annals of Clinical Biochemistry* 1987; **24**: 119–32.

Chapter 8

Diehl AM. Alcoholic liver disease. *Medical Clinics of North America* 1989; **73**: 815–30.

Editorial. Gilbert's syndrome — more questions than answers. *Lancet* 1987; **ii**: 1071.

Hayes PC, Bouchier IAD. Liver function tests: their uses and limitations. *Clinical Chemistry and Enzymology Communications* 1989; **2**: 23–34.

Johnson PJ. Role of the standard 'liver function tests' in current clinical practice. *Annals of Clinical Biochemistry* 1989; **26**: 463–71.

Laker MF. Liver function tests. *British Medical Journal* 1990; **301**: 250–1.

Seidel D. Lipoproteins in liver disease. *Journal of Clinical Chemistry and Clinical Biochemistry* 1987; **25**: 541–51.

Sherlock S, Dooley J. *Diseases of the Liver and Biliary System* (Ninth Edition). Oxford: Blackwell Scientific Publications, 1992.

Stibler H. Carbohydrate-deficient transferrin in serum: a new marker of potentially harmful alcohol consumption reviewed. *Clinical Chemistry* 1991; **37**: 2029–37.

Stremmel W, Meyerrose K-W, Niederau C, Hefter H, Kreuzpaintner G, Strohmeyer G. Wilson's disease. *Annals of Internal Medicine* 1991; **115**: 720–6.

Walshe JM. Diagnosis and treatment of presymptomatic Wilson's disease. *Lancet* 1988; **ii**: 435–7.

Chapter 9

Bakir A, Williams RH, Shayakh M, Dunea G, Dubin A. Biochemistry of the uremic syndrome. *Advances in Clinical Chemistry* 1992; **29**: 62–120.

Batlle DC. Renal tubular acidosis. *Medical Clinics of North America* 1983; **67**: 859–78.

Cohen EP, Lemann J. The role of the laboratory in evaluation of kidney function. *Clinical Chemistry* 1991; **37**: 785–96.

Gabriel R. Time to scrap creatinine clearance? *British Medical Journal* 1986; **293**: 1119–20.

Mandal AK, Lee AH (Editors). Renal disease. *Medical Clinics of North America* 1990; **74**: 859–1083.

Narayanan S. Renal biochemistry and physiology: pathophysiology and analytical perspectives. *Advances in Clinical Chemistry* 1992; **29**: 121–57.
van Aswegen CH, du Plessis DJ. A biochemical approach to renal stone formation. *Advances in Clinical Chemistry* 1992; **29**: 263–72.
Waller KV, Ward KM, Mahan JD, Wismatt DK. Current concepts in proteinuria, *Clinical Chemistry* 1989; **35**: 755–65.

Chapter 10

Hodgson HJF, Maton PN. Carcinoid and neuroendocrine tumours of the liver. *Bailière's Clinical Gastroenterology* 1987; **1**: 35–61.
King CE, Toskes PP. The use of breath tests in the study of malabsorption. *Clinics in Gastroenterology* 1983; **12**: 591–610.
Mignon M, Bonfils S. Diagnosis and treatment of Zollinger–Ellison syndrome. *Baillière's Clinical Gastroenterology* 1988; **2**: 677–98.
Scharpe S, Iliano L. Two indirect tests of exocrine pancreatic function evaluated. *Clinical Chemistry* 1987; **33**: 5–12.
Toskes PP. Biochemical tests in pancreatic disease. *Current Opinions in Gastroenterology* 1991; **7**: 709–13.

Chapter 11

Betteridge DJ. Reactive hypoglycaemia. *British Medical Journal* 1987; **295**: 286–7.
Hatem M, Anthony F, Hogston P, Rowe DJF, Dennis KJ. Reference values for 75 g oral glucose tolerance test in pregnancy. *British Medical Journal* 1988; **296**: 676–8.
Jarrett RJ. Gestational diabetes: a non-entity? *British Medical Journal* 1993; **306**: 37–8.
Kitabchi AE, Murphy MB. Diabetic ketoacidosis and hyperosmolar hyperglycemic non-ketotic coma. *Medical Clinics of North America* 1988; **72**: 1545–63.
Lester E. The clinical value of glycated haemoglobin and glycated plasma proteins. *Annals of Clinical Biochemistry* 1989; **26**: 213–19.
Rowe DJF, Dawnay A, Watts GF. Microalbuminuria in diabetes mellitus: review and recommendations for the measurement of albumin in urine. *Annals of Clinical Biochemistry* 1990; **27**: 297–312.
Schade DS, Eaton RP. Diabetic ketoacidosis — pathogenesis, prevention and therapy. *Clinics in Endocrinology and Metabolism* 1983; **12**: 321–38.
Townsend JC. Increased albumin excretion in diabetes. *Journal of Clinical Pathology* 1990; **43**: 3–8.
WHO Expert Committee on Diabetes Mellitus, Second Report. WHO Technical Report Series 646. Geneva: World Health Organization, 1980.
Wiener K. The diagnois of diabetes mellitus, including gestational diabetes. *Annals of Clinical Biochemistry* 1992; **29**: 481–93.
Winocour PH. Microalbuminuria. *British Medical Journal* 1992; **304**: 1196–7.
Yudkin JS, Alberti KGMM, McLarty DG, Swai ABM. Impaired glucose tolerance. Is it a risk factor for diabetes or a diagnostic ragbag? *British Medical Journal* 1990; **301**: 397–401.

Chapter 12

Bhatnagar D, Durrington PN. Clinical value of apolipoprotein measurement. *Annals of Clinical Biochemistry* 1991; **28**: 427–37.
Castelli WP, Garrison RJ, Wilson PWF, Abbott RD, Kalousdian S, Kannel WB. Incidence of coronary heart disease and lipoprotein cholesterol levels. *Journal of the American Medical Association* 1986; **256**: 2835–8.
International Collaborative Study Group. Metabolic epidemiology of plasma cholesterol. Mechanisms of variation of plasma cholesterol within populations and between populations. *Lancet* 1986; **ii**: 991–6.

Martin MJ, Hulley SB, Browner WS, Kuller LH, Wentworth D. Serum cholesterol, blood pressure and mortality: implications from a cohort of 361,662 men. *Lancet* 1986; **ii**: 933–6.

O'Brien BJ. *Cholesterol and Coronary Heart Disease: Consensus or Controversy?* London: Office of Health Economics, 1991.

Scott J. Lipoprotein (a). *British Medical Journal* 1991; **303**: 663–4.

Shepherd J, Packard CJ. The pathogenesis of hyperlipoproteinaemia. *Scottish Medical Journal* 1986; **31**: 154–61.

Chapter 13

Elin RJ. Assessment of magnesium status. *Clinical Chemistry* 1987; **33**: 1965–70.

Fisken RA, Heath DA, Somers S, Bold AM. Hypercalcaemia in hospital patients. *Lancet* 1981; **i**: 202–7.

Gray TA, Paterson CR. The clinical value of ionised calcium assays. *Annals of Clinical Biochemistry* 1988; **25**: 210–19.

Leading article. PTHrP: endocrine and autocrine regulator of calcium. *Lancet* 1991; **i**: 146–8.

Levine MA. Laboratory investigation of disorders of the parathyroid glands. *Clinics in Endocrinology and Metabolism* 1985; **14**: 257–72.

Logue FC, Beastall GH, Fraser WD, O'Reilly DStJ. Intact parathyroid hormone assays. *British Medical Journal* 1990; **300**: 210–11.

Moseley JM. Parathyroid hormone-related protein of humoral hypercalcemia of malignancy. *Advances in Clinical Chemistry* 1990; **28**: 219–42.

Ryan MF. The role of magnesium in clinical biochemistry: an overview. *Annals of Clinical Biochemistry* 1991; **28**: 19–26.

Stewart AF, Broadus AE. Parathyroid hormone-related proteins. *Journal of Clinical Endocrinology and Metabolism* 1990; **71**: 1410–14.

Wood PJ. The measurement of parathyroid hormone. *Annals of Clinical Biochemistry* 1992; **29**: 11–21.

Chapter 14

Elder GH, Smith SG, Smyth SJ. Laboratory investigation of the porphyrias. *Annals of Clinical Biochemistry* 1990; **27**: 395–412.

Fell GS. Lead toxicity: problems of definition and laboratory evaluation. *Annals of Clinical Biochemistry* 1984; **21**: 453–60.

Holland HK, Spivak JL. Hemochromatosis. *Medical Clinics of North America* 1989; **73**: 831–45.

Peters TJ, Pippard MJ. Disorders of iron metabolism. In Cohen RD, Lewis B, Alberti KGMM, Denham AM (Editors) *The Metabolic and Molecular Basis of Acquired Disease.* London: Baillière Tindall, 1990: 1870–84.

Chapter 15

Aggett PJ. Physiology and metabolism of essential trace elements. *Clinics in Endocrinology and Metabolism* 1985; **14**: 513–43.

George CF (Chairman). Intravenous nutrition. In *British National Formulary* **24**. London: British Medical Association, 1992: 342–5.

Goldstein SA, Elwyn DH. The effect of injury and sepsis on fuel utilization. *Annual Reviews of Nutrition* 1989; **9**: 445–73.

Lentner C (Editor). Nutritional standards. In *Geigy Scientific Tables* **1**. Basle: Ciba-Geigy Ltd, 1981: 237–9.

Marshall WJ, Mitchell PEG. Total parenteral nutrition and the clinical chemistry laboratory. *Annals of Clinical Biochemistry* 1987; **24**: 327–36.

Shenkin A. Clinical aspects of vitamin and trace element metabolism. *Baillière's Clinical Gastroenterology* 1988; **2**: 765–98.

Shizgal HM. Parenteral and enteral nutrition. *Annual Reviews in Medicine* 1991; **42**: 549–65.

Woolfson AMJ (Editor). *Biochemistry of Hospital Nutrition*. Edinburgh: Churchill Livingstone, 1986.

Chapter 16

Cameron JS, Simmonds HA. Uric acid, gout and the kidney. *Journal of Clinical Pathology* 1981; **34**: 1245–54.

Devgun MS, Dhillon HS. Importance of diurnal variations on clinical value and interpretation of serum urate measurements. *Journal of Clinical Pathology* 1992; **45**: 110–13.

Scott JT. Asymptomatic hyperuricaemia. *British Medical Journal* 1987; **294**: 987–8.

Chapter 17

Bone HG. Diagnosis of the multiglandular endocrine neoplasias. *Clinical Chemistry* 1990; **36**: 711–18.

Ekins R. The free hormone hypothesis and measurement of free hormones. *Clinical Chemistry* 1992; **38**: 1289–93.

Franklyn JA. Syndromes of thyroid hormone resistance. *Clinical Endocrinology* 1991; **34**: 237–45.

Gow SM, Kellett HA, Seth J, Sweeting VM, Toft AD, Beckett GJ. Limitations of new thyroid function tests in pregnancy. *Clinica Chimica Acta* 1985; **152**: 325–33.

John R. Screening for congenital hypothyroidism. *Annals of Clinical Biochemistry* 1987; **24**: 1–13.

Kaplan MM, Hamburger JI. Non-thyroidal causes of abnormal thyroid function test data. *Journal of Clinical Immunoassay* 1989; **12**: 90–9.

Nicoloff JT, Spencer CA. The use and misuse of the sensitive thyrotropin assays. *Journal of Clinical Endocrinology and Metabolism* 1990; **71**: 553–8.

Thomas, SHL, Sturgess I, Wedderburn A, Wylie J, Croft DN. Clinical versus biochemical assessment in thyroxine replacement therapy: a retrospective study. *Journal of the Royal College of Physicians of London* 1990; **24**: 289–91.

Chapter 18

Burke CW. Adrenocortical insufficiency. *Clinics in Endocrinology and Metabolism* 1985; **14**: 947–76.

Clayton RN. Diagnosis of adrenal insufficiency: the short tetracosactrin test can almost always replace the insulin stress test. *British Medical Journal* 1989; **298**: 271–2.

Cutler CB, Laue L. Congenital adrenal hyperplasia due to 21-hydroxylase deficiency. *New England Journal of Medicine* 1990; **323**: 1806–13.

Findling JW. The Cushing syndromes. *New England Journal of Medicine* 1989; **321**: 1677–8.

Harvey JM, Beevers DG. Biochemical investigation of hypertension. *Annals of Clinical Biochemistry* 1990; **27**: 287–96.

James V (Editor). *The Adrenal Gland* (Second Edition). New York: Raven Press, 1992.

Leading article. CRH test in the 1990s. *Lancet* 1990; **ii**: 1416.

Rosano TG, Swift TA, Hayes LW. Advances in catecholamine and metabolite measurements for diagnosis of pheochromocytoma. *Clinical Chemistry* 1991; **37**: 1854–67.

Ross NS, Aron DC. Hormonal evaluation of the patient with an incidentally discovered adrenal mass. *New England Journal of Medicine* 1990; **323**: 1401–5.

Swales JD. Primary aldosteronism: how hard should we look? *British Medical Journal* 1983; **287**: 702–3.

Trainer PJ, Grossman A. The diagnosis and differential diagnosis of Cushing's syndrome. *Clinical Endocrinology* 1991; **34**: 317–30.

White PC, New MI, Dupont B. Congenital adrenal hyperplasia. *New England Journal of Medicine* 1987; **316**: 1519–24 and 1580–6.

Chapter 19

Abboud CF. Laboratory diagnosis of hypopituitarism. *Mayo Clinic Proceedings* 1986; **61**: 35–48.

Gillies G, Grossman A. The CRFs and their control: chemistry, physiology and clinical implications. *Clinics in Endocrinology and Metabolism* 1985; **14**: 821–43.

Ho KY, Evan WS, Thorner MO. Disorders of prolactin and growth hormone secretion. *Clinics in Endocrinology and Metabolism* 1985; **14**: 1–33.

Imura H. ACTH and related peptides: molecular biology, biochemistry and regulation of secretion. *Clinics in Endocrinology and Metabolism* 1985; **14**: 845–66.

Leading article. Hyperprolactinaemia: when is a prolactinoma not a prolactinoma? *Lancet* 1987; **ii**: 1002–4.

Robinson AG. Disorders of anti-diuretic hormone secretion. *Clinics in Endocrinology and Metabolism* 1985; **14**: 55–89.

Chapter 20

Barth JH. Hirsute women: should they be investigated? *Journal of Clinical Pathology* 1992; **45**: 188–92.

Butt WR, Blunt SM. The role of the laboratory in the investigation of infertility. *Annals of Clinical Biochemistry* 1988; **25**: 601–9.

Chamberlain G. Detection and management of congenital abnormalities–I. *British Medical Journal* 1991; **302**: 949–50.

Chamberlain G. Checking for fetal well-being — II. *British Medical Journal* 1991; **302**: 900–2.

Chard T. What is happening to placental function tests? *Annals of Clinical Biochemistry* 1987; **24**: 435–9.

Crawfurd M d'A. Prenatal diagnosis of common genetic disorders. *British Medical Journal* 1988; **297**: 502–6.

Ehrmann DA, Rosenfield RL. An endocrinologic approach to the patient with hirsutism. *Journal of Clinical Endocrinology and Metabolism* 1990; **71**: 1–4.

Evans JG (Chairman). King's Fund forum consensus statement: screening for fetal and genetic abnormality. *British Medical Journal* 1987; **295**: 1551–3.

Fotherby K. Oral contraceptives and lipids. *British Medical Journal* 1989; **298**: 1049–50.

Franks S. Primary and secondary amenorrhoea. *British Medical Journal* 1985; **290**: 815–19.

Lilford RJ. The rise and fall of chorion villus sampling. *British Medical Journal* 1991; **303**: 936–7.

Reynolds TM. Practical problems in Down syndrome screening. *Communications in Laboratory Medicine* 1992; **2**: 31–8.

Wang C, Swerdloff RS. Evaluation of testicular function. *Baillière's Clinical Endocrinology and Metabolism* 1992; **6**: 405–34.

Westergaard JG, Teisner B, Grudzinskas JG. Biochemical assessment of placental function — late pregnancy. *Clinics in Obstetrics and Gynaecology* 1986; **13**: 571–91.

Wu FCW, Bancroft JHJ. Male infertility. *British Medical Journal* 1985; **290**: 1417–20.

Chapter 21

Campbell AGM, McIntosh N (Editors). *Textbook of Paediatrics* (Fourth Edition). Edinburgh: Churchill Livingstone, 1992.

Clayton BE, Round JM (Editors). *Chemical Pathology and the Sick Child*. Oxford: Blackwell Scientific Publications, 1984.

Green A. *Guide to Diagnosis of Inborn Errors of Metabolism in District General Hospitals*. Association of Clinical Pathologists Broadsheet **120**, London: British Medical Association, 1989.

Haan EA, Danks DM. Clinical investigation of suspected metabolic disease. In Barson AJ (Editor) *Laboratory Investigation of Fetal Disease*. Bristol: John Wright, 1981: 410–28.

Heeley AF, Bangert SK. The neonatal detection of cystic fibrosis by measurement of immunoreactive trypsin in blood. *Annals of Clinical Biochemistry* 1992; **29**: 361–76.

Hobbs JR. Displacement bone marrow transplantation and immunoprophylaxis for genetic diseases. *Advances in Internal Medicine* 1988; **33**: 81–118.

Holton JB. Diagnosis of inherited metabolic diseases in severely ill children. *Annals of Clinical Biochemistry* 1982; **19**: 389–95.

Isherwood DM, Fletcher KA. Neonatal jaundice: investigation and monitoring. *Annals of Clinical Biochemistry* 1985; **22**: 109–28.

John R. Screening for congenital hypothyroidism. *Annals of Clinical Biochemistry* 1987; **24**: 1–12.

MacLennan WJ. Screening elderly patients. *British Medical Journal* 1990; **300**: 694–5.

MacLennan WJ, Peden NR. *Metabolic and Endocrine Problems in the Elderly*. Berlin: Springer-Verlag, 1989.

Medical Research Council Steering Committee for the MRC/DHSS Phenylketonuria Register. Routine neonatal screening for phenylketonuria in the United Kingdom 1964–78. *British Medical Journal* 1981; **282**: 1680–4.

Modell B. Biochemical neonatal screening. *British Medical Journal* 1990; **300**: 1667–8.

MRC Working Party on Phenylketonuria. Phenylketonuria due to phenylalanine hyrdoxylase deficiency: an unfolding story. *British Medical Journal* 1993; **306**: 115–9.

Rudd BT. Growth, growth hormone and the somatomedins: a historical perspective and current concepts. *Annals of Clinical Biochemistry* 1991; **28**: 542–55.

Schonberg D. Diagnosis of growth hormone deficiency. *Baillière's Clinical Endocrinology and Metabolism* 1992; **6**: 527–46.

Scriver CR, Beaudet AL, Sly W, Valle, D (Editors). *The Metabolic Basis of Inherited Disease*. New York: McGraw-Hill, 1989.

Chapter 22

Davies KE (Editor). *Application of Molecular Genetics to the Diagnosis of Inherited Disease*. London: Royal College of Physicians, 1990.

Emery AEH, Rimoin DL. *Principles and Practice of Medical Genetics* (Second Edition). Edinburgh: Churchill Livingstone, 1990.

Rees A. DNA markers in the hyperlipidaemias and atherosclerosis. *Journal of the Royal College of Physicians of London* 1987; **21**: 51–4.

Ross DW. *Introduction to Molecular Medicine*. New York: Springer-Verlag, 1992.

Weatherall DJ. *The New Genetics and Clinical Practice* (Third Edition). Oxford: Oxford University Press, 1992.

Wenham P. DNA-based techniques in clinical biochemistry. *Annals of Clinical Biochemistry* 1992; **29**: 598–624.

Chapter 23

Davson H, Welch K, Segal MB. *The Physiology and Pathophysiology of the Cerebrospinal Fluid*. Edinburg: Churchill Livingstone, 1987.

Giles PD, Wroe SJ. Cerebrospinal fluid oligoclonal IgM in multiple sclerosis: analytical problems and clinical limitations. *Annals of Clinical Biochemistry* 1990; **27**: 199–207.

Ratnaike S, Klipatrick T, Tress B. Cerebrospinal fluid biochemistry in the diagnosis of multiple sclerosis. *Annals of Clinical Biochemistry* 1990; **27**: 195–8.

Thompson EJ, Keir G. Laboratory investigation of cerebrospinal fluid proteins. *Annals of Clinical Biochemistry* 1990; **27**: 425–35.

Chapter 24

Annesley TM. Special considerations for geriatric therapeutic drug monitoring. *Clinical Chemistry* 1989; **35**: 1337–41.
Gough TA (Editor). *The Analysis of Drugs of Abuse.* Chichester: John Wiley, 1991.
Hallworth MJ. Audit of therapeutic drug monitoring. *Annals of Clinical Biochemistry* 1988; **25**: 121–8.
Pippenger CE. Therapeutic drug monitoring in the 1990s. *Clinical Chemistry* 1989; **35**: 1348–51.
Reynolds DJM, Aronson JK. Making the most of plasma drug concentration measurements. *British Medical Journal* 1993; **306**: 48–51.
Simpson D, Greenwood J, Jarvie DR, Moore FML. Experience of a laboratory service for drug screening in urine. *Scottish Medical Journal* 1993; **38**: 20–6.

Chapter 25

Lowe D. How to do it: set a multiple choice question (MCQ) examination. *British Medical Journal* 1991; **302**: 780–2.
Harden RMcG, Brown TA, Biran LA, Dallas Ross WP, Wakeford RE. Multiple choice questions: to guess or not to guess. *Medical Education* 1976; **10**: 27–32.
Hubbard JP, Clemans WV. *Multiple-choice Examinations in Medicine.* London: Henry Kimpton, 1961.
Sanderson PH. The 'don't know' option in MCQ examinations. *British Journal of Medical Education* 1973; **11**: 216–20.

Appendix B

Campion EW. A retreat from SI units. *New England Journal of Medicine* 1992; **327**: 49.
McQueen MJ. SI Unit Pocket Guide. Chicago: American Society of Clinical Pathologists, 1990.
Nylenna M, Smith R. Americans retreat on SI units. *British Medical Journal* 1992; **305**: 268. Also see subsequent correspondence.
World Health Organisation. *The SI for the Health Professions.* Geneva: WHO, 1977.

Index

Page numbers in **bold** indicate principal references.

abbreviations   xi
abetalipoproteinaemia   192
abnormal results   21, 27–34
accuracy (of an analysis)   21
acetoacetate   15, 173
acetone   15, 173
acetyl cholinesterase   317–18, 375
N-acetyl-β-D-glucosaminidase   138–9
achlorhydria   146, 238
acid phosphatase   80, 101–2
acid–base balance   **57–71**
 in chronic renal failure   137
 interpretation of results   63–5
 investigating   58–60
 mixed disturbances   60–2, 64–5, 371
 treatment of disturbances   69–70
 specimen collection   59
 see also acidosis; alkalosis
acidification tests (urine)   131–2
acidosis   49
 hyperchloraemic   66
 hyperkalaemia and   52
 hypokalaemia and   51
 ketone bodies and   173
 lactic   173–4
 metabolic   60, 62, 63, 70, 138, 172–6
 plasma calcium and   201
 renal tubular   132
 respiratory   60, 61, 63, 69, 70
acrodermatitis enteropathica   232
acromegaly   297
ACTH *see* adrenocorticotrophin
acute intermittent porphyria   223
acute phase response   92–3
addiction (drugs)   373–4
Addison's disease   53, 278–9
 adrenal antibodies in   283
 screening tests   279–81
adenosine phosphoribosyltransferase   243
admission screening   4
adrenal cortex
 investigation of patients on steroid
  treatment   283–4
 tumours   276–8, 284–6
  chemical test results in   277–8
  hormonal test results in   273, 276, 277
adrenal hyperplasia

congenital   286–90
 hirsutism and   311–12
adrenal medulla tumours
 phaeochromocytoma   290–2, 339
adrenal steroid hormone synthesis and
  secretion regulation   267–70
adrenaline
 hypokalaemia and   50
 measurement in phaeochromocytoma
  291
adrenocortical hyperfunction investigation
  271–8
adrenocortical hypofunction investigation
  278–84
adrenocorticotrophin   267, 295–6
 aldosterone secretion and   269
 cortisol release by   267–9
 in Cushing's syndrome   276
 in plasma   270, 277–8
  in adrenocortical hyperfunction   273
  in adrenocortical hypofunction   282
 secretion regulation   267–9
adrenogenital syndrome *see* adrenal
  hyperplasia, congenital
AFP *see* α-fetoprotein
agammaglobulinaemia   96
age effects on reference ranges *see* reference
  ranges
ALA   221
alanine aminotransferase (ALT)   78
 in liver disease   115, 118
 in pyridoxine deficiency   237
albumin
 effects on plasma calcium   200
 fluid balance disorders   46
 genetic variants   260
 glycated   172
 levels in nutritional disturbances   239,
  334–5
 in liver disease   113, 118–23
 plasma   46, **87–9**, 315
 thyroid function tests (effects on)   253,
  260
 transport functions   86–7, 108, 200–1,
  232, 251, 253, 260
 in urine   14, 172
alcohol effect on plasma lipids   187, 192

alcohol (ethanol)   116, 121–2, 191–2, 232, 371–2
alcoholic liver disease   122
    porphyria and   223
alcoholism mimicking Cushing's syndrome   264
aldosterone
    hyperaldosteronism   284–6
    secretion   39, 269–70
alkaline phosphatase   78–80
    in bone disease   202
    in the elderly   340
    in liver disease   107, 115, 118–20, 122
    in pregnancy   315
    reference ranges   79, 322
    as tumour marker   102
alkalosis   49, 50
    hypokalaemia and   51
    metabolic   60, 62, 63–4, 70, 277, 285, 371
    plasma calcium and   201, 207
    respiratory   60, 61, 63–4, 70–1, 207
aluminium toxicity   375
amenorrhoea   308–10
amino acid
    absorption   155
    disorders in neonates   324
    in liver disease   116
    in nutrition   230, 240
    transport defects   134, 155
amino acidurias   132–4
5-aminolaevulinate (ALA) synthase
    increase   220, 223
    lead poisoning and   226–7
ammonia   116, 325
ammonium chloride test   131
amniocentesis   317–19
amniotic fluid
    acetyl cholinesterase   317–18
    bilirubin   319
    α-fetoprotein (AFP)   317
    lecithin   318–19
    pre-natal diagnosis   327–8
amylase   80–1
    in duodenal contents   151
    in plasma   80, 123, 149
    in urine   149–50
anaemia
    folate deficiency   237
    haemolytic   74, 89, 111, 117
    iron deficiency   219
    sickle cell   355
analbuminaemia   89
analytical factors
    causing errors in measurement   21–3
    effects on reference ranges   27
androgens   303
    excess in CAH   287–8, 311
angiotensin   39, 285
anion gap   65–6
anion transport (hepatic)   108–13

antibodies   93–100
    adrenal   283
    islet cell   168
    liver   117
    thyroid   260, 263
anticoagulants see coagulation factors
anticonvulsants (therapeutic monitoring)   369
antidiuretic hormone (ADH) see arginine vasopressin
α_1-antitrypsin see α_1-protease inhibitor
apolipoproteins   183–5, 190–2
arginine vasopressin (AVP)   300–1
    disorders in renal disease   129–30
    inappropriate secretion   42–3, 44, 48, 56, 301
    secretion, water balance and   37–8, 41
arterial disease, hyperlipidaemia and   192–4
arterial specimens, for acid–base analysis   59
ascites   113, 122
ascorbic acid   238–9
Asher's catechism   2
aspartate aminotransferase (AST)   77
    in liver disease   115, 118
    in myocardial infarction   82–5
assessment (of diagnostic tests)   28–33
asthma attack (blood gases)   68, 70
atheroma, risk estimation of   362
atrial natriuretic peptides   40
audit   9–11
auto-immune disease   96–7, 168–9, 260, 263, 283

bacterial colonization of small intestine   157–9
balance (metabolic)
    acid–base   57–71
    calcium   195–6
    fluid and electrolyte   55
    potassium   48–9
    sodium   35–40
    water   35–40
Bartter's syndrome   51
BB isoenzyme (creatine kinase)   76
'bedside biochemistry'   17–20, 170, 319
Bence Jones protein   14, 97–9
betamethasone see dexamethasone suppression test
between-individual variation in test results   25
bicarbonate
    acid–base disturbances (arterial bicarbonate)   **57–65**
    CSF   365
    renal excretion   132–4
    total CO_2 (venous bicarbonate, mainly)   60–1, 65–6
    treatment   69–70, 174, 207
bile   106–7, 108
bile acids

fat absorption and   155–6
in plasma   112–13
biliary disease   159
bilirubin
  in amniotic fluid   319
  measurement in plasma   17, 109, 333
  metabolism and excretion   108–13
  reference ranges in children   322
  tests in urine   12, 15, 109, 117–18
bilirubinometers   17
biological variation   24–7
bisalbuminaemia   89
blood
  in faeces, testing for   15–16
  glucose   163–4
    analysers   17, 170
  lead   226
  oxygen transport   67
  porphyrins   224
blood specimens
  analysis in ward and clinic areas   17–20
  collection, drug therapy and   367–8
  collection and preservation   5–8
  collection following myocardial
    infarction   83–4
  collection for acid–base measurements
    59
  collection from children   321–2
  for glucose analysis   164
  working with   19
blood buffers   57
blood-gas analysers   17
blunders (in test results)   23
bone
  alkaline phosphatase   79, 102, 202
  disease   202–5, 207–13, 215
    in chronic renal failure   137, 212–13
    in the elderly   342–3
    hypercalcaemia and   207
    metabolic   210–13
    raised alkaline phosphatase levels in   80
  turnover, calcium and   195
    parathyroid hormone and   196
brain damage   76, 373
breath tests   157–8
  [^{14}C]-glycocholate   157–8
  hydrogen   155
  triglyceride   157
  [^{14}C]-xylose   157
bromsulphthalein test   113
BT-PABA–[^{14}C]-PABA tests   152–3
buffers   57

C-peptide, insulinoma and   177–8
C-reactive protein   87, 92–3
CA 15-3, CA 19-9, CA 125   104
calcidiol see 25-hydroxycholecalciferol
calciferol see vitamin D
calcitonin   199
  in medullary carcinoma of thyroid   264

calcitriol   197–9
calcium   **195–213**
  absorption defects   160
  balance   195–6
  intracellular   199
  ionized   196, 201
  levels in chronic renal failure   137
  metabolism, abnormal   **200–13**
  in plasma   99, 200–1
    in acute pancreatitis   150
    in children   331–2, 338
    hormonal control of   196–9
    in hyperparathyroidism   137, 204, 211
    in hypoparathyroidism   207, 209
    malignant disease   202–3
    MEN syndromes   205, 265
    renal disease   138, 212–13
    thyroid disorders and   264
  reference ranges in children   322
  requirements   195
  stones, renal   141–2
  urine excretion studies   204
calculi, renal   141–3, 247
carbohydrate
  absorption   154, 157, 229
  antigens (tumour)   104
  in diet   229
  disorders in neonates   179–80, 324
  metabolism, disorders of   **162–81**
    in liver disease   116
    oral contraceptives and   312
carbon dioxide
  in plasma   57–66, 68–71
    total CO_2 55, 65–6, 68
      in hyperglycaemic coma   175
      in hyperparathyroidism   204
      in renal tubular acidosis   132
carbonic anhydrase   57, 133
carboxyhaemoglobin   228
carcinoembryonic antigen (CEA)   102–3
carcinoid syndrome   161
carcinoid tumours   160–1
carcinoma see tumours
cardiac failure, hyponatraemia and   44
case-finding programmes   3
  see also screening
catecholamines   290–2, 339
cellobiose : mannitol ratio   158
central nervous system, metabolic disorders
    and   364
cerebrospinal fluid examination   364–6
ceruloplasmin   87, 92
  in liver disease   114
children
  convulsions   330–2
  failure to thrive   334–6
  immunoglobulins in   95
  inherited metabolic disorders   323–30
  poisoning   373
  raised alkaline phosphatase levels in   79
  reference ranges   322

short stature   336–8
specimen collection   321–2
see also neonates
chloride in plasma   47, 65–6
anion gap   65–6
chloride in sweat   335
cholecalciferol   197–9
cholecystokinin (CCK)   145
-pancreozymin test   150–1
cholestasis   119, 121, 123
cholestatic hyperbilirubinaemia   110, 111
cholesterol   **182–94**
plasma levels   187–8
in the elderly   340
reduction of   193–4
screening   18, 193
cholinesterase   81–2
in liver disease   114
pesticide poisoning   375
choriocarcinoma   314
chorion villus biopsy   327
chorionic gonadotrophin (human, hCG)
257, 313–14
chromatograpy in neonates   325
chromium deficiency   232–3
chronic obstructive airways disease   69
chylomicrons   183, 185, 189
cirrhosis of liver   120
α_1-protease deficiency   91, 355
CK-MB isoenzyme *see* creatine kinase and
isoenzymes
clearance tests (renal)   126
clonidine test (short stature)   337
coagulation factors   113–14, 236
coagulation tests, liver disease   113–14,
118
coeliac disease   337–8
collagen measurement, liver disease   116
colloid osmotic pressure   37
colorectal carcinoma, CEA levels in   103
coma
hypoglycaemic   177
ketotic hyperglycaemic   172–3
non-ketotic hyperglycaemic   174
combined hyperlipidaemia (familial)   190
complement-fixing antibodies   263
concentration tests (renal)   128–31
connecting peptide (C-peptide, insulin)   163,
177–8, 331
Conn's syndrome   284
contraceptives, oral   312–13
convulsions, in children   330–2
copper
deficiency   231
levels in Wilson's disease   120–1
transport   92
coproporphyria, hereditary   224
Cori types (glycogen storage diseases)   179,
324, 326
coronary heart disease   82, 187–8, 192–4
corpus luteum   306–7, 311

corticotrophin-releasing hormone (CRH)
267, 295
stimulation test   277, 296
cortisol   **267–90**
-binding globulin   268–9
free   271
in plasma and serum   270
in hyperadrenalism   272–8
in hypoadrenalism   279–84
urinary   271, 274
creatine kinase and isoenzymes   76–7
activity   73
isoforms   76, 82
levels following myocardial infarction   28–
31, 82–5
muscle disease and   77
creatinine
clearance   126
in the elderly   339–40
in plasma   46–7, 99, 124
reference ranges in children   322
in renal disease   124–6
CRH stimulation test   277, 296
Crigler–Najjar syndrome   112
cryoglobulins   98
Cushing's syndrome   271–8
confirmatory tests   274–6
CRH stimulation test   277, 296
determining the cause of   276–7
hypokalaemia and   51, 277
screening tests   272–4
cyanocobalamin   238
cyclic AMP (urinary)   210
cystic fibrosis
in children   323, 335–6
Molecular Biology   358, 360
cystine stones, renal   142
cystinosis   134
cystinuria   134, 323
cytotoxic drug treatment
(hyperuricaemia)   248

DDAVP test   129–30
de Ritis ratio   107 (note)
dehydration   40–1, 45–6
in diabetic coma   172–5
impaired ability to concentrate urine   129–
31
7-dehydrocholesterol   198
dehydro*epi*androsterone sulphate, hirsutism
311–12
demyelinating disease (CSF changes)   366
11-deoxycorticosterone   290
11-deoxycortisol   278, 279
dexamethasone suppression test
high-dose   276–7
low-dose   273
diabetes insipidus   130–1, 301
diabetes mellitus   **164–76**
classification   168–70

diagnostic criteria   165–6
in the elderly   342
genetics and   362
gestational   169–70
glucose tolerance test   166–8
hyperkalaemia and   53
idiopathic   168–9
metabolic complications of   172–5
pregnancy and   169–70, 315
screening for   4
secondary   169
therapy, monitoring in   17, 170–2
diabetic ketoacidosis   172–6
diagnosis, use of tests   1, 21, 28–31, 33–4
dialysis dementia   212, 375
dibucaine numbers   82
diet
    effect on concentrations of analytes
        in blood   6, 24, 125, 127, 167, 187–8,
            243
        in urine   161, 291
    iron in   216
    principal constituents in   229–30
    trace elements   230–3
    vitamin D deficiency and   208–9
    vitamins in   233–5
    see also nutrition
digestive tract   144–61
digoxin
    monitoring   368–9
    poisoning, hyperkalaemia and   53
1 : 25-dihydroxycholecalciferol (DHCC)
    197–9
    therapy   213
    see also vitamin D
24 : 25-dihydroxycholecalciferol   198–9
5α-dihydrotestosterone   304
diquat toxicity   375
disaccharide tolerance tests   154–5
disease
    prevalence   30–2
    screening for rare diseases   32–3
diuretic therapy   42, 51, 135, 248
diurnal variation effect on specimens   6, 24,
    217
DNA   346
    'fingerprint'   358
    gene cloning   348–52
    polymerase chain reaction   359–60
    restriction endonucleases and other
        enzymes   346–8
    restriction fragment length polymorphisms
        355, 356–8
    sequencing   352–4
    Southern blotting   354–5
dopamine   40, 297, 339
Down syndrome, screening   318
drugs
    abuse   373–4
    effect on test results   6, 24, 125, 244, 259,
        291, 297–8

enzyme induction   122
    metabolites   368–9
    screening for misuse   372–4
    side-effects on liver   122
    therapy and glucose tolerance   169
        causing hypercalcaemia   207
        causing hypocalcaemia   210
        causing plasma thyroid hormone
            abnormalities   259
        monitoring   1–2, 367–70
        for reducing cholesterol levels   194
    toxicity monitoring   368, 370–4
    urine appearance   13
Dubin–Johnson syndrome   112
Duchenne muscular dystrophy   77, 323
dwarfism   336–7
dysgammaglobulinaemia   96

ECG, enzyme tests and 85
'ectopic' hormone production   101, 276,
    277
electrolyte
    content of intravenous feed   241
    tests in adrenocortical hypofunction   283
'electrolyte group' of tests   4, 55, 127
electrophoresis
    isoenzymes   74, 318
    lipoproteins   189, 192
    serum protein   87, 98–9, 114
    urine protein   97–9
emergency requests (out of hours)   9, 17–
    20, 370–2
emphysema   68–9, 90–1
endocrine disorders, hypercalcaemia and
    207·
enolase   102
enterohepatic circulation   106, 108–9, 156,
    194
enzymes
    activity units   73
    amniotic fluid   317–18
    of clinical importance   74–82
    faecal   336
    involved in lipid transport   185
    plasma tests   **72–85**
        in liver disease   114–15, 118–23
        in myocardial infarction   28–31, 82–5
        selecting   72–3
    as tumour markers   101–2
epilepsy, treatment monitoring   369–70
errors in analytical results   33
    audit   10, 19
    blunders   23
    false-negative results   16, 30
    false-positive results   16, 28, 30–1
erythrocyte
    porphyrins   222, 227
    transketolase   236
erythropoietic porphyria
    congenital   222

essential fatty acids   182, 230, 240
ethanol
liver disease   80, 116, 121–2
overdose   371–2
examination questions   **376–408**
multiple-choice questions   378–406, 409–10
short answer questions   406–8
exercise
cholesterol levels and   187
effects on test results   24, 72, 125
exomphalos, prenatal diagnosis   317, 318
exophthalmic Graves' disease   253, 263
extracellular fluid
balance   35–45
hydrogen ion concentration   57
extra-laboratory tests   17–20, 193, 319
exudate   123

faeces
acidity   155
electrolytes   158, 160
fat content   156, 160
occult blood   15–16
pH in malabsorption   155
porphyrins   224
specimen collection and preservation   9, 156
trypsin   336
water content   35, 158
failure to thrive, children   334–6
false-positive rates   28
Fanconi syndrome   134
fat
absorption   155–7
in diet   229–30
causing raised alkaline phosphatase levels in plasma   79
in faeces   156, 160
fat-soluble vitamin deficiency   234, 235–6
vitamin K deficiency   113–14, 236
see also vitamin D, deficiency
fatty acids   182, 229
female
gonadal function   **306–12**
infertility   309, 310–11
ferritin   217–20
in pregnancy   315–16
ferrochelatase   220, 226
fetal abnormalities, prenatal diagnosis of   316–19
fetal monitoring during labour   319
fetoplacental unit, pregnancy and   313–16
α-fetoprotein (AFP)   87, 91–2, 102, 103
prenatal diagnosis   316–17
fluid
balance   **35–48**, 55–6, 128–31
deprivation test in renal disease   130
replacement   55, 174, 241
fluorescein dilaurate test   153

fluoride numbers   82
folic acid   237–8
follicle stimulating hormone   293–5
amenorrhoea and   309–10
male gonadal function   303–6
menstrual disorders and infertility   306–11
ovarian dysfunction   309–12
formiminoglutamate   238
Franklin's disease   98
free fatty acids   230
fructosamine assay   172
fructose intolerance, hereditary   180
fructosuria, essential   180

G-cell hyperplasia   148–9
galactorrhoea   297
galactosaemia   179–80, 323–5, 330
screening for   330
'side-room' tests   13–14, 324–5
gamma-glutamyl transferase (GGT)   80
in liver disease   115, 118–20, 122
reference ranges for children   322
ganglioneuroblastoma in children   339
gastric fluid loss, hypokalaemia and   51
gastrin   145–7
in plasma   147–9
gastrinoma   147–9
gastrointestinal peptides   145
gastrointestinal tract disease   **144–61**
Gaussian distribution curves   22, 26
gene cloning   348–52
gene probe diagnosis   360–2
genetic counselling   326
genetic disorders in children   323–30
genetic polymorphism   89, 90
genomic clone   348
genotypes (cholinesterase)   81–2
Geriatrics, Clinical Biochemistry in   **339–44**
gestational diabetes mellitus   169–70
giantism   297
Gilbert's syndrome   111–12, 334
globulin (plasma) classification   87
glomerular filtration rate   40, 124–5
glomerular proteinuria   139–40
glomerulonephritis   140–1
glucagon   162
test in short stature   337
glucocorticoids   162, **267–90**
deficiency, water retention and   43
glucose   **162–80**
analysis in blood or plasma   163–8
in diabetes   168–71
for hyperglycaemic coma   174–5
home-monitoring of blood and urine glucose   14, 17, 164, 170
in hypoglycaemia   176–8
in intestinal absorption tests   154–5
blood levels
in the elderly   340

in neonates 331
in CSF 365
metabolism, hormonal control 162–3
tolerance test 165, 166–8
in Cushing's syndrome 278
thyroid disorders and 264
glucose-dependent insulinotrophic
peptide 145, 163
glucosuria 14
renal 134, 168
glutamic oxaloacetic transaminase *see*
aspartate aminotransferase
glutamic pyruvic transaminase *see* alanine
aminotransferase
glycated haemoglobin 18, 171
plasma proteins 172
[^{14}C]-glycocholate breath test 157–8
glycogen storage diseases 178–9, 324, 326
glycoprotein antigens 104
glycosuria 14
in neonates 179–80, 324–5
gonadal failure 295
gonadal function
female 306–12
male 303–6
gonadal neoplasms 100, 104, 306, 312,
314
gonadotroph adenoma 295
gonadotrophin-releasing hormone 294–5,
303, 306–7
Gn-RH test 295
gonadotrophins (FSH, LH) 294–5, 303–10
(human) chorionic (hCG) 306, 313–14
gout
primary 246–8
secondary 248
Graves' disease *see* hyperthyroidism
growth
disorders in children 336–8
hormone 293, 296–7
deficiency in children 337
guanine 243, 244
Guthrie test 329
gynaecomastia in males 306

haem metabolism 108–10, 220–6
haematin 228
haemochromatosis 219–20
primary (idiopathic) 220
haemoglobin 67, 108–10
abnormal derivatives of 227–8
glycated 171
haemolysis during venepuncture 7
haemosiderin 217
haptoglobin 87, 89–90
Hartnup disease 134, 155, 323
Hashimoto's thyroiditis 263
health and safety code for blood specimen
handling 19
heart disease 28–31, 82–5

plasma cholesterol and 18, 187–8, 192–
4
'heart-specific' lactate dehydrogenase 75,
82–4
heavy chains (immunoglobulin) 93–4
heavy chain disease 98
Helicobacter pylori and gastric urease 149
Henderson equation 58
Henderson–Hasselbalch equation 58
hepatic anion transport 108–13
hepatic disorders, API levels in 91
hepatic fibrosis, tests for 116
hepatic transport of bilirubin etc. 106, 108–
13
hepatic transport systems 106, 108
hepatic *see also liver entries*
hepatitis
acute 74, 77–8, 110, 114–15, 118–19
chronic 79–80, 114–15, 118–19, 121
neonatal 334
hepatocellular carcinoma 103, 119
hepatocellular hyperbilirubinaemia 110–11
hepatocytes 105–6
hepatolenticular degeneration 120–1
hepatoma 123
herbicide toxicity 375
HGPRT deficiency 248
high density lipoproteins (HDL) 183–9
arterial disease and 192–3
hirsutism in females 311–12
histidine load test (folate deficiency) 238
homovanillic acid 339
hormones as tumour markers 100–1
human chorionic gonadotrophin (hCG)
pregnancy and 313–14
test 306
human placental lactogen 314
hydatidiform mole (hCG production) 314
hydrogen ion
blood 57–64, 319
faecal 160
urine 15, 131–2
hydrogen test in breath 155
4-hydroxy, 3-methoxy mandelic acid
(HMMA) 290–1, 339
4-hydroxy, 3-methoxy phenylacetic acid 339
β-hydroxy-β-methylglutaryl-coenzyme A
reductase (cholesterol synthesis)
185, 194
3-hydroxybutyrate 173
hydroxybutyrate dehydrogenase 75, 82–4
1α-hydroxycholecalciferol 213
25-hydroxycholecalciferol 198–9, 209
11-hydroxycorticosteroids 43
see also cortisol
5-hydroxyindole acetic acid 160–1
5-hydroxyindole-secreting tumours 160–1
1α-hydroxylase, renal (vitamin D
metabolism) 198–9, 208
11β-hydroxylase defect 289–90, 323
21-hydroxylase defect 287–9, 311, 323

17α-hydroxyprogesterone and congenital
  adrenal hyperplasia 287–90, 311–
  12
5-hydroxytryptamine, 5-hydroxytryptophan
  (carcinoids) 160–1
hygiene for blood specimen collection 6–7
hyper-α-lipoproteinaemia 191
hyperacidity (gastric) 145–8
hyperaldosteronism
  hypokalaemia and 51
  primary 51, 284–6
  secondary 44, 51, 113, 285–6
hyperbilirubinaemia **109–12**, 117–23
  cholestatic 111, 119–21
  congenital 111–12
  hepatocellular 110–11, 118–19
  neonatal 333–4
  pre-hepatic 109–10
hypercalcaemia 202–7
  causes 203
  in children 338
  familial hypocalciuric 207
  tumours and 202–3
hypercalciuria 141–2
  in children 338
hyperchloridaemia 66
hypercholesterolaemia 189–94, 264
  primary 189–90
  screening for 18, 193
  treatment 193–4
hypergammaglobulinaemia 95–100
  investigation of paraproteinaemia 98–9
hyperglycaemia **164–75**, 323
  glucose tolerance test 166–70
  hyperglycaemic coma 172–5
hypergonadotrophic hypogonadism 305–6
hyperinsulinism, functional (of infancy) 331
hyperkalaemia 49, 52–4
  artefact 56
  in renal disease 135
hyperkalaemic familial periodic paralysis 53
hyperlipidaemia **189–94**
  arterial disease and 192–4
  familial combined 190
  pseudohyponatraemia 45
  secondary 191–2
  treatment 193–4
hyperlipoproteinaemias 189–92
hypermagnesaemia 214
hypernatraemia 45–6
hyperparathyroidism
  primary 203–6, 214–15
    MEN syndromes 265
    screening for 4
  secondary 137, 208
  tertiary 137, 207
hyperphenylalaninaemia 329–30
hyperphosphataemia 202
hyperprolactinaemia 297
hyperpyrexia, malignant 77
hypertension

in Conn's syndrome 284
gout and 248
in phaeochromocytoma 290, 291
hyperthyroidism 255–6, 294
  management 261
  in pregnancy 314–15
  screening for 4, 343–4
  thyroid auto-antibodies 263
  TRH test 294
hypertriglyceridaemia 122, 190–4
  familial 190
hyperuricaemia 100, 122, 179, **244–6**
  in pre-eclampsia 316
hyperventilation 61–2, 207
hypoalbuminaemia 89
hypoaldosteronism
  adrenocortical insufficiency, 278–83
  congenital adrenal hyperplasia 286–90
  hyperkalaemia and 53
hypobetalipoproteinaemia 192
hypocalcaemia 207–10
  acute pancreatitis 150
  chronic renal failure 137
  neonatal 332
hypochloridaemia 66
hypocholesterolaemia 192
hypogammaglobulinaemia 95
hypoglycaemia 175–8
  neonatal 331
  see also insulin-hypoglycaemia tests
hypogonadism 295
  in males 304–6
hypokalaemia 49, 52
  in 'ectopic' ACTH production 277
  and hyperaldosteronism 284–5
hypokalaemic familial periodic
    paralysis 50–1
hypolipidaemia, secondary 192
hypolipoproteinaemia 189–91, 192
hypomagnesaemia 213–14
  neonatal 332
hyponatraemia 41–5
  artefact 45
  AVP excess 44
hypoparathyroidism 209–10
  neonatal 332
hypophosphataemia 202, 208–9
  amino aciduria and 134
hypophosphatasia 209
hypopituitarism 300
hypoproteinaemia 44, 88, 89, 95–6, 113,
    315
  malnutrition 334–5
hypothalamic hormones **293–9**
hypothalamic–pituitary–adrenal axis **267–
    84**
  adrenocortical hyperfunction 271–8
  adrenocortical hypofunction 278–84
  stress test of 275–6
hypothalamic–pituitary–gonadal axis 303–
    4, 306–11

hypothalamic–pituitary–thyroid axis 251–2
hypothyroidism 256
  management 261–3
  in neonates 3, 32, 323, 330
  screening
    in the elderly 343–4
    thyroid auto-antibodies 363–4
  TRH test 294
hypotriglyceridaemia 192
hypouricaemia 246
hypoxaemia 68–9
hypoxanthine-guanine phosphoribosyl-
    transferase deficiency 243, 248

ileal disease 156–8
  bypass 194
immunoglobulins 87, **93–100**
  CSF 366
  disorders of synthesis 95–8
  in liver disease 114
  mouse, antibodies to 260
immunoreactive trypsin 151–2, 336
imprecision (of analyses) 22–3
inappropriate secretion of
  AVP (ADH) 42–3
  other hormones 100–1, 278
inborn errors of metabolism *see* inherited
    metabolic disorders
indican, urinary 157
individual variation 24–6, 187
induction of enzymes 80, 115
industrial chemical toxicity 374–5
infection, hypergammaglobulinaemia and 96
infertility
  in females 309–11
  in males 304–6
infiltrations (liver) 120
inherited metabolic disorders **323–30**
  carbohydrate metabolism 178–80, 324–
    6, 330
  congenital adrenal hyperplasia 286–90,
    311–12
  incidence 323
  phenylketonuria 32, 328–30
  screening 3, 32–3, 327–30
injury
  acute phase response 92–3
  creatine kinase 76
  metabolic response to 55–6, 268
insulin
  diabetes mellitus and 164, 168–9, 172–3
  effects on cellular metabolism 50, 162–4
  hypoglycaemia 175–8
  secretion 162–3
  therapy 50, 174–6
insulin-hypoglycaemia tests
  in adrenocortical hyperfunction 275–6
  in adrenocortical hypofunction 282–3
  in assessing vagotomy 146–7
  in pituitary disease 282–3, 296–7

  in children 337
insulinoma 177–8
intensive care units, chemical analyses 17–
  20
intermediate density lipoproteins 183, 184
international units of enzyme activity 73
interpretation (of results) 21–3
intestinal malabsorption 144, 154–60, 209
intestinal mucosal disease 159
intestinal permeability 158
intracellular fluid balance 35–8
intravenous feeding 239–42
iodide, iodine 249–50
iodotyrosines 249–50, 263
ion difference (anion gap) 65–6
ion-selective electrode systems 17
iron-binding capacity, total 219, 315
iron metabolism **216–20**
  deficiency 219
  malabsorption 160
  overload 219–20
  in plasma 217–18
    in pregnancy 315–16
ischaemic heart disease, plasma cholesterol
    levels and 187–8, 192–4
isoenzymes 74
  acid phosphatase 80, 101–2
  alkaline phosphatase 78, 102, 315
  creatine kinase 76, 82–5
  lactate dehydrogenase 74–6, 82–4
  tumour-specific 102
  see also individual enzyme entries
isoforms (creatine kinase) 76, 82

jaundice 109–12, 117–21
  neonatal 333–4
  in pregnancy 316
  'side-room' tests 13, 109

kernicterus 333
Keshan disease 231–2
ketoacidosis, diabetic 172–3, 174–5
ketone bodies 15, 173
ketotic, hyperglycaemic coma 172–5
kidney *see* renal entries
Klinefelter syndrome 295, 305–6
kwashiorkor 192, 334–5

lactate 66, 173
lactate dehydrogenase 74–5
  in myocardial infarction 82–5
lactic acidosis 173–4, 179
lactoferrin 152
lactose tolerance test 154–5
lactosuria 14, 170, 180
LDL and LDL-cholesterol 184, 186–8,
  190–3, 264, 312

see also low density lipoproteins and LDL-
    cholesterol
lead poisoning   226
lecithin, amniotic fluid   318–19
lecithin cholesterol acyltransferase   185
Lesch–Nyhan syndrome   248
leucocyte ascorbate   238
light chain disease   97, 98–9
light chains (immunoglobulin)   93–4
Lignac–Fanconi disease   134
lipids   182–3
    abnormalities of metabolism   **186–94**
        in liver disease   117
        oral contraceptives and   312
    storage diseases   326
    transport in blood   183–5
lipoprotein lipase   185, 189
    deficiency   191
lipoproteins   183–5
    lipoprotein X   117
    metabolism   185–6
    primary hyperlipoproteinaemias   189–91
lithium treatment (monitoring)   368, 369
liver disease   **105–23**
    albumin in   113, 118–20
    alkaline phosphatase in   79, 102, 115,
        118–20
    bilirubin metabolism in   109–12, 117–20,
        122–3
    cirrhosis   120
    copper metabolism and   120–1
    GGT in   80, 115, 118–20, 122
    hypergammaglobulinaemia in   96, 114
    infiltrations   119–20
    porphyria and   222–4
    α₁-protease inhibitor deficiency and   91
    vitamin D deficiency and   209
    see also hepatic entries
'liver function tests'   107–17
    thyroid disorders and   264
low density lipoproteins (LDL) and LDL-
        cholesterol   183–4, 186, 362
    arterial disease and   192–4
    primary hyperlipoproteinaemias   190–4
    steroid contraceptives and   312
    thyroid disorders and   191, 264
Lp(a)   184
    arterial disease and   192
Lundh test   151–2
luteinizing hormone   294–5
    female gonadal function and   306–11
    male gonadal function and   ' 303–6

'M' (monoclonal) components   97
macro-amylasaemia   150
α₂-macroglobulin   87, 92
macroglobulinaemia, Waldenström's   97
magnesium metabolism   213–14
malabsorption   154–60
    of vitamins   209

male gonadal function   303–6
    hypogonadism and infertility   304–6
    sex differentiation disorders   306
malignant disease see tumours
malnutrition in children   334–6
maltose tolerance test   154–5
manganese deficiency   233
marasmus   334
maternal serum α-fetoprotein   317, 318
MB isoenzyme (creatine kinase)   76, 82–5
meals (effects on results of analyses)
    blood analyses   6, 79, 124, 127, 167
    urine analyses   161, 291
mean value (statistical)   22–3
medullary carcinoma (thyroid)   264–5
melanocyte-stimulating hormone   295,
        298–9
MEN syndromes   205–6, 265
Mendelian disorders   323
meningitis (CSF changes)   365
Menkes' disease   231
menstrual cycle
    disorders   306–7
    effects on test results   24, 217, 307
metabolic bone disease   210–13
metabolic disorders, inherited see inherited
        metabolic disorders
metabolic response to trauma   55–6, 92–3
metadrenaline   290, 339
metal poisons   226–7, 374–5
metanephrine   290, 339
methaemalbumin in plasma in acute
        pancreatitis   150
methaemoglobinaemia   227–8
methanol poisoning   371
methylmalonic acid   238
metyrapone test   278
'microalbuminuria'   172
β₂-microglobulin   87, 92, 99
milk–alkali syndrome   207
mineralocorticoid deficiency   **278–84**
    hyperkalaemia and   53, 283
mobilizing lipase   185
Molecular Biology   **346–63**
molybdenum deficiency   233
mucopolysaccharidoses   323, 326
multiple endocrine neoplasia (MEN)
        syndromes   205–6, 265
multiple myeloma   97–100, 203
multiple sclerosis, CSF proteins   366
muscle diseases, creatine kinase and   77
myeloproliferative disorders, gout and   248
myocardial infarction
    creatine kinase in   28–31, 82–5
    other plasma enzyme tests in   82–5

NAG (renal transplant)   138
Nagao isoenzyme   102
National External Quality Assurance
        Schemes   10

natriuresis 48
'near-patient' chemical measurements 17–20, 170, 319
negative feedback control 196–7, 252, 267–8, 304, 307
neonates **321–34**
  congenital adrenal hyperplasia 286–90
  convulsions 330–2
  hyperbilirubinaemia in 333–4
  inherited metabolic disorders 178–80, 323–30
    index case 324–5
    screening for disease 3, 32, 323–30
    specimen collection 321–2, 325–6
    urine testing 14, 15, 324–5
neoplastic disease see tumours
nephrotic syndrome 89, 140, 191
neural tube defects 316–17
neuroblastoma 339
neurone-specific enolase 102
niacin 237
nicotinic acid test in Gilbert's syndrome 112
nitrogen metabolism in liver disease 116
'non-endocrine' tumours 101
'non-thyroidal illness' 257–9
noradrenaline 291
'normal range' 27
normetadrenaline, normetanephrine 290
nucleic acids 243, **346–60**
nucleotide synthesis 243–4
nutrition **229–42**
  biochemical assessment of status 239
  inadequate, in the elderly 341
  intravenous feeding 239–42
  nutrition team 242
  support 239–42
  see also diet; malnutrition in children
nychthemeral rhythm
  ACTH 270, 296
  cortisol 268–9
    loss of 274–5

objectives (educational) vii
obstructive jaundice see cholestasis
occult blood (faeces) 15–16
occupational hazards (chemical) 374–5
oedema 43–4, 46
oestrogens, plasma 306–11
  in amenorrhoea and infertility 309–11
  menstrual cycle and 306–7
  in pregnancy 314
oligonucleotide probes 352
oliguria 48, 136
oncotic pressure, plasma 37
organic solvents (toxicity) 375
organophosphate toxicity 375
osmolality 36–7, 47
  plasma 47, 56
  urine 47–8
    in renal disease 128–9

osmolarity 36–7
osmostat 43
osmotic gap in malabsorption 160
osteocalcin 199, 211
osteoclastic activating factors 203
osteodystrophy, renal 212–13
osteomalacia 209
  in the elderly 343
osteoporosis 210–11
ovarian cysts 312
ovarian dysfunction 307–12
oxalate stones, renal 142
oxygen
  oximetry 17, 67–70, 319
  transport 67

Paediatric Clinical Biochemistry **321–39**
  see also children; neonates
Paget's disease 211, 342–3
pancreatic disease 149–53, 159
  acute pancreatitis 81, 149–50
  chronic pancreatitis 150–3, 159
  diabetes 169
pancreolauryl test 153
paracetamol overdose 370–1
paralysis
  hyperkalaemic familial periodic 53
  hypokalaemic familial periodic 50–1
paraproteinaemia 97–9
paraquat toxicity 375
parathyroid hormone (PTH) 196–7, 204–5
  PTH-related protein 203
  tumour localization 205
parathyroidectomy 205
patient identification (PID) system 5
patients
  identification of specimens 5
  non-compliance with treatment 368
  posture, effects on test results 7, 24
  screening for disease 2–5
PBG deaminase 222
P_{CO_2} 57–65, 68–9
pentagastrin test 145–6
pentosuria, essential 180
peptic ulcer 145–9
peptides, gastrointestinal 144–5
per cent oxygen saturation 67–8
pernicious anaemia 146, 238
pesticide toxicity 375
pH
  of blood 57–9, 319
  of urine 15, 131–2
phaeochromocytoma 290–2, 339
phenylalanine metabolism 328–9
phenylketonuria 323, 328–30
  screening for 3, 32, 329–30
phenytoin, treatment monitoring 369
phosphate
  plasma levels 201–2
    in chronic renal failure 137

in renal osteodystrophy 212
reference ranges in children 322
urine 138, 204
phospholipids 182–3
photosensitivity (porphyrias) 221, 223, 225
pituitary
anterior 293–9
function tests 294–6, 300
in adrenal dysfunction 253, 278
investigation of disease 299–300
posterior 300–1
plasma
bicarbonate 57–65
bilirubin transport in 108
enzyme tests in diagnosis 72–85
in liver disease 114–15
lipid and lipoprotein disorders 182–94
osmolality 36, 47, 56
proteins
abnormalities 86–104, 113–14
glycated 172
oral contraceptives and 312–13
reference ranges in children 322
volume 41, 315
see individual enzymes, proteins etc. and also blood; serum
plasmid, cloning with 349–52
pleural fluid 123
Po_2 67–9
poisoning 226, 228, 370–4
in children 373
polycystic ovary syndrome 310, 312
polydipsia 129–31, 164, 301
polygenic disorders 362–3
polymerase chain reaction 359–60
polymyositis, creatine kinase and 77
polyuria 47–8
diabetes mellitus 164
in renal disease 129–31, 301
porphyrias **220–6**
chemical investigation of 224–6
lead poisoning 226–7
positive test results, predictive value 28
post-operative management
fluid 55–6
nutritional support 239–42
posture (effect on tests) 7, 24, 167
orthostatic proteinuria 140
potassium
balance **48–55**
content of intravenous feed 241
excretion 135
plasma levels in ectopic ACTH production 277
in hyperaldosteronism 285
in hyperglycaemic coma 174–5
in renal failure 136–7
reference ranges in children 322
urine, 51, 54, 135
pre-albumin 87, 91, 260, 341
precision of tests 22–3

predictive value of tests 28–33
pre-eclampsia 316
pregnancy
AFP levels in 317–18
alkaline phosphatase in 78–9
diabetes mellitus and 169–70, 315
fetoplacental unit and 313–16
maternal complications 315–16
thyroid status in 257
pregnanetriol in CAH 288–9
prenatal diagnosis of fetal abnormalities 316–19, 327–8
prevalence (of disease) 30–2
procollagen measurement in liver disease 116
progesterone 307
in infertility 310–11
pro-insulin 163
prolactin 297–8
in amenorrhoea 309
prolactinoma 298
pro-opiomelanocortin 295–6
procainamide monitoring 369
pro-vitamin D 198
prostate-specific antigen 103–4
prostatic acid phosphatase 101–2
α_1-protease inhibitor (API) 87, 90–1
deficiency detection 91, 355, 360–1
protein
in CSF 365–6
in diet 230
malabsorption 160
in plasma, abnormalities of **86–104**
in liver disease 113–14
lipoproteins 183–6, 189–90
oral contraceptives and 312–13
in pregnancy 313–14, 315
total 88
transport functions 86
tests in urine 14
protein-energy malnutrition in children 334–5
proteinuria
Bence Jones 98–9
in diabetes mellitus 172
in pregnancy 316
in renal disease 139–41
'side-room' tests 14, 139, 172
prothrombin 87, 113–14
protoporphyria 222
protoporphyrin, zinc 227
pseudocholinesterase 81
pseudohyperkalaemia 54
pseudohyponatraemia 45
pseudohypoparathyroidism 209–10
in children 338
psychogenic diabetes insipidus 130–1
pulmonary emphysema 68–9
API levels in 90–1
purine metabolism disorders 243–8
pyridoxine 237

quality of analytical results   10, 20, 33

race (effect on blood constituents)   25, 187
reactive hypoglycaemia   176
record-keeping for blood analysed by clinical
    staff   19
reducing substance tests in urine   14
reference ranges   25–7, 411–12
    effects of age   25, 79, 95, 187, 188, 308
    in the elderly   339–41
    in Paediatrics   322
    sex differences   187, 188, 218, 243, 304,
        308
Regan isoenzyme   102
remnant hyperlipoproteinaemia   191
renal concentration tests   129–31
renal disease   **124–43**
    hyperkalaemia and   53, 135
    hypernatraemia and   134–5
    hypokalaemia and   51, 135
    hyponatraemia and   43–4, 135
    proteinuria and   139–41
    screening for   4
    vitamin D deficiency and   209
    water retention and   43
renal failure
    acute   135–7
    chronic   137–9
renal glucosuria   166–8
renal osteodystrophy   212–13
renal stones   141–3
renal transplantation   138–9
renal tubular acidosis   132
renin activity, plasma, in
        hyperaldosteronism   285–6
renin–angiotensin–aldosterone system   39,
        269–70
reports of results   **21–34**
    audit   10–11
requests for investigations   **1–11**
    audit   10–11
    urgent   9, 17, 370
respiratory distress syndrome,
        neonatal   332–3
respiratory insufficiency   68–9, 70
restriction endonucleases   346–8
restriction fragment length
        polymorphisms   355, 356–8
    hypervariable regions and   358
reverse T3   249
reverse transcriptase   347
Reye's syndrome in children   338
riboflavin   236
rickets   209
    neonatal   332
Rotor syndrome   112

salicylate overdose   371
salvage pathway (nucleotides)   243

Sanger DNA sequencing   352–4
sarcoidosis, hypercalcaemia and   206–7
scoline apnoea   81–2
screening
    in the elderly   341–4
    of neonates   328–30
    tests   2–5
        for adrenal hyperfunction   272–4
        for adrenocortical hypofunction   279–
            81
        for alcohol abuse   122
        for colorectal cancer   15–16, 103
        for cystic fibrosis   336
        for diabetes mellitus   14, 342
        for Down syndrome   318
        for drug misuse   372–4
        for glycosuria   14
        for hypercalcaemia   4, 203
        for hypercholesterolaemia   18, 193
        for neural tube defects   316–18
        for phenylketonuria   329–30
        for rare metabolic diseases   32–3, 327,
            328–30
        for thyroid disease   330, 343–4
Scriver test   329
scurvy   238–9
secretin   145
    test for gastrinoma   148–9
secretin/CCK-PZ test   150–1
selenium deficiency   231–2
self-poisoning   370–2
sensitivity of tests   28, 73, 85
serial tests   23–4
serological tests
    Addison's disease   283
    liver disease   117
    thyroid disease   263–4
serotonin   160
serum
    cortisol   270
        in Addison's disease   279–80
        in Cushing's syndrome   271–6, 277
    immunoreactive trypsin   151–2
    parathyroid hormone   204–5
    protein electrophoresis   98
        in liver disease   114
sex, effect on reference ranges   187, 188,
        218, 243, 304, 308
sex differentiation disorders in males   306
sex hormone-binding globulin   303, 311
sex hormones
    female   307–11
    male   303–6
short stature in children   336–8
SI units   ix–x, 411–13
'sick cell syndrome'   44
'sick euthyroid syndrome'   257–9
'side-room' tests   **12–20**
    on blood   17–18, 170
    on faeces   15–16
    on urine   12–15, 117–18, 164, 170, 172

skin hygiene before blood specimen
     collection   6
sodium   **35–48**
  balance   35–40
    disorders   40–6
  content of intravenous feed   241
  in faeces   35, 160
  in sweat   335
  in urine   39–41, 43–4, 48, 134–5
solvent
  abuse   373
  toxicity   375
Southern blotting   354–5
specific gravity testing of urine   15, 129
specificity of tests   28 (footnote), 73, 85
specimen collection   5–9
  audit   10
  CSF   364
  from neonates and children   321–2, 325–6
  for plasma lipid studies   188–9
  for serum cortisol   270
  and transport for acid–base analysis   59
  see also under blood; faeces; urine
spermatogenesis control   303
'stagnant gut' syndrome   156, 157
standard deviation   22–3
steatorrhoea   156, 159
Stein–Leventhal syndrome   312
stercobilinogen   108
steroid contraceptives, metabolic effects
     of   217, 312–13
steroid hormones   **267–90, 303–12**
  adrenocortical function tests during steroid
     treatment   283–4
  in pregnancy   314
stomach   **145–9**
  content testing in overdose of drugs   372
stones, renal   141–3
stress
  glucocorticoid response to   268
  tests see insulin-hypoglycaemia tests
subfertility   304–6, 307–11
sucrose tolerance test   154–5
sugar (glucose) see glucose
sulphaemoglobin   228
sweat test in children   335–6
Synacthen tests   280–1, 281–2
syndrome of inappropriate secretion of
     ADH   42–3, 44, 48, 56, 301
Système International units   ix–x, 411–3

T3-thyrotoxicosis   256
tall stature, in children   336
Tangier disease   192
Taq polymerase   306
teratoma   103, 314
testicular feminization syndrome   306
testosterone
  in females   311–12

  in males   303–5
tetany   207
tetracosactrin tests of adrenal
     hypofunction   280–1, 281–2
therapeutic drug monitoring   **367–70**
thiamin   236
thrombolytic therapy, myocardial
     infarction   82–3
thyroglobulin   249–50, 263
thyroid enzymes   249–50, 263
thyroid function   **249–66**
  in disease
    auto-immune disease   260, 263–4
    carcinoma, follicular   263
    medullary carcinoma   264–5
    subclinical primary   256
    see also hyperthyroidism;
       hypothyroidism
  function tests in the elderly   243–4
  hormones in pregnancy   257, 314–15
  investigations   252–9, 263–4
    selective use   254–5
  'non-thyroidal illness'   257–9
  regulation of   252
  results interpretation
    hyperthyroidism   255–6
    hypothyroidism   256
  'sick euthyroid syndrome'   257–8
  treatment management
    hyperthyroidism   261
    hypothyroidism   261–3
thyroid-stimulating hormone   252, 294
  in disease   254–7, 259–63
  in the elderly   343–5
  reference ranges in children   322
thyroid-stimulating immunoglobulins   263
thyrotroph adenoma   294
thyrotrophin-receptor antibodies   263
thyrotrophin-releasing hormone   252, 294
  TRH test   294
thyroxine (T4)   249–63
  in plasma   250–63
    binding to proteins   250–1, 254, 257
    abnormal binding   259–60
    free T4   251–3, 254, 255–63
    free T4 index   253–4
    reference ranges in children   322
    total T4   250–1, 254, 255–63
    treatment   261–3
thyroxine-binding globulin   87, 250–1
  abnormal TBG   260
thyroxine-binding protein
     abnormalities   259–60
tonicity (or osmolality)   36–7
total CO_2 65–6
  in diabetic coma   174–5
  in hyperparathyroidism   204
  in renal tubular acidosis   131–2
total iron-binding capacity   219
total parenteral nutrition   239–42
toxaemia of pregnancy   316

toxicology tests 368, **370–4**
trace elements
  in diet 230–3
  toxicity 375
training in blood specimen collection 19
transaminases *see* alanine aminotransferase;
    aspartate aminotransferase
transcortin 268–9
transferrin 87, 219
  desialated, in liver disease 116
transketolase, erythrocyte 236
transplants (renal) 138
transport proteins 86
  see also individual proteins
transudate 123
trauma
  acute phase response 92–3
  creatine kinase 76
  metabolic response to 55–6, 268
TRH test 294
tri-iodothyronine (T3) **249–50, 254–62**
  in plasma
    binding to proteins 250–1, 254, 257
     abnormal binding 259–60
    free T3 252–3, 254, 255–62
    total T3 254–62
  reverse 249–50
  thyrotoxicosis 256
tricyclic antidepressants 369
triglycerides 182, 229
  arterial disease and 192
  breath test 157
  in lipoproteins 183–6
    abnormalities 188–92
  measurement 186–7, 188–9
trophoblast tumours 314
trypsin, immunoreactive 336
tryptophan load test 237
tubular function in kidney **128–35**
  proteinuria 141
tumour markers **99–104**
  antigens 102–4
  in ectopic ACTH production 277
tumours 100–4
  adrenal 276–8, 284–6
  bone metastases 101–2, 202–3
  bronchus 103
  colorectal 15–16, 103
  gonads 104, 312
  hepatoma and hepatic secondary
    deposits 103, 119–20
  liver 102, 103, 119
  pancreas 177–8
  prostate 101–2, 103–4
  teratoma 103, 314
  thyroid, medullary carcinoma 264–5
  trophoblast 314

units of measurement ix–x, 73, 379, 411–
    13
uraemia 127–8

uraemic toxins in chronic renal failure 138
urate **243–8**
  excretion 246
  gout 246–8
  in plasma 99, 122, 179, 243–6
    in pregnancy 316
  stones, renal 142
urea
  cycle defects in neonates 323–4
  in plasma 46–7, 126–7
    in liver disease 116, 120
    in renal disease 127–8
  in urine
    in renal disease 128
  total parenteral nutrition (assessing
    nitrogen requirements) 241–2
urease activity in stomach 149
urine
  abnormal colours 13
  acidification tests 131–2
  albumin 14, 172
  amylase 149–50
  bilirubin 15, 108–9, 117–19
  calcium 197, 204
  catecholamines 290–1, 339
  cortisol 271
    free cortisol 274
  formiminoglutamate 238
  glucose 14, 164
  indican 157
  'microalbuminuria' 172
  osmolality 36, 47–8
    in renal disease 128–9
  pH 15, 131–2
  phosphate 134, 204
  porphobilinogen 224
  potassium 54, 135
  protein electrophoresis 98–9
  'side-room' tests 12–15, 109
  sodium 48, 134–5
  specific gravity 15, 129
  specimen collection and preservation 8–9
  thiamin 236
  urea 128, 242
urobilinogen 15, 108–9, 117–19
using laboratory results 33

vanillyl mandelic acid *see* 4-hydroxy,
    3-methoxy mandelic acid (HMMA)
variation in test results
  analytical 21–3
  biological and pathological causes 24–8
  serial testing 23–4
variegate porphyria 224
vasoactive intestinal peptide 145, 158
vasopressin (DDAVP) test 129–31
venepuncture technique 6–7, 11, 200
Verner–Morrison syndrome 158
very low density lipoproteins 182, 183–5
  in hyperlipoproteinaemias 190–2
  metabolism 185–6

viral hepatitis *see* hepatitis
virilism in females 311–12
vitamin D 197–9, 234, 235
  deficiency 208–9
  excess 206
  malabsorption 209
  neonatal rickets 332
  in renal osteodystrophy 212
vitamin deficiencies
  fat-soluble vitamins (A, E, K) 234, 235–6
    see also vitamin D
  water-soluble vitamins
    ascorbic acid 234, 238–9
    B group 234, 236–8
    thiamin 234, 236
vitamins **232–9**
  content in intravenous feed 241
  in children 335
  fat malabsorption and 156
  fat-soluble 235–6
  water-soluble 236–9
  see also vitamin deficiencies
von Gierke's disease 179, 248

Waldenström's macroglobulinaemia 97
ward and clinic-based chemical analyses 17–20

water
  balance 35–8
    disorders 40–6
  intoxication, acute 55–6
  reabsorption (intestinal) 158
well-population screening 2–3
Werner's syndrome 205
WHO classifications
  diabetes mellitus 165
  primary hyperlipoproteinaemias 189–91
Williams syndrome 338
Wilson's disease 120–1
within-individual variation in results 24–5

xanthine
  oxidase deficiency 246
  stones, renal 142
xanthinuria 233
xanthochromia (CSF) 365
xylose absorption test 154
[^{14}C]-xylose breath test 157

zinc
  deficiency 232
  protoporphyrin, in erythrocytes 227
Zollinger–Ellison syndrome 147–8